Digestive and Hepatic Aspects of the Rheumatic Diseases

Editor

LIRON CAPLAN

RHEUMATIC DISEASE CLINICS OF NORTH AMERICA

www.rheumatic.theclinics.com

Consulting Editor
MICHAEL H. WEISMAN

February 2018 • Volume 44 • Number 1

ELSEVIER

1600 John F. Kennedy Boulevard • Suite 1800 • Philadelphia, Pennsylvania, 19103-2899
http://www.theclinics.com

RHEUMATIC DISEASE CLINICS OF NORTH AMERICA Volume 44, Number 1
February 2018 ISSN 0889-857X, ISBN 13: 978-0-323-58291-9

Editor: Lauren Boyle
Developmental Editor: Casey Potter

Rheumatic Disease Clinics of North America (ISSN 0889-857X) is published quarterly by Elsevier Inc., 360 Park Avenue South, New York, NY 10010-1710. Months of issue are February, May, August, and November. Business and editorial offices: 1600 John F. Kennedy Boulevard, Suite 1800, Philadelphia, PA 19103-2899. Periodicals postage paid at New York, NY and additional mailing offices. Subscription prices are USD 355.00 per year for US individuals, USD 706.00 per year for US institutions, USD 100.00 per year for US students and residents, USD 419.00 per year for Canadian individuals, USD 880.00 per year for Canadian institutions, USD 465.00 per year for international individuals, USD 880.00 per year for international institutions, and USD 230.00 per year for Canadian and foreign students/residents. To receive student/resident rate, orders must be accompanied by name of affiliated institution, date of term, and the *signature* of program/residency coordinator on institution letterhead. Orders will be billed at individual rate until proof of status received. Foreign air speed delivery is included in all *Clinics* subscription prices. All prices are subject to change without notice. **POSTMASTER:** Send address changes to *Rheumatic Disease Clinics of North America,* Elsevier Health Sciences Division, Subscription Customer Service, 3251 Riverport Lane, Maryland Heights, MO 63043. **Customer Service: 1-800-654-2452 (US and Canada). From outside of the US and Canada: 314-447-8871. Fax: 314-447-8029. For print support,** e-mail: **JournalsCustomerService-usa@elsevier.com. For online support, e-mail: JournalsOnline Support-usa@elsevier.com.**

Reprints. For copies of 100 or more of articles in this publication, please contact the Commercial Reprints Department, Elsevier Inc., 360 Park Avenue South, New York, New York, 10010-1710; Tel.: +1-212-633-3874, Fax: +1-212-633-3820, and E-mail: reprints@elsevier.com.

Rheumatic Disease Clinics of North America is covered in *MEDLINE/PubMed (Index Medicus), Current Contents/Clinical Medicine, Science Citation Index, ISI/BIOMED,* and *EMBASE/Excerpta Medica.*

Contributors

CONSULTING EDITOR

MICHAEL H. WEISMAN, MD
Cedars-Sinai Chair in Rheumatology, Director, Division of Rheumatology, Professor of Medicine, Cedars-Sinai Medical Center, Distinguished Professor, David Geffen School of Medicine at UCLA, Los Angeles, California, USA

EDITOR

LIRON CAPLAN, MD, PhD
Section Head, Rheumatology, Chief, Medicine Service, VA Rocky Mountain Network, Denver, Colorado, USA; Associate Professor, University of Colorado School of Medicine, Aurora, Colorado, USA

AUTHORS

ERIC ANDERSON, MD
Denver Veterans Affairs Medical Center, University of Colorado School of Medicine, Denver, Colorado, USA

BRIAN N. BREWER, MD
Resident Physician PGY3, Department of Internal Medicine, Augusta University-University of Georgia, Athens, Georgia, USA

LIRON CAPLAN, MD, PhD
Section Head, Rheumatology, Chief, Medicine Service, VA Rocky Mountain Network, Denver, Colorado; Associate Professor, University of Colorado School of Medicine, Aurora, Colorado, USA

LAURA C. CAPPELLI, MD, MHS
Assistant Professor of Medicine, Division of Rheumatology, Johns Hopkins Medicine, Baltimore, Maryland, USA

AYKUT FERHAT ÇELIK, MD
Professor of Medicine, Division of Gastroenterology, Department of Internal Medicine, Cerrahpasa Faculty of Medicine, Istanbul University, Istanbul, Turkey

ETHAN CRAIG, MD, MHS
Rheumatology Fellow, Division of Rheumatology, Johns Hopkins Medicine, Baltimore, Maryland, USA

TRACY M. FRECH, MD, MS
Department of Internal Medicine, Division of Rheumatology, The University of Utah, VA Salt Lake Health Care System, Salt Lake City, Utah, USA

CHIRANJEEVI GADIPARTHI, MD, MPH
Division of Gastroenterology and Hepatology, The University of Tennessee Health Science Center, Memphis, Tennessee, USA

NEEL GAKHAR, MD
Denver Veterans Affairs Medical Center, University of Colorado School of Medicine, Denver, Colorado, USA

ELENA GENERALI, MD
Division of Rheumatology and Clinical Immunology, Humanitas Research Hospital, Rozzano, Milan, Milan, Italy

MERRILL ERIC GERSHWIN, MD
Division of Rheumatology, Allergy, and Clinical Immunology, University of California, Davis, Davis, California, USA

AMNEET HANS, MD
University of Colorado School of Medicine, Aurora, Colorado, USA

GULEN HATEMI, MD
Professor of Medicine, Division of Rheumatology, Department of Internal Medicine, Cerrahpasa Faculty of Medicine, Istanbul University, Istanbul, Turkey

IBRAHIM HATEMI, MD
Professor of Medicine, Division of Gastroenterology, Department of Internal Medicine, Cerrahpasa Faculty of Medicine, Istanbul University, Istanbul, Turkey

MOHAMMAD K. ISMAIL, MD, AGAF
Division of Gastroenterology and Hepatology, The University of Tennessee Health Sciences Center, Memphis, Tennessee, USA

DIANE L. KAMEN, MD, MSCR
Associate Professor of Medicine, Division of Rheumatology and Immunology, The Medical University of South Carolina, Charleston, South Carolina, USA

KRISTINE A. KUHN, MD, PhD
Assistant Professor, Department of Medicine, University of Colorado School of Medicine, Denver, Colorado, USA

DIANE MAR, MD
Department of Internal Medicine, University of Colorado, Denver, Colorado, USA

BAHARAK MOSHIREE, MD, MS-CI
Professor of Medicine, Director of Motility, Division of Gastroenterology, Carolinas HealthCare System, Charlotte, North Carolina, USA

YEVGENIY POPOV, DO, MPH
Internal Medicine Resident, Department of Medicine, University of Massachusetts Medical School, Worcester, Massachusetts, USA

KYLE POTTS, MD
Associate Professor of Medicine/Rheumatology, Denver Veterans Affairs Medical Center, University of Colorado School of Medicine, Aurora, Colorado, USA

KAREN SALOMON-ESCOTO, MD
Clinical Associate Professor of Medicine, Rheumatology Division, University of Massachusetts Medical School, Worcester, Massachusetts, USA

RICHARD A. SCHATZ, MD
Fellow, Division of Gastroenterology and Hepatology, The Medical University of South Carolina, Charleston, South Carolina, USA

CARLO SELMI, MD, PhD
Division of Rheumatology and Clinical Immunology, Humanitas Research Hospital, Rozzano, BIOMETRA Department, University of Milan, Milan, Italy

COURTNEY STULL, MD
Denver Veterans Affairs Medical Center, University of Colorado School of Medicine, Denver, Colorado, USA

PATRICK R. WOOD, MD
Fellow, VA Rocky Mountain Network, University of Colorado School of Medicine, Aurora, Colorado, USA

Contents

Vasculitis is an inflammatory condition that targets the blood vessels, which may occur in isolation or as a component of a systemic inflammatory condition. Although many of the vasculitides can directly affect the organs of the gastrointestinal system, some types exhibit a proclivity for certain gastrointestinal and hepatic organs. Often a patient presents with nonspecific symptoms, delaying the diagnosis and treatment of the underlying vasculitis. Vasculitis can also present with severe manifestations, such as upper gastrointestinal bleeds and bowel perforation. It is important to identify the signs and symptoms of vasculitis in the gastrointestinal system and institute appropriate treatment.

Although classification criteria for systemic sclerosis (SSc) do not incorporate gastrointestinal tract (GIT) manifestations often present in this disease, the GIT is the most common internal organ involved. Pathophysiology of GIT involvement is thought to be similar to that of other organs in SSc, with fibroproliferative vascular lesions of small arteries and arterioles, increased production of profibrotic growth factors, and alterations of innate, humoral, and cellular immunity. These processes result in neuropathy progressing to myopathy with eventual fibrosis. Proper diagnostics and therapeutics for SSc-GIT involvement require the treating physician to have an understanding of an integrated approach and potential medication adverse effects.

A variety of gastrointestinal adverse drug reactions are seen in nearly all conventional antirheumatic medications, ranging from nausea to life-threatening drug-induced liver injury. Rheumatologists should be particularly familiar with hepatotoxicity associated with long-term methotrexate use, and the range of unique hepatic, biliary, and pancreatic manifestations associated with azathioprine. Hepatitis B virus reactivation is the most serious gastrointestinal disease risk associated with many biological therapies, particularly rituximab. Gastrointestinal perforation may be a specific concern for agents directed at interleukin-6 pathways, and some reports have raised the question of whether interleukin-17 inhibition may elevate inflammatory bowel disease risk.

chronic intestinal pseudoobstruction, celiac disease, and inflammatory bowel disease, have been described. Comprehensive cancer screening is warranted soon after the diagnosis of inflammatory myopathies because of high risk of occult malignancies. Elevated levels of aminotransferases may suggest muscular injury rather than hepatic dysfunction. Knowledge regarding the systemic involvement of inflammatory myopathies can assist in timely diagnosis of these complex disorders.

Fibromyalgia (FM) has historically been associated with several diseases in gastroenterology and hepatology. The most substantiated evidence pertains to irritable bowel syndrome (IBS). The pathogeneses of FM and IBS remain unclear, but it is likely related to dysregulation within the brain-gut axis, resulting in a hyperalgesic state. IBS and FM share other similarities, including a female predominance, fatigue, insomnia, and susceptibility to psychiatric state. These common manifestations and pathogeneses serve as a foundation for overlapping, multidisciplinary treatment modalities.

Sjogren syndrome (SS) is a lymphocyte-mediated, infiltrative autoimmune disorder characterized by the destruction of exocrine glands leading to secretory dysfunction. The typical manifestations include xerostomia and xerophthalmia; however, extensive gastrointestinal involvement is increasingly being recognized, emphasizing the variable and systemic nature of SS.

The association of inflammatory arthritis with intestinal pathology extends back more than 100 years. This association is now supported by epidemiologic studies demonstrating an elevated prevalence of inflammatory bowel disease in spondyloarthritis and vice versa, compared with the general population. Genetic and intestinal microbiome studies have further linked these diseases. Although diabetes and nonalcoholic fatty liver disease disproportionately affect individuals with psoriatic arthritis, diseases of the esophagus, stomach, pancreas, and liver are not particularly common in spondyloarthritis. Clinicians should be aware of the differential diagnosis and the appropriate diagnostic tools available when evaluating digestive and hepatic disorders in spondyloarthritis.

Gastrointestinal (GI) symptoms are common among patients with systemic lupus erythematosus (SLE), although only rarely are they caused by active organ system involvement from SLE itself. Rapid diagnosis and appropriate treatment of lupus enteritis and other GI manifestations of SLE are critical, because of the potential for organ and life-threatening complications. The 3 main variants of lupus enteritis are lupus mesenteric vasculitis, intestinal pseudoobstruction, and protein-losing enteropathy. These GI manifestations and others in patients with SLE are reviewed here.

RHEUMATIC DISEASE CLINICS
OF NORTH AMERICA

THE CLINICS ARE AVAILABLE ONLINE!
Access your subscription at:
www.theclinics.com

Foreword

Digestive and Hepatic Aspects of the Rheumatic Diseases

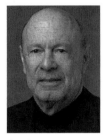

Michael H. Weisman, MD
Consulting Editor

Liron Caplan has done a remarkable job in assembling state-of-the-art articles that carefully describe the importance of the gastrointestinal tract (GIT) in our rheumatic disease patients. These articles highlight digestive and liver involvement regarding diagnosis, pathogenesis, management, and prognosis. In the setting of systemic vasculitis, GIT signs and symptoms often represent more severe disease, making early diagnosis and treatment imperative. The GIT is the most common internal organ involved in scleroderma and by its very nature demands attention. In systemic lupus erythematosus or rheumatoid arthritis, the GIT may represent comorbidities or other conditions that must be sorted out for the overall proper management of these diseases. Upper airway involvement and the ever-present issue of malignancy make the GIT a key feature to address in myopathies. The challenges we face when ulceration occurs in Bechet disease are carefully described in this issue. The relationship between inflammatory bowel disease and axial spondyloarthritis is becoming more critical as we make advances in genetic, biological, and mechanical triggers for both conditions. Our gastrointestinal colleagues tell us that SpA is just another extraintestinal manifestation of inflammatory bowel disease.

As we achieve success in treating our diseases with biologic and non-biologic means there may be some very unpleasant risks to the GIT that must be carefully monitored. Autoimmune liver diseases can be both diagnostic and therapeutic conundrums; our article represents a very thoughtful approach to disease recognition, pathogenesis, and management. Fibromyalgia and functional gastrointestinal diseases overlap, and our article provides a critical approach to diagnosis and management. Finally, Sjogren disease is no stranger to the GIT, and extensive manifestations are becoming increasingly recognized. Up to now, rheumatology clinicians and investigators find the GIT to be a "black box" of problems to be encountered in both the

Rheum Dis Clin N Am 44 (2018) xiii–xiv
https://doi.org/10.1016/j.rdc.2017.10.002
0889-857X/18/© 2017 Published by Elsevier Inc.

inpatient and the outpatient settings. Dr Caplan has made an outstanding effort to clear the air and provide an excellent background upon which to move forward.

Michael H. Weisman, MD
Division of Rheumatology
Cedars-Sinai Medical Center
8700 Beverly Boulevard
Los Angeles, CA 90024, USA

E-mail address:
Michael.Weisman@cshs.org

Preface

The Intersection of Autoimmunity, Arthritis, and the Alimentary Canal

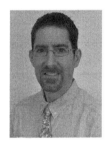

Liron Caplan, MD, PhD
Editor

As guest editor, I find it a privilege and a pleasure to introduce the current issue of *Rheumatic Disease Clinics of North America* to readers. This issue focuses on digestive and hepatic considerations among the various rheumatic diseases. Thanks to the generosity, expertise, and skill common to a large number of authors, this offering addresses a broad selection of the rheumatic diseases. I would like to personally thank all the contributors.

The development of this issue also engendered a unique opportunity for rheumatologists and gastroenterologists from across the globe to contribute their diverse perspectives through collaboration. It represents what is possible when we act collectively and exemplifies the collegial spirit of the scientific and medical community.

For the most part, the articles herein are arranged by specific rheumatic disease, and the subject matter within each article is organized according to the anatomy of the gastrointestinal system. The content from these articles provides a veritable differential diagnosis for digestive and hepatic organ involvement, as summarized in **Table 1**.

Table 1 is not intended as an exhaustive list, but does serve to highlight key gastrointestinal manifestations and aspects for consideration by rheumatologists, gastroenterologists, and general practitioners.

I am deeply indebted to Dr Michael Weismann, who provided the opportunity to act as guest editor, encouragement when I lagged, and counsel regarding the scope and potential contributors to this journal. Michael is a cherished and formidable asset to the rheumatology community. Also, I offer my profound admiration and gratitude to the staff of the *Rheumatic Disease Clinics of North America*, who are equal parts talented and patient.

Rheum Dis Clin N Am 44 (2018) xv–xvii
https://doi.org/10.1016/j.rdc.2017.10.001
0889-857X/18/© 2017 Published by Elsevier Inc.

rheumatic.theclinics.com

Table 1
Digestive and hepatic aspects of the rheumatic diseases, and the corresponding article number

Organ	Involvement	Article number(s)/Topic
Oral cavity	Perioral fibrosis	2 (systemic sclerosis)
	Sicca	2 (systemic sclerosis), 9 (Sjogren)
	Oropharyngeal dysphagia	7 (inclusion body myositis), 10 (spondyloarthritis), 11 (systemic lupus)
	Ulcerations	1 (vasculitis, Kawasaki disease), 3 (disease-modifying drugs, methotrexate), 4 (Behçet disease), 10 (spondyloarthritis), 11 (systemic lupus)
Esophagus	Gastroesophageal reflux	2 (systemic sclerosis)
	Esophagitis	2 (systemic sclerosis), 4 (Behçet disease)
	Patulous esophagus/ dysmotility	2 (systemic sclerosis), 9 (Sjogren)
Stomach	Gastric antral vascular ectasia	1 (vasculitis, systemic lupus), 2 (systemic sclerosis)
	Dysmotility	2 (systemic sclerosis), 6 (rheumatoid arthritis, secondary amyloid), 9 (Sjogren)
	Gastric cancer	7 (dermatomyositis)
	Ulcerations	4 (Behçet disease)
Small intestine	Small intestinal bacterial overgrowth	2 (systemic sclerosis)
	Telangiectasia	2 (systemic sclerosis)
	Malabsorption	2 (systemic sclerosis)
	Vasculitis	1 (Takayasu/polyarteritis nodosa/IgA-associated), 6 (rheumatoid arthritis), 11 (systemic lupus)
	Dysmotility	2 (systemic sclerosis), 6 (rheumatoid arthritis, secondary amyloid), 7 (dermatomyositis/polymyositis)
	Mesenteric thromboses	11 (systemic lupus)
	Abdominal serosis	11 (systemic lupus)
	Crohn	10 (spondyloarthritis)
	Perforation	3 (disease modifying drugs, tofacitinib/tocilizumab)
Liver/gall baldder	Primary biliary cholangitis	2 (systemic sclerosis), 5 (autoimmune liver disease), 9 (Sjogren)
	Felty syndrome	6 (rheumatoid arthritis)
	Primary sclerosing cholangitis	2 (systemic sclerosis), 5 (autoimmune liver disease)
	Steatohepatitis	7 (dermatomyositis/polymyositis), 10 (spondyloarthritis)
	Autoimmune hepatitis	5 (autoimmune liver disease)
	Vasculitis	1 (vasculitis, polyarteritis nodosum)
	Hepatotoxicity	3 (disease-modifying drugs, methotrexate)
	Viral hepatitis reactivation	3 (disease-modifying drugs, rituximab/tumor necrosis factor inhibitors)
Pancreas	Pancreatitis	9 (Sjogren), 3 (disease-modifying drugs, azathioprine), 11 (systemic lupus)
	Diabetes	10 (spondyloarthritis, psoriatic)
Colon	Constipation	2 (systemic sclerosis)
	Pseudo-obstruction	2 (systemic sclerosis), 7 (polymyositis), 11 (systemic lupus)
	Crohn disease	7 (dermatomyositis/polymyositis), 10 (spondyloarthritis)
	Ulcerative colitis	7 (dermatomyositis/polymyositis), 10 (spondyloarthritis)
	Vasculopathy	7 (dermatomyositis)
	Ulcerations	4 (Behçet disease)
	Irritable bowel syndrome	8 (fibromyalgia)
Anus	Fecal incontinence	2 (systemic sclerosis)
	Rectal prolapse	2 (systemic sclerosis)
	Ulcerations	10 (spondyloarthritis), 11 (systemic lupus)

Finally and most sincerely, I would like to express my gratitude to my muse, editor, and beloved companion, Eliana Caplan, whose support makes all things possible.

I ask the indulgence of the *Rheumatic Disease Clinics of North America* readers for any oversights and errors included in these articles.

Liron Caplan, MD, PhD
Denver Veterans Affairs Medical Denver
University of Colorado
School of Medicine
1775 Aurora Court–B115
Aurora, CO 80045, USA

E-mail address:
liron.caplan@ucdenver.edu

Gastrointestinal and Hepatic Disease in Vasculitis

Eric Anderson, MD, Neel Gakhar, MD, Courtney Stull, MD,
Liron Caplan, MD, PhD*

KEYWORDS

- Vasculitis • Granulomatosis with polyangiitis • Polyarteritis nodosa
- Antineutrophil cytoplasmic antibody–associated vasculitis • Kawasaki disease
- Gastrointestinal diseases • Mouth diseases • Esophageal diseases

KEY POINTS

- Vasculitis can affect every organ of the gastrointestinal system.
- Vasculitis often presents with nonspecific symptoms, including gastrointestinal bleeding, and should be included in the differential when initial work-up fails to find an obvious source of gastrointestinal symptoms.
- Gastrointestinal involvement in the setting of systemic vasculitis often represents more severe disease making early diagnosis and treatment imperative.

INTRODUCTION

The vasculitides are a group of disorders that cause inflammation of blood vessels. They can be classified according to the size of the arteries affected (small, medium, and large), etiology (primary vs secondary), and extent of involvement (localized vs

Conflicts of Interest: All authors declare no conflicts of interest in this article, including financial, consultant, institutional, and other relationships that might lead to bias or a conflict of interest. Guarantor of the Article: Liron Caplan, MD, PhD.
Financial Support: There was no financial or grant support for this study. Dr L. Caplan is supported by VA HSR&D IIR 14-048-3 and the Michelson Fund at the University of Colorado Foundation.
Author Contributions: E. Anderson, N. Gakhar, C. Stull, and L. Caplan were responsible for drafting, critical revision, and approval of the final article. All authors were involved in the final approval of the version of the article submitted and have agreed to be accountable for all aspects of the work. The views expressed in this article are those of the authors and do not necessarily reflect the position or policy of the Department of Veterans Affairs.
Potential Competing Interests: None.
Denver Veterans Affairs Medical Center, University of Colorado School of Medicine, Denver, CO, USA
* Corresponding author. Denver Veterans Affairs Medical Center, University of Colorado School of Medicine, 1775 Aurora Court, B115, Aurora, CO 80045.
E-mail address: liron.caplan@ucdenver.edu

systemic). If untreated, this group of diseases can potentially cause life-threatening complications with significant morbidity. Therefore, it is vital that clinicians identify and treat this group of diseases effectively. Unfortunately, the scientific basis for summarizing the digestive and hepatic involvement by vasculitides is largely limited to case reports and case series.

This article examines the different types of vasculitis that may affect each anatomic component of the gastrointestinal system. The initial section summarizes the nomenclature, classification, and diagnostic criteria for some of the vasculitides. The epidemiology of vasculitis is addressed and then individual sections are dedicated to anatomic components of the gastrointestinal system, touching on the particular types of vasculitis known to affect each gastrointestinal organ. These sections address the presentation, pathophysiology, and treatment of vasculitis affecting each organ system.

If affected by vasculitis, the oral mucosa and esophagus are typically involved with Kawasaki disease (KD) or the antineutrophil cytoplasmic antibody (ANCA)-associated vasculitides (AAVs). These include granulomatosis with polyangiitis (GPA), eosinophilic GPA (EGPA), and microscopic polyangiitis (MPA). The stomach may also be affected by the AAV and by leukocytoclastic vasculitis (LCV), in particular, immunoglobulin A–associated vasculitis (IgAV), formerly known as Henoch-Schönlein purpura. The small intestine, large intestine, and mesentery can be affected by Takayasu arteritis (TA), LCV, AAV, polyarteritis nodosa (PAN), giant cell arteritis (GCA), systemic lupus erythematosus (SLE)-associated vasculitis, and rheumatoid arthritis–associated vasculitis (RAAV). The liver and gall bladder are typically affected by PAN and single-organ vasculitis (SOV), but there are numerous reports of involvement from other vasculitides as well, including GCA. Finally, the pancreas can also be involved with GPA and SOV. Behcet's disease will not be addressed here, as there is a dedicated article to this vasculitis and its gastrointestinal manifestations (see Ibrahim Hatemi and colleagues' article, "Gastrointestinal Involvement in Behçet Disease," in this issue). SLE-associated vasculitis is only briefly mentioned, for the same reason.

NOMENCLATURE, CLASSIFICATION CRITERIA, AND DIAGNOSTIC CRITERIA

GPA represents a necrotizing vasculitis typically affecting small and medium-sized vessels. It commonly involves the respiratory tract and kidneys, where it causes a necrotizing glomerulonephritis. In 1990, the American College of Rheumatology (ACR) established classification criteria for Wegener granulomatosis, the eponym previously assigned to GPA.[1] These criteria include the following:

- Nasal or oral inflammation
- Abnormal chest radiograph with infiltrates or nodules
- Urinary sediment with microhematuria (greater than 5 white blood cells per high-power field)
- Granulomatous inflammation on biopsy of artery or arteriole

Two or more of these criteria confer an 88.2% sensitivity and 92% specificity for establishing a diagnosis of GPA.[2]

EGPA is also a necrotizing vasculitis that affects small and medium-sized vessels, which is associated with asthma and eosinophilia. The ACR established 6 criteria to classify EGPA and they are as follows:

- Asthma
- Eosinophilia (more than 10% of circulating leukocytes)
- Paranasal sinusitis
- Pulmonary infiltrates on radiographs

- Histologic proof of vasculitis with extravascular eosinophils
- Mononeuritis multiplex or polyneuropathy

If 4 or more of these criteria are present, there is an 85% sensitivity and 99.7% specificity for the diagnosis of EGPA.[3]

MPA is defined in the Chapel Hill Consensus Conference criteria,[1,3] but reliable classification criteria for this condition are still not available. Distinguishing MPA from GPA typically depends on the failure to demonstrate granulomata on tissue biopsy.

LCV refers to a small-vessel vasculitis involving the skin and can be associated with many of the vasculitides, including IgA vasculitis, GPA, and EGPA. Diagnosis often requires a biopsy of skin lesions, with histopathology typically revealing "polymorphonuclear neutrophils in and around vessel wells with signs of activation, degranulation, and death of neutrophils illustrated by leukocytoclasia."[4] Presence of palpable purpura with LCV on pathology in conjunction with abdominal pain should prompt further investigation of the precise vasculitis responsible.[4]

IgAV is a small vessel vasculitis primarily affecting the skin, kidneys, and gastrointestinal system. It is characterized by IgA deposits in the vessel wall. Classification criteria have been released jointly by the European League Against Rheumatism, Paediatric Rheumatology International Trials Organisation, and Paediatric Rheumatology European Society.[5] These criteria require

- Purpura or petechiae *AND* 1 of the following 4 criteria:
  - Abdominal pain
  - Arthritis or arthralgia
  - Renal involvement
  - LCV with predominant IgA deposits or proliferative glomerulonephritis with predominant IgA deposits.

The sensitivity and specificity of these criteria for adults were 99.2% and 86.0%, respectively.[6]

KD consists of a medium-sized vessel vasculitis that primarily affects children. Diagnostic criteria for KD have been published by the American Heart Association, which suggest that patients must have a fever lasting at least 5 days with 4 of the 5 following criteria[7]:

- Bilateral bulbar conjunctival injection without exudate
- Oral mucous membrane changes (fissured lips, injected pharynx, or strawberry tongue)
- Erythema of palms or soles, edema of feet, or periungual desquamation
- Polymorphous rash
- Cervical lymphadenopathy, with at least 1 lymph node greater than 1.5 cm in diameter.

PAN is a medium to small vessel vasculitis that affects the kidneys, skin, muscles, joints, nerves, and gastrointestinal system. There are 10 criteria that can help classify PAN; they are as follows:

- Weight loss greater than or equal to 4 kg
- Livedo reticularis
- Testicular pain/tenderness
- Myalgias
- Mononeuropathy or polyneuropathy
- Diastolic blood pressure greater than 90 mm Hg
- Elevated serum urea nitrogen or serum creatinine

- Presence of hepatitis B
- Arteriographic abnormality
- Presence of granulocyte or mixed leukocyte infiltrate in arterial wall biopsy

The individual is classified with PAN if 3 or more of these are present.[8]

TA is a large vessel vasculitis that is defined by granulomatous inflammation of the aorta and its major branches.[3] Multiple definitions, diagnostic criteria, and classification criteria have been developed for TA over the past 30 years.[9] Given the lack of specificity in laboratory markers for TA, MRI, ultrasound, and fludeoxyglucose F18–PET have all been shown to help diagnosis and monitor disease progress.[10]

GCA, or temporal arteritis, usually presents as a large vessel vasculitis that affects the cranial arteries in older persons. The pathology reveals transmural inflammation with disruption of the internal lamina caused by infiltrating multinucleated giant cells, lymphocytes, and macrophages. Classification criteria[11] include

- Age greater than 50
- New onset of headache
- Abnormality of temporal artery (temporal artery tenderness, decreased pulsation)
- Raised erythrocyte sedimentation rate (ESR) ($\geq$50 mm/h)
- Abnormal arterial biopsy (vasculitis with predominantly mononuclear cell infiltration or granulomatous inflammation with evidence of giant cells)

A case may be classified as GCA when 3 or more criteria are positive.

A diagnosis of RAAV simply requires a patient to have an existing diagnosis of rheumatoid arthritis in addition to having pathologic findings of vasculitis inciting tissue damage or ischemia.[12,13] It affects small and medium-sized vessels.

SLE is a systemic and chronic inflammatory disease that can affect almost any organ in the body. Disease susceptibility seems to occur through a combination of environmental exposures and multiple genetic loci, resulting in abnormalities of apoptosis, humoral autoimmunity, and hypocomplementemia. SLE may present with an associated vasculitis that can affect vessels of every gauge, though small vessels are most frequently implicated.[14]

EPIDEMIOLOGY

The overall incidence of GPA is approximately 1.9 per 100,000.[15] Age of onset is typically between 35 years to 55 years of age.[16] EGPA may be more common than GPA, with prevalence of up to 3 persons per 100,000.[17]

In a hospital-based study performed in the Czech Republic, the incidence of KD was estimated to be approximately 5.5 cases per 100,000 persons under the age of 17. For PAN, a study performed in a suburb of Paris estimated prevalence to be approximately 3 cases per 100,000 people.[18]

The Czech study estimated the incidence of IgAV to be 10.2 per 100,000 in children under the age of 17.[19] For adults with IgA vasculitis, results from a recent survey of 260 patients showed the average age of diagnosis approximately 50 years of age.[20] TA seems to affect between 0.26 and 0.64 people per 100,000 and is more frequent in those with Asian descent.[21,22]

VASCULITIS OF THE ORAL MUCOSA AND ESOPHAGUS

KD is distinguished by prominent oral manifestations. A study performed in Turkey, for example, noted that of 24 children with KD, close to 90% exhibited oral mucosal manifestations.[23] Apart from KD, GPA and EGPA are the 2 most common vasculitides that can manifest both in the oral mucosa and esophagus. Of those afflicted by GPA, approximately 6% to 13% develop oral manifestations.[24]

Physical Examination/Presentation

KD frequently presents with oral involvement, including fissured, erythematous, crusting, or swollen lips, and strawberry tongue.[23] Exudative pharyngitis with discrete oral vesicles and ulcers is also possible.

Diagnosis of AAV is often delayed because individuals with these conditions often present with nonspecific and diverse symptoms. Patients with GPA typically have nonspecific symptoms, such as fevers, chills, night sweats, and weight loss, and can also present with hemoptysis and acute renal failure rather than oral symptoms. In a study examining 34 patients with GPA, however, 9 developed gastrointestinal symptoms that included oral ulcerations, gingival hyperplasia, dyspepsia, vomiting, diarrhea, and abdominal pain.[25] In particular, gingival hyperplasia (also known as strawberry gingivitis) can be one of the presenting signs of GPA.[26] Although not strictly components of the classification criteria, saddle nose deformity, serosanguinous discharge from the nose, and palpable purpura and ulcerative lesions on the extremities may contribute to the clinical picture of GPA. Cases of EGPA have been reported that presented with dysphagia and an upper gastrointestinal bleed and cutaneous findings, such as nasal polyposis, leukocytoclastic angiits, and livedo reticularis.[27]

Pathophysiology/Serologic Testing

ESR, C-reactive protein (CRP), ferritin, and white blood cell count can be elevated in KD,[28] whereas both GPA and EGPA demonstrate varying degrees of antineutrophil cytoplasmic antibody positivity. Between 82% and 94% of patients with GPA have been shown to be ANCA positive.[29] Although the exact pathophysiologic basis for ANCA remains in dispute, between 40% and 60% of patients with EGPA demonstrate ANCA positivity.[30] Laboratory evaluation of GPA may reveal elevated ESR and CRP.[31] Positive staining or enzyme-linked immunosorbent assays may indicate the presence of antibody-recognizing protease 3.[32] EGPA-associated eosinophilic esophagitis can be diagnosed via endoscopically obtained biopsy.[33]

Treatment

KD can have potentially devastating effects on the cardiovascular system, including coronary artery aneurysm. Intravenous immune globulin with or without aspirin has been shown to reduce the likelihood of developing these complications.[34]

Similarly, if left untreated, GPA and EGPA can be catastrophic for patients. A diagnosis of GPA without treatment carries up to a 90% mortality within the first 2 years.[35] The initial treatment of choice depends on the severity of the disease and degree of organ involvement. For nonsevere disease, initial treatment is usually glucocorticoids with a traditional disease-modifying antirheumatic drug. Although methotrexate might be a reasonable option in milder disease without involvement of the oral mucosa, the potential of this agent to produce oral ulcers makes it a less ideal agent. In severe disease, the biologics tocilizumab and rituximab and the chemotherapeutic alkylating agent cyclophosphamide may be appropriate. If remission is achieved, the patient and provider may elect to pursue maintenance therapy with azathioprine, mycophenolate, rituximab, or methotrexate.

Initial treatment of EGPA is typically systemic glucocorticoids. With regard to gastrointestinal involvement in EGPA, a case report has described a patient with EGPA who presented with dysphasia whose symptoms improved with corticosteroids.[27] Anti–interleukin (IL)-5 therapy has shown promise in small trials in the treatment of complications from eosinophilia in EGPA and may be used to treat eosinophilic esophagitis.[36] The Five-Factor Score can be used to estimate mortality risk and therefore determine if additional treatment is justified in EGPA and PAN. The score system is as follows[37]:

- Age greater than 65 years
- Cardiac insufficiency
- Renal insufficiency (with stable serum creatinine of 1.7)
- Gastrointestinal involvement
- Absence of ear, nose, and throat manifestations (their presence is associated with lower mortality)

Visceral involvement is a particularly strong predictor of outcome. A score of 1 is assigned if only 1 of these criteria is present and a score of 2 is assigned if 2 or more are present.[38] For scores greater than or equal to 2, treatment with cyclophosphamide has been demonstrated to confer a mortality benefit.[39] Once remission is achieved with cyclophosphamide, methotrexate and azathioprine may be used for maintenance therapy.

VASCULITIS OF THE STOMACH

SLE-associated vasculitis, PAN, IgAV, EGPA, and GPA have all been implicated, albeit infrequently, in vasculitis of the stomach. SLE has also been associated with the occurrence of gastric antral vascular ectasia, which presents with a classic watermelon stomach lesion.[40]

SOV of the stomach is rare. A single case of isolated obliterative gastric vasculitis mimicking gastric cancer has been reported.[41] In this case, there was no clinical or radiographic evidence of primary or secondary vasculitis; the diagnosis occurred on pathologic examination only after gastric resection was performed for suspected gastric cancer in the setting of chronic abdominal pain and suspicious esophagogastroduodenoscopy (EGD) and esophageal ultrasound findings.

EGPA has been reported to mimic gastric neoplasm.[42–44] In the first case, a 42-year-old woman presented with upper gastrointestinal symptoms of vomiting, hematemesis, weight loss, and loss of appetite. Subsequent EGD showed an infiltrating lesion from the body of the stomach to the antrum with mucosal biopsies returning a result of "normal." A gastrojejunostomy with biopsy showed findings consistent with EGPA rather than malignancy. The patient was treated with corticosteroids and the gastric lesion resolved.[42] In the second case,[44] an EGD raised the specter of gastric malignancy in an individual with nasal polyps, rhinitis, and asthma. The gastrectomy specimen demonstrated that EGPA vasculitis may occur in the deeper layers of the gastric wall, highlighting the limitations of biopsy obtained via EGD. The last case occurred after carbimazole treatment of Graves disease. Diagnosis was confirmed on biopsy with clinical and morphologic features resolving within a couple months after discontinuation of the drug.[43]

Finally, Zheng and colleagues[45] reported a case of GPA affecting the stomach lining. In this case, a 31-year-old Chinese woman presented with abdominal distention, pain, weight loss, intermittent fever, fatigue, and oral and lip ulcers. On laboratory evaluation, cytoplasmic ANCA was positive and EGD showed a diffusely thickened gastric wall with many ulcers. Biopsy revealed granulomatous formation and many neutrophils and lymphocytes, allowing the diagnosis of GPA. Her symptoms improved with corticosteroids and cyclophosphamide.

VASCULITIS OF THE INTESTINES AND MESENTERY

There are many vasculitides than can affect the intestines and mesentery. TA and the AAV are considered the most likely vasculitides to be associated with IBD.[46]

PAN, AAV, IgAV, SLE-associated vasculitis, TA, RAAV, and GCA have all been associated with mesenteric ischemia. Only approximately 5% to 10% of those with AAV involve the mesentery.[47] On the other hand, approximately 33% of cases of TA,[47] 50% to 60% of PAN,[47] and 40% to 50% of IgA vasculitis involve the mesentery.[47]

Lupus enteritis is the most common cause of persistent abdominal pain in patients with SLE, although the precise prevalence of biopsy-demonstrated vasculitis in patients with enteritis remains unclear. In 1 study of 175 SLE patients, 22% of patients with enteritis presented with abdominal pain.[48] Approximately 0% to 10% of SLE cases involve the mesentery.[47]

Fewer than 15 cases of GCA involving the mesentery have been reported in the past 40 years.[49] This entity presents with symptoms of bowel ischemia but is distinguished from other forms of vasculitis by the presence of giant cells and granulomas on histology as well as concurrent clinical manifestations (sudden loss of vision and so forth, which are indicative of GCA).

An estimated 1% to 10% of RAAV cases involves the mesentery.[47] RAAV can also be responsible for bowel ischemia and ulcerations, arteritis of liver, spleen, and pancreas.[12] Elevated ESR and CRP as well as thrombocytosis are classic laboratory abnormalities accompanying RAAV. Most patients also tend to have positive serologies, whether rheumatoid factor, anticyclic citrullinated peptide antibodies, or, less frequently, antinuclear antibodies and ANCA positivity.

Physical Examination/Presentation

When vasculitis affects the bowel and mesentery, it often presents with nonspecific symptoms, such as nausea, vomiting, diarrhea, rectal bleeding, and fever.[46] Symptoms are caused by vascular compromise and not surprisingly can mimic symptoms of embolic bowel ischemia with abdominal pain that is out of proportion to examination findings. In a review of 62 patients with gastrointestinal vasculitis attributed to PAN, MPA, GPA, EGPA, and RAAV, the following symptoms were reported[50]:

- Abdominal pain, 97%
- Nausea/vomiting, 34%
- Diarrhea, 27%
- Hematochezia or melena, 16%
- Gastroduodenal ulcers, 27% (seen on EGD)
- Peritonitis, 15%
- Perforation, 16%

PAN can also cause microaneurysms of the mesenteric artery, which can be distinguished on CT angiography or MRI.[51] There has been at least 1 case report of GPA presenting initially with upper gastrointestinal bleed.[52]

In EGPA, gastrointestinal symptoms of abdominal pain, diarrhea, or gastrointestinal bleeding occurred in 20% of patients,[53] with more recent studies documenting 25% to 30% involvement over time.[29,54] Mortality secondary to gastrointestinal involvement is approximately 8% (usually from gastrointestinal bleeding or bowel perforation).

Treatment

Corticosteroids are the treatment of choice for TA, but if there are significant aneurysmal changes of the mesenteric vasculature, revascularization may be required.[55]

Corticosteroids also remain the first-line choice in treating IgA vasculitis, with recent study showing noninferiority of adding cyclophosphamide.[20] High-dose corticosteroids are also effective for treatment of lupus enteritis.[48] Patients with signs of intestinal hemorrhage from GPA may need surgical intervention.[25] RAAV is associated with a higher mortality rate than rheumatoid arthritis without signs of vasculitis. Therefore, a patient with RAAV that involves the bowel or mesentery warrants aggressive treatment with high-dose corticosteroids along with rituximab or cyclophosphamide.[56]

VASCULITIS OF THE HEPATOBILIARY SYSTEM

Vasculitis in the gallbladder can be divided in to 2 categories: (1) SOV or (2) part of a larger systemic vasculitis. The distinction between these processes is important to recognize because the pathophysiology, management, and prognosis can differ greatly between them. A 2014 analysis of 61 patients with vasculitis involving the gallbladder found 67% of cases consistent with systemic vasculitis and 33% with SOV.[57]

Vasculitis in the gallbladder is classified as SOV if there is no disease beyond the gallbladder after at least 6 months of follow-up. This entity is considered distinct from systemic vasculitis involving the gallbladder.

Vasculitis in the gallbladder is considered part of a systemic vasculitis when a biopsy reveals vasculitis at an anatomic site outside of the gallbladder. When the gallbladder is involved as part of a systemic vasculitis, the most commonly implicated etiology is PAN. Analyses of patients with PAN describes the occurrence of cholecystitis in 2% to 17% of clinically observed patients and up to 40% of autopsied patients.[50] Although PAN is the most common systemic vasculitis associated with gallbladder disease, AAV (MPA, EGPA, and GPA), autoimmune disease–associated (SLE, rheumatoid arthritis, and systemic sclerosis), cryoglobulinemic vasculitis, IgAV, and GCA are all vasculitides that have been associated with gallbladder involvement.

Liver involvement in vasculitis usually represents a clinically inconsequential component of what is otherwise a serious systemic disease. That is, the liver disease of vasculitis tends to be subclinical and is not recognized as a major cause of morbidity or mortality. Nonetheless, there are case reports of clinically significant hepatic manifestations of vasculitis, including ischemic hepatitis and hepatic infarction, most commonly associated with PAN.[50] Minor clinical hepatic involvement has been reported in many systemic vasculitides, including AAV, autoimmune, IgA vasculitis, GCA, and cryoglobulinemia. Although cryoglobulinemia accompanies liver disease as a component of chronic hepatitis C virus infection, its manifestations are primarily extrahepatic.[58] An analysis of 62 patients with systemic small and medium vessel vasculitides with gastrointestinal involvement, identified hepatic microaneurysms in patients with PAN (both hepatitis B virus related and non–hepatitis B virus related) and EGPA who also had microaneurysms of renal, mesenteric, and/or splenic arteries.[50] A review of PAN in the gastrointestinal tract notes liver involvement in 16% to 56% of patients, although again stressing that clinical manifestations related to liver disease are rare.[59] A Japanese autopsy series noted arteritis in 21% of livers from patients with SLE.[60]

Presentation Examination/Presentation

The presentation of vasculitis involving the gallbladder differs depending on the etiology. When part of a systemic vasculitis, the signs and symptoms characteristic of the underlying vasculitis typically occur before or concurrent with biliary symptoms. The most common biliary symptoms may be described as those of an acalculous chole-cystitis from arteritis involving the gallbladder wall.[57] Rare but recognized complications of gallbladder vasculitis second to PAN include biliary strictures and intracholecystic hemorrhage from rupture of cystic arteries into the gallbladder lumen.[59]

SOV of the gallbladder is typically discovered only after routine cholecystectomy performed for gallstone-associated cholecystitis or recurrent right upper quadrant pain. Unlike systemic vasculitis involving the gallbladder, SOV of the gallbladder is rarely associated with systemic symptoms, with the noted exception of fever, and is more frequently associated with isolated abdominal pain.[57]

When the liver is involved in systemic vasculitides, it is, by definition, one of several involved organs. As a result, patients tend to present with general abdominal pain and systemic symptoms. Hepatomegaly has been identified in patients with SLE vasculitis, hepatitis B virus–associated PAN, and cryoglobulinemia.[50] Hepatic arteriography in patients with PAN can show corkscrew vessels and distal microanuerysms that form in the weakened portions of affected vessel walls (hepatic arteries).[59] Rare hepatic complications of PAN involving hepatic arteries include liver infarction and acute liver failure as well as subcapsular or intrahepatic hemorrhage from rupture of hepatic microaneurysms.[59]

Pathophysiology/Serologic Testing

Vasculitis in the gallbladder occurs when inflammatory leukocytes in vessel walls lead to reactive damage to mural structures. Histologically, vasculitis in the gallbladder, whether part of a systemic or single-organ process, is typically a nongranulomatous necrotizing vasculitis of medium-sized vessels. Additional histologic features that have been noted in gallbladder vasculitis include acute and healed vasculitic lesions and aneurysm formation.[57] Vasculitis of small and medium arteries that supply small bile ducts can cause intrahepatic sclerosing cholangitis, which is characterized by periductal inflammation and ductal proliferation.[59]

As might be predicted, systemic vasculitis in the gallbladder tends to be associated with higher ESR than SOV in the gastrointestinal tract. When vasculitis is confined to the gallbladder, autoimmune serologies are typically negative/normal.

In the liver, the most common serologic abnormality is nonspecific elevated liver function tests (ie, transaminitis). A recent study investigating liver involvement in AAV revealed liver function test abnormalities in approximately half the cases of active AAV. Among the AAVs, significantly higher levels of alanine aminotransferase, gamma-glutamyltransferase (GGT), and alkaline phosphatase were seen in patients with GPA compared with MPA or EGPA. On the other hand, bilirubin was significantly increased in patients with active EGPA but not active GPA or MPA.[61] The same study did not demonstrate any association of liver function test abnormalities with antibodies to proteinase-3 or myeloperoxidase. Histologically, there are reports of granulomatous liver involvement in GPA and GCA[29,62,63] and necrotizing vasculitis in liver biopsy specimens of patients with PAN.[59]

Treatment

For gallbladder involvement, there is a difference in prognosis and therefore management of systemic vasculitis compared with the single-organ phenomenon. If the etiology of gallbladder vasculitis is a systemic vasculitis (most often PAN), potent immunosuppressants are warranted. With the most common etiology of systemic gallbladder vasculitis, PAN, the treatment includes glucocorticoids and cyclophosphamide. Compared with SOV, systemic vasculitis of the gallbladder is associated with a higher mortality.[57] For SOV of the gallbladder, surgery is often sufficient to achieve a cure. Because the process is confined to the gallbladder, there is no indication for systemic anti-inflammatory or immunosuppressive therapy and patients tend to do very well after surgery.

In cases of AAV-associated liver vasculitis, liver function test elevations tend to normalize after initiation of therapy, without progression of liver disease or the incitement of autoimmune hepatic disease. Although GGT is commonly associated with hepatic cells, it is also present in renal, pancreatic, and other tissues. Increased GGT in GPA is associated with pulmonary and pulmonary-renal involvement as well as a longer time to remission.[61] Similarly, in a 2006 retrospective analysis of prognostic factors in small vessel vasculitis, there was an adverse prognosis for survival with liver function test elevations.[64]

VASCULITIS OF THE PANCREAS

Multiple vasculitides have been associated with pancreatic involvement, albeit rarely. A case series of 62 patients with vasculitic involvement of the gastrointestinal tract found that acute pancreatitis was diagnosed in only 3 of the 62 patients.[50]

Presentation Examination/Presentation

Pancreatitis and pancreatic masses are the major manifestations of vasculitis of the pancreas. GPA,[65,66] PAN,[67,68] SLE-associated vasculitis,[69] AAV,[70] and IgAV[71] have all been associated with pancreatic involvement.

Yokoi and colleagues[68] conducted a literature review summarizing the known cases of PAN and GPA presenting as a pancreatic mass. They report that affected patients had a median age of 62 (range 44–66) with a male predominance (5:3 ratio). In terms of ethnicity, 3 patients were Japanese, 2 were white, and 1 was of Jewish extraction. Symptoms included abdominal pain, fever, otitis media, and, rarely, jaundice. All lesions were found 2 cm to 3 cm in diameter and were typically in the head of the pancreas. The vasculitis-associated masses had similar presentations despite different underlying vasculitides; they were hypodense and hypoechoic with poorly defined enhancement on CT. Most patients were diagnosed after surgery or autopsy.

Pathophysiology/Serologic Testing

Diagnosis of pancreatic involvement from vasculitis is challenging, given that many patients may have normal lipase and amylase despite presenting with classic epigastric pain with radiation to the back. Nevertheless, amylase might be an early diagnostic clue that points to the occurrence of IgAV.[71] Pancreatic neoplasm often represents the initial concern when a pancreatic mass is initially identified. Patients with pancreatic mass and fever, however, should also prompt consideration for vasculitis as a part of the differential diagnosis. In 1 case of a patient with pancreatitis-like symptoms, an MRI study revealed a pancreatic mass. A subsequent biopsy, however, demonstrated histologic findings of vasculitis with fibrinoid necrosis, granulomas, and giant cells, resulting in a diagnosis of GPA.[66]

Treatment

Early introduction of glucocorticoids and a cytotoxic agent was effective in the review by Yokoi, but a delay in treatment initiation could result in a rapid deterioration to fatal necrotizing vasculitis.[68] Other investigators have reported a severe clinical course prior to management with immunosuppression, but rapid improvement and lack of symptoms at 6 months after azathioprine and glucocorticoids.[66]

SUMMARY

The vasculitides can affect any part of the gastrointestinal system. It is important for clinicians to be aware of their generally nonspecific presentation, need to include vasculitis in the list of differential diagnosis, and requirement for appropriate immunosuppression. Further research with more rigorous study designs is required to expand the knowledge base within this field of medicine.

REFERENCES

1. Jennette JC, Falk RJ, Bacon PA, et al. 2012 revised International Chapel Hill consensus conference nomenclature of vasculitides. Arthritis Rheum 2013; 65(1):1–11.
2. Leavitt RY, Fauci AS, Bloch DA, et al. The American College of Rheumatology 1990 criteria for the classification of Wegener's granulomatosis. Arthritis Rheum 1990;33(8):1101–7.
3. Jennette JC, Falk RJ, Andrassy K, et al. Nomenclature of systemic vasculitides. Proposal of an international consensus conference. Arthritis Rheum 1994;37(2): 187–92.
4. Gota C. Overview of cutaneous small vessel vasculitis. In: Matteson EL, Callen J, editors. UpToDate. Alphen aan den Rijn (Netherlands): Wolters Kluwer; 2016. Available at: https://www.uptodate.com/contents/overview-of-cutaneous-small-vessel-vasculitis. Accessed August 12, 2017.
5. Ozen S, Pistorio A, Iusan SM, et al. EULAR/PRINTO/PRES criteria for Henoch-Schonlein purpura, childhood polyarteritis nodosa, childhood Wegener granulomatosis and childhood Takayasu arteritis: Ankara 2008. Part II: Final classification criteria. Ann Rheum Dis 2010;69(5):798–806.
6. Hocevar A, Rotar Z, Jurcic V, et al. IgA vasculitis in adults: the performance of the EULAR/PRINTO/PRES classification criteria in adults. Arthritis Res Ther 2016;18:58.
7. Newburger JW, Takahashi M, Gerber MA, et al. Diagnosis, treatment, and long-term management of Kawasaki disease: a statement for health professionals from the Committee on rheumatic fever, endocarditis, and kawasaki disease, council on cardiovascular disease in the young, American Heart Association. Pediatrics 2004;114(6):1708–33.
8. Lightfoot RW Jr, Michel BA, Bloch DA, et al. The American College of Rheumatology 1990 criteria for the classification of polyarteritis nodosa. Arthritis Rheum 1990;33(8):1088–93.
9. de Souza AW, de Carvalho JF. Diagnostic and classification criteria of Takayasu arteritis. J Autoimmun 2014;48-49:79–83.
10. Andrews J, Mason JC. Takayasu's arteritis–recent advances in imaging offer promise. Rheumatology (Oxford) 2007;46(1):6–15.
11. Hunder GG, Bloch DA, Michel BA, et al. The American College of Rheumatology 1990 criteria for the classification of giant cell arteritis. Arthritis Rheum 1990; 33(8):1122–8.
12. Bartels CM, Bridges AJ. Rheumatoid vasculitis: vanishing menace or target for new treatments? Curr Rheumatol Rep 2010;12(6):414–9.
13. Scott DG, Bacon PA, Tribe CR. Systemic rheumatoid vasculitis: a clinical and laboratory study of 50 cases. Medicine (Baltimore) 1981;60(4):288–97.
14. Barile-Fabris L, Hernandez-Cabrera MF, Barragan-Garfias JA. Vasculitis in systemic lupus erythematosus. Curr Rheumatol Rep 2014;16(9):440.

15. Watts RA, Lane SE, Scott DG, et al. Epidemiology of vasculitis in Europe. Ann Rheum Dis 2001;60(12):1156–7.
16. Lane SE, Watts RA, Shepstone L, et al. Primary systemic vasculitis: clinical features and mortality. QJM 2005;98(2):97–111.
17. Eustace JA, Nadasdy T, Choi M. Disease of the month. The Churg Strauss Syndrome. J Am Soc Nephrol 1999;10(9):2048–55.
18. Mahr A, Guillevin L, Poissonnet M, et al. Prevalences of polyarteritis nodosa, microscopic polyangiitis, Wegener's granulomatosis, and Churg-Strauss syndrome in a French urban multiethnic population in 2000: a capture-recapture estimate. Arthritis Rheum 2004;51(1):92–9.
19. Dolezalova P, Telekesova P, Nemcova D, et al. Incidence of vasculitis in children in the Czech republic: 2-year prospective epidemiology survey. J Rheumatol 2004;31(11):2295–9.
20. Audemard-Verger A, Pillebout E, Guillevin L, et al. IgA vasculitis (Henoch-Shonlein purpura) in adults: diagnostic and therapeutic aspects. Autoimmun Rev 2015;14(7):579–85.
21. Numano F, Kobayashi Y. Takayasu arteritis–beyond pulselessness. Intern Med 1999;38(3):226–32.
22. Roberts JR, Monteagudo LA, Shah PA, et al. Takayasu arteritis. In: Diamond HS, editor. Medscape. New York: WebMD; 2016. Available at: http://emedicine.medscape.com/article/332378-overview.
23. Ozdemir H, Ciftci E, Tapisiz A, et al. Clinical and epidemiological characteristics of children with kawasaki disease in Turkey. J Trop Pediatr 2010;56(4):260–2.
24. Ponniah I, Shaheen A, Shankar KA, et al. Wegener's granulomatosis: the current understanding. Oral Surg Oral Med Oral Pathol Oral Radiol Endod 2005;100(3):265–70.
25. Masiak A, Zdrojewski L, Zdrojewski Z, et al. Gastrointestinal tract involvement in granulomatosis with polyangiitis. Prz Gastroenterol 2016;11(4):270–5.
26. Hanisch M, Frohlich LF, Kleinheinz J. Gingival hyperplasia as first sign of recurrence of granulomatosis with polyangiitis (Wegener's granulomatosis): case report and review of the literature. BMC Oral Health 2016;17(1):33.
27. Park J, Im S, Moon SJ, et al. Churg-strauss syndrome as an unusual cause of dysphagia: case report. Ann Rehabil Med 2015;39(3):477–81.
28. Lee KY, Rhim JW, Kang JH. Kawasaki disease: laboratory findings and an immunopathogenesis on the premise of a "protein homeostasis system". Yonsei Med J 2012;53(2):262–75.
29. Guillevin L, Cohen P, Gayraud M, et al. Churg-Strauss syndrome. Clinical study and long-term follow-up of 96 patients. Medicine (Baltimore) 1999;78(1):26–37.
30. Conron M, Beynon HL. Churg-Strauss syndrome. Thorax 2000;55(10):870–7.
31. Kubaisi B, Abu SK, Foster CS. Granulomatosis with polyangiitis (Wegener's disease): an updated review of ocular disease manifestations. Intractable Rare Dis Res 2016;5(2):61 9.
32. Schonermarck U, Lamprecht P, Csernok E, et al. Prevalence and spectrum of rheumatic diseases associated with proteinase 3-antineutrophil cytoplasmic antibodies (ANCA) and myeloperoxidase-ANCA. Rheumatology (Oxford) 2001;40(2):178–84.
33. Assmann G, Molinger M, Pfreundschuh M, et al. Gastrointestinal perforation due to vasculitis at primary diagnosis of eosinophilic granulomatosis with polyangiitis (EGPA) despite a high dose glucocorticosteroids treatment. Springerplus 2014;3:404.

34. Furusho K, Kamiya T, Nakano H, et al. High-dose intravenous gammaglobulin for kawasaki disease. Lancet 1984;2(8411):1055–8.
35. Hoffman GS, Kerr GS, Leavitt RY, et al. Wegener granulomatosis: an analysis of 158 patients. Ann Intern Med 1992;116(6):488–98.
36. Wechsler ME, Akuthota P, Jayne D, et al. Mepolizumab or placebo for eosinophilic granulomatosis with polyangiitis. N Engl J Med 2017;376(20):1921–32.
37. Guillevin L, Pagnoux C, Seror R, et al. The Five-Factor Score revisited: assessment of prognoses of systemic necrotizing vasculitides based on the French Vasculitis Study Group (FVSG) cohort. Medicine (Baltimore) 2011;90(1):19–27.
38. Gayraud M, Guillevin L, Le TP, et al. Long-term followup of polyarteritis nodosa, microscopic polyangiitis, and Churg-Strauss syndrome: analysis of four prospective trials including 278 patients. Arthritis Rheum 2001;44(3):666–75.
39. Bourgarit A, Le TP, Pagnoux C, et al. Deaths occurring during the first year after treatment onset for polyarteritis nodosa, microscopic polyangiitis, and Churg-Strauss syndrome: a retrospective analysis of causes and factors predictive of mortality based on 595 patients. Medicine (Baltimore) 2005;84(5):323–30.
40. Cojocaru M, Cojocaru IM, Silosi I, et al. Manifestations of systemic lupus erythematosus. Maedica (Buchar) 2011;6(4):330–6.
41. Will U, Gerlach R, Wanzar I, et al. Isolated vasculitis of the stomach: a novel or rare disease with a difficult differential diagnosis. Endoscopy 2006;38(8):848–51.
42. Premaratna R, Saparamadu A, Samarasekera DN, et al. Eosinophilic granulomatous vasculitis mimicking a gastric neoplasm. Histopathology 1999;35(5):479–81.
43. Seve P, Stankovic K, Michalet V, et al. Carbimazole induced eosinophilic granulomatous vasculitis localized to the stomach. J Intern Med 2005;258(2):191–5.
44. Stolte M, Jatzwauk P, Bethke B. The Churg-Strauss syndrome: diagnosed for the first time in a gastrectomy specimen. Z Gastroenterol 2013;51(6):573–5.
45. Zheng Z, Ding J, Li X, et al. Gastric presentation (vasculitis) mimics a gastric cancer as initial symptom in granulomatosis with polyangiitis: a case report and review of the literature. Rheumatol Int 2015;35(11):1925–9.
46. Weiss GM. Gastrointestinal involvement in systemic vasculitis. Rheumatology Network. Norwalk (CT): UBM Medica; 2016. Available at: http://www.rheumatologynetwork.com/news/gastrointestinal-involvement-systemic-vasculitis.
47. Koster MJ, Warrington KJ. Vasculitis of the mesenteric circulation. Best Pract Res Clin Gastroenterol 2017;31(1):85–96.
48. Lee CK, Ahn MS, Lee EY, et al. Acute abdominal pain in systemic lupus erythematosus: focus on lupus enteritis (gastrointestinal vasculitis). Ann Rheum Dis 2002;61(6):547–50.
49. Annamalai A, Francis ML, Ranatunga SK, et al. Giant cell arteritis presenting as small bowel infarction. J Gen Intern Med 2007;22(1):140–4.
50. Pagnoux C, Mahr A, Cohen P, et al. Presentation and outcome of gastrointestinal involvement in systemic necrotizing vasculitides: analysis of 62 patients with polyarteritis nodosa, microscopic polyangiitis, Wegener granulomatosis, Churg-Strauss syndrome, or rheumatoid arthritis-associated vasculitis. Medicine (Baltimore) 2005;84(2):115–28.
51. Jee KN, Ha HK, Lee IJ, et al. Radiologic findings of abdominal polyarteritis nodosa. AJR Am J Roentgenol 2000;174(6):1675–9.
52. Tavakkoli H, Zobeiri M, Salesi M, et al. Upper gastrointestinal bleeding as the first manifestation of Wegener's granulomatosis. Middle East J Dig Dis 2016;8(3):235–9.
53. Comarmond C, Pagnoux C, Khellaf M, et al. Eosinophilic granulomatosis with polyangiitis (Churg-Strauss): clinical characteristics and long-term followup of the

383 patients enrolled in the French Vasculitis Study Group cohort. Arthritis Rheum 2013;65(1):270–81.

54. Moosig F, Bremer JP, Hellmich B, et al. A vasculitis centre based management strategy leads to improved outcome in eosinophilic granulomatosis and polyangiitis (Churg-Strauss, EGPA): monocentric experiences in 150 patients. Ann Rheum Dis 2013;72(6):1011–7.

55. Hunder GG. Treatment of Takayasu arteritis. In: Matteson EL, editor. UpToDate. Alphen aan den Rijn (Netherlands): Wolters Kluwer; 2016. Available at: https://www.uptodate.com/contents/overview-of-cutaneous-small-vessel-vasculitis. Accessed August 12, 2017.

56. Whelan P. Treatment of rheumatoid vasculitis. In: Matteson EL, editor. UpToDate. Alphen aan den Rijn (Netherlands): Wolters Kluwer; 2017. Available at: https://www.uptodate.com/contents/overview-of-cutaneous-small-vessel-vasculitis. Accessed August 12, 2017.

57. Hernandez-Rodriguez J, Tan CD, Rodriguez ER, et al. Single-organ gallbladder vasculitis: characterization and distinction from systemic vasculitis involving the gallbladder. An analysis of 61 patients. Medicine (Baltimore) 2014;93(24):405–13.

58. Apstein MD. Gastrointestinal manisfestations of vasculitis. In: Merkel PA, editor. UpToDate. Alphen aan den Rijn (Netherlands): Wolters Kluwer; 2016. Available at: http://www.uptodate.com. Accessed June 1, 2017.

59. Ebert EC, Hagspiel KD, Nagar M, et al. Gastrointestinal involvement in polyarteritis nodosa. Clin Gastroenterol Hepatol 2008;6(9):960–6.

60. Matsumoto T, Yoshimine T, Shimouchi K, et al. The liver in systemic lupus erythematosus: pathologic analysis of 52 cases and review of Japanese autopsy registry data. Hum Pathol 1992;23(10):1151–8.

61. Willeke P, Schluter B, Limani A, et al. Liver involvement in ANCA-associated vasculitis. Clin Rheumatol 2016;35(2):387–94.

62. Lee S, Childerhouse A, Moss K. Gastrointestinal symptoms and granulomatous vasculitis involving the liver in giant cell arteritis: a case report and review of the literature. Rheumatology (Oxford) 2011;50(12):2316–7.

63. Holl-Ulrich K, Klass M. Wegener s granulomatosis with granulomatous liver involvement. Clin Exp Rheumatol 2010;28(1 Suppl 57):88–9.

64. Pavone L, Grasselli C, Chierici E, et al. Outcome and prognostic factors during the course of primary small-vessel vasculitides. J Rheumatol 2006;33(7):1299–306.

65. Chawla S, Atten MJ, Attar BM. Acute pancreatitis as a rare initial manifestation of Wegener's granulomatosis. A case based review of literature. JOP 2011;12(2):167–9.

66. Valerieva Y, Golemanov B, Tzolova N, et al. Pancreatic mass as an initial presentation of severe Wegener's granulomatosis. Ann Gastroenterol 2013;26(3):267–9.

67. Flaherty J, Bradley EL III. Acute pancreatitis as a complication of polyarteritis nodosa. Int J Pancreatol 1999;25(1):53–7.

68. Yokoi Y, Nakamura I, Kaneko T, et al. Pancreatic mass as an initial manifestation of polyarteritis nodosa: a case report and review of the literature. World J Gastroenterol 2015;21(3):1014–9.

69. Hatemi I, Hatemi G, Celik AF. Systemic vasculitis and the gut. Curr Opin Rheumatol 2017;29(1):33–8.

70. Iida T, Adachi T, Tabeya T, et al. Rare type of pancreatitis as the first presentation of anti-neutrophil cytoplasmic antibody-related vasculitis. World J Gastroenterol 2016;22(7):2383–90.

71. Frigui M, Lehiani D, Koubaa M, et al. Acute pancreatitis as initial manifestation of adult Henoch-Schonlein purpura: report of a case and review of literature. Eur J Gastroenterol Hepatol 2011;23(2):189–92.

Gastrointestinal and Hepatic Disease in Systemic Sclerosis

Tracy M. Frech, MD, MS[a],*, Diane Mar, MD[b]

KEYWORDS

- Scleroderma • Systemic sclerosis • Therapeutics • Gastrointestinal diseases
- Mouth diseases • Esophageal diseases • Stomach diseases • Liver diseases

KEY POINTS

- The gastrointestinal tract (GIT) is the most commonly involved internal organ in systemic sclerosis (SSc).
- GIT management involves an integrated approach of patient education for lifestyle modification, medical therapies, and ancillary services for nutrition support.
- Medical therapeutics for SSc have several important considerations that require an understanding of potential adverse effects.

EPIDEMIOLOGY

Systemic sclerosis (SSc, scleroderma) is a connective tissue disease characterized by vasculopathy, fibrosis, and immune dysfunction with a prevalence varying from 30 to 443 per million population.[1] SSc classification criteria[2] do not incorporate the gastrointestinal tract (GIT) manifestations that are often present in this disease, despite the fact that GIT involvement produces substantial morbidity and is the most commonly involved internal organ in SSc.[3] The GIT is the presenting disease feature in 10% of SSc, occurs during disease course in up to 95% of individuals, and is responsible for 6% to 12% of mortality in SSc patients.[4] Malabsorption, gastroesophageal reflux (GERD), nausea, vomiting, diarrhea, and constipation are some of the GIT complications that occur in

Funding Source: This work was supported by awards from the National Institutes of Health (K23AR067889) and the US Department of Veterans Affairs (I01 CX001183). The content is solely the responsibility of the authors and does not necessarily represent the official views of the National Institutes of Health or the Department of Veterans Affairs.
Disclosures: The authors have no conflict of interest to disclose.
[a] Department of Internal Medicine, Division of Rheumatology, University of Utah, Salt Lake Veterans Affair Medical Center, Salt Lake City, UT, USA; [b] Department of Internal Medicine, University of Colorado, Denver, 12631 East 17th Avenue, Aurora, CO 80045, USA
* Corresponding author. 4b200 SOM 30 North, 1900 East, Salt Lake City, UT 84132.
E-mail address: tracy.frech@hsc.utah.edu

Rheum Dis Clin N Am 44 (2018) 15–28
https://doi.org/10.1016/j.rdc.2017.09.002
0889-857X/18/© 2017 Elsevier Inc. All rights reserved.

rheumatic.theclinics.com

this population, and despite varying degrees of disease severity from mouth to anus, SSc GIT involvement significantly impairs quality of life in almost all patients.[5,6] Severe GIT involvement in up to 8% of SSc patients is associated with a high morbidity and poorer outcome.[7,8]

PATHOGENESIS AND PATHOPHYSIOLOGY

The specific pathogenesis of GIT involvement is complex and not adequately understood, but neuropathy progressing to myopathy with eventual fibrosis has been proposed.[8] The pathophysiology of GIT involvement is thought to parallel other organ involvement in SSc with fibroproliferative vascular lesions of small arteries and arterioles, increased production of various profibrotic growth factors, and alterations of innate, humoral, and cellular immunity.[9,10] Although the role of immune dysfunction has not been adequately characterized, environmental factors may trigger the initial endothelial cell injury, which results in release of reactive oxygen species, chemokines, and cytokines that activate and recruit chronic inflammatory cells, including T- and B-lymphocytes and macrophages.[8]

Animal models for SSc described in the literature demonstrate that there are several induced and spontaneous systems mimicking certain inflammatory, immunologic, or fibrotic aspects of the disease, which provide contexts in which to study various aspects of this complex disorder.[11] However, the most extensive GIT work has been done in the transgenic (TG) mouse strain TβRIIΔk-fib, which is characterized by ligand-dependent upregulation of transforming growth factor-β (TGF-β) signaling. Quantitative polymerase chain reaction results of TG GIT fibroblasts showed evidence of upregulated collagen transcription and noncanonical TGF-β signaling pathways.[12]

The concept of GIT cell-mediated immunity in SSc is supported by biopsy specimens that demonstrate an increase in endothelial/lymphocyte activation leading to a pronounced increase in the $CD4^+/CD8^+$ ratio, and type 2 helper (Th2) polarization.[13] The classic Th2 cytokines interleukin (IL)-4 and IL-13 are not only profibrotic but also upregulate humoral immunity by inducing immunoglobulin production.[14] Of interest, immunoglobulins isolated from the serum of SSc patients interfere with cholinergic-mediated contraction of the GIT, a phenomenon that is most intense early in the disease and more extensive later in the disease, when both smooth muscle and myenteric neurons are involved.[15–17] These circulating antimuscarinic 3 receptor autoantibodies block cholinergic neurotransmission by inhibition of acetylcholine release and thus the ability of the smooth muscle in the GIT to respond to stimuli. As fibroblasts become activated into myofibroblasts by TGF-β, excess collagen is produced, which causes structural damage and also impaired motility. The result of these processes is a dysfunctional GIT, which contributes to Barrett esophagus, gastroparesis, malabsorption, and fecal incontinence.

ANATOMIC DISTRIBUTION OF INVOLVEMENT
Oral Cavity

Oral involvement in SSc may include perioral fibrosis, sublingual frenulum thickening, or secondary Sjogren syndrome, all of which can predispose patients to malnutrition because of reduction of oral aperture and intake.[18,19] Dental changes because of bone reabsorption may affect mastication and result in tooth loss.[20]

Esophagus

In SSc patients, the esophagus is the most commonly affected organ of the GIT, occurring in up to 90% of patients and resulting in symptoms of heartburn, regurgitation, and dysphagia.[21] However, up to 30% of SSc patients may have asymptomatic esophageal involvement; thus, establishing a diagnosis of GIT involvement in an SSc patient (particularly early in the disease course) may present a challenge for the physician.[22] Decreased peristalsis in the lower two-thirds of the esophagus with associated reduction of lower esophageal sphincter tone is classically defined as a patulous esophagus on imaging in SSc patients. Esophageal dysmotility is more severe in SSc patients with a longer disease duration and is associated with interstitial lung disease due to microaspiration.[23,24] This latter association is particularly important to note, because chronic cough and asthma may be attributed to GERD and warrants assessment. Long-standing GERD is associated with both stricture formation and Barrett esophagus, which is a risk factor for esophageal adenocarcinoma.[21]

Stomach

Stomach involvement in SSc includes gastric antral vascular ectasia (GAVE) and gastroparesis. Most patients with GAVE present with iron-deficiency anemia; however, GAVE itself may be the presenting SSc disease feature.[25] Although the pathogenesis of GAVE has been proposed to be similar to that of the immune-mediated development of telangiectases, further studies are needed to understand autoantibody associations.[26] In SSc, gastroparesis is due to autonomic dysfunction in the stomach, which causes impaired gastric compliance and delayed gastric emptying. Up to 50% of SSc patients complain of early satiety, nausea, bloating, and abdominal pain.[27]

Small Intestine

The second most commonly involved aspect of the GIT is the small intestine. Reduction in gastric acid and hypomotility of the small bowel may result in small intestinal bacterial overgrowth (SIBO), which occurs in up to 50% of SSc patients.[28] Other small intestine manifestations, including pneumatosis cystoides intestinalis and pseudo-obstruction, are also thought to be related to motor impairment due to decreased smooth muscle contractility.[29,30] Jejunal diverticula may occur in areas of muscle atrophy.

Liver

The most common liver disease associated with SSc is primary biliary cirrhosis (PBC), which is also associated with an anticentromere autoantibody. The prevalence of PBC in SSc has been reported to be 2% to 22% and increases when antimitochondrial antibodies, MIT3, and gp100 are used for diagnosis.[31] The prognosis of SSc-PBC is better than that of PBC alone, with a slower progression to end-stage liver disease.[32] Overlap conditions with autoimmune hepatitis, idiopathic portal hypertension, intrahepatic portal hypertension due to nodular regenerative hyperplasia, and primary sclerosing cholangitis have been reported in SSc.[33–35]

Colon

Colonic involvement is present in 20% to 50% of SSc patients[27] and is typically due to a reduction in colonic motility and prolonged transit due to an impaired gastrocolic response.[36–38] Severe constipation may result in fecal impaction. Other complications of colonic involvement in SSc may include megacolon, transverse and sigmoid colonic volvulus, telangiectasia, stenosis, as well as "wide mouth" diverticula and stercoral ulceration.[39] Intestinal pseudo-obstruction is a clinical syndrome that may complicate SSc; it is characterized by obstructive symptoms in the absence of a mechanical cause and is thought to be due to impaired colonic propulsion.[36]

Anus

Anorectal involvement occurs in 50% to 70% of SSc patients, with fecal incontinence affecting up to 40% of patients.[40] Internal anal sphincter smooth muscle changes due to neuropathy or myopathy with resultant impaired inhibitory response are thought to be the cause of fecal incontinence in SSc.[41–43]

DIAGNOSTIC EVALUATION
Oral Cavity

Irrespective of sicca symptoms, regular dental care is indicated because mandibular resorption, dental loss, and possible increase in tongue carcinoma have been reported in SSc.[20,44,45] Assessment of oropharyngeal dysphagia and aspiration risk should be considered in SSc patients because the lower pharynx may be involved in SSc.[46,47]

Esophagus

Esophageal symptoms may include volume reflux, nausea, vomiting, heartburn, and dysphagia. The first line of investigation for esophageal symptoms in SSc is generally esophagogastroduodenoscopy (EGD), which can be diagnostic for esophagitis attributable to causes such as eosinophilic or candidiasis as well as (pre-) cancerous changes, and therapeutic for esophageal strictures.[21,48] If stricture formation is suspected, a barium swallow can identify severity. The impact of GERD on symptoms can be assessed by pH monitoring, a procedure often done on antireflux medications to assess therapeutic efficacy. The effect of peristalsis on symptoms can be assessed by impedance that can be performed alone or in combination with pH monitoring. Manometry is used to diagnosis motility disorders by measuring pressure profiles in the esophagus. High-resolution esophageal manometry has further enhanced the ability to study motility in much greater detail by providing pressure measurements at more levels along the esophagus.[3]

Stomach

Abdominal pain and distention are often treated empirically as SIBO before any formal investigation because of the high costs, invasiveness, inconvenience to patients, lack of standardization, and sampling error associated with testing. However, if these symptoms fail to respond to antibiotics, further investigation should be pursued.[21] Diagnostic tests for SIBO include culture of duodenal aspirate during EGD and the hydrogen breath test. If gastroparesis is suspected, a gastric emptying study is indicated before initiation of prokinetics.[48] An SSc patient with an iron deficiency anemia requires an EGD for identification and treatment of GAVE.

Small Intestine

Capsule endoscopy may also be used to evaluate the esophagus, small bowel, and colon with possible identification of occult gastrointestinal bleeding from GAVE. Additional testing of small bowel complications in SSc may include qualitative fecal fat if exocrine pancreatic insufficiency is considered or measurement of fat-soluble vitamins if malabsorption is suspected.[49]

Colon

An abdominal radiograph or computed tomography (CT) scan of the abdomen is often obtained to assess for intestinal pseudo-obstruction in patients with severe abdominal pain associated with distention. Stool studies, including testing for *Clostridium difficile*, may be indicated for patients with diarrhea. Colonoscopy can identify telangiectasia and is indicated in SSc over the age of 50 for malignancy screening.

Anus

Anorectal manometry can be used to assess fecal incontinence in SSc; however, manometric changes may appear before clinical symptoms appear,[50] highlighting the challenge of ordering invasive testing. Magnetic resonance defecography is a noninvasive test that uses MRI to obtain images at various stages of defecation to evaluate how well the pelvic muscles are working and provide insight into rectal function. A balloon expulsion test is a procedure that places a fluid-filled balloon into the rectum in order to measure expulsion time and assess whether the rectoanal inhibitory reflex is intact, meaning that the internal anal sphincter demonstrates appropriate transient relaxation in response to rectal distention.

Malnutrition

The risk for malnutrition is reported in the range of 18% to 56% among SSc populations screened by questionnaire and bioelectrical impedance analysis[51,52]; thus, patients should be screened at diagnosis and annually.[53] Unfortunately, traditional markers of nutritional status, including current body mass index and serum albumin, do not seem to be good indicators of malnutrition in SSc.[54,55] Nonetheless, once identified, malnutrition should be closely monitored and effectively treated[53] (**Table 1**).

Table 1
Systemic sclerosis gastrointestinal tract involvement and testing

Organ	Involvement	Diagnostic Evidence	Citation
Oral cavity	Perioral fibrosis Sicca Oropharyngeal dysphagia	Perioral tethering and sublingual frenulum thickening on examination Barium swallow with fluoroscopy Mandibular resorption on radiography	Veale et al,[18] 2016; Frech et al,[19] 2016; Rajapakse et al,[46] 1981; Rajapakse,[47] 2016
Esophagus	GERD Esophagitis Stricture Barrett esophagus Patulous esophagus	EGD pH monitoring Modified barium swallow Impedance monitoring Manometry	Hansi et al,[21] 2014; Raja et al,[56] 2016
Stomach	GAVE Dysmotility	EGD Gastric-emptying study	Ebert,[36] 2008; Nagaraja et al,[48] 2015
Small intestine	SIBO Telangiectasia Malabsorption	Hydrogen breath testing Capsule endoscopy Fecal fat quantification	Sallam et al,[27] 2006
Liver	PBC	Antimitochondrial antibody Liver biopsy	Kumar et al,[8] 2017; Assassi et al,[31] 2009
Colon	Constipation Pseudo-obstruction	Colonoscopy Abdominal radiograph or CT	Sallam et al,[27] 2006
Anus	Fecal incontinence Rectal prolapse	Manometry Defecography Balloon expulsion test	Richard et al,[40] 2017

PHYSICAL EXAMINATION FINDINGS

The physical examination for assessment of GIT manifestations can be rather nonspecific; however, there are a few notable findings specific to SSc that are worth highlighting. The oral examination can identify patients that will benefit from ancillary services from speech and swallow therapists as well as dentists and orthodontists[18,19] (**Fig. 1**). Irrespective of the GIT involvement, cutaneous telangiectases may be a clinical biomarker for pulmonary vascular disease and thus are an important physical examination feature.[57]

An abdominal examination is always important to perform in SSc patients. A low threshold for abdominal imaging is indicated for assessment of pseudo-obstruction.[58] Anorectal examination may reveal rectal prolapse and direct appropriate referral.

MANAGEMENT OF GASTROINTESTINAL MANIFESTATIONS

GIT management involves an integrated approach of patient education for lifestyle modification, medical therapies, and ancillary services for nutrition support.[21] Patient questionnaires may be used to identify symptoms and assess the social and psychological contribution to symptoms; therefore, they are an important aspect of clinical decision making.[59] The Patient-Reported Outcomes Measurement Information System GIT symptom item bank contains 60 items that capture 8 gastrointestinal (GI)-specific symptom scales and is available at no cost with minimal respondent burden.[60]

Behavioral Considerations and Interventions

Most GIT symptoms in SSc are managed through supportive therapies and symptom control, of which behavioral modification is an important component. For example, sicca syndromes in SSc patients often lead to cavities and ulcerations; thus, adequate hydration and routine dental hygiene are important factors in maintaining oral health.[61] Microstomia can be managed through rehabilitation therapies, such as orofacial stretching programs. However, the long-term efficacy of adaptive oral hygiene devices and orofacial exercise is unclear. Yuen and colleagues[62,63] explored orofacial exercise programs, which showed a 2.8-mm difference at 3 months, but no difference at 6 months. The lack of effect at 6 months may be related to poor adherence to the program, because it required about 30 min/d of orofacial exercises.

Lifestyle modifications are an important aspect of GERD management and include maintaining a healthy weight and avoiding alcohol and tobacco products. Not eating more than 3 hours before reclining and elevation of the head of the bed while sleeping may also help reduce acid symptoms.[64] Dietary modification to identify food intolerance associations with functional GIT symptoms may be helpful.[65] In particular, if gastroparesis is present, a low-residue diet with frequent small meals can reduce

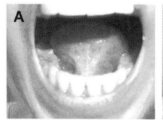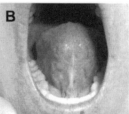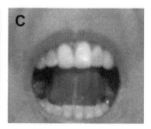

Fig. 1. Systemic sclerosis oral physical examination findings: (A) frenulum thickening, (B) telangiectases, and (C) reduced oral aperture.

symptoms. Adequate hydration and minimizing constipating medications are an important aspect of constipation management. Increased fiber intake should be used cautiously in patients with concurrent SIBO.[48] Behavioral therapies such as pelvic floor exercises may help patients with fecal incontinence.

Patients who have difficulty maintaining normal oral nutrition will benefit from educational support from a dietician. Multivitamin replacement should be guided by laboratory testing.[48] Patients with a reduced oral aperture may benefit from education regarding mechanically soft food as well as consultation with an oral surgeon. Patients with intestinal pseudo-obstruction often require hospitalization for bowel rest, intravenous fluids, and correction of electrolyte abnormalities. Patients with intestinal failure may require total parenteral nutrition, as postpylori jejunal tube feeding becomes more difficult with small bowel involvement.[66]

Promotility Therapeutics

Motility of the entire GI tract can be affected in SSc. Avoidance of drugs that can impair motility is a first step in management. Drugs such as anticholinergics, opiates, and nondihydropyridine calcium channel blockers (often used for Raynaud management) can be responsible for dysmotility in SSc patients. Thus, an active medication administration review is an important step at all SSc patient visits. Opiate antagonists, such as methylnaltrexone, alvimopan, and naloxone, can be used concurrently to help reverse dysmotility effects of opiates.[66] If opiates must be used for pain management, tramadol has fewer effects on motility, and methadone may have a better side-effect profile.[66]

Metoclopramide is presently the only US Food and Drug Administration (FDA) -approved medication for treatment of gastroparesis. However, the FDA requires a boxed warning and risk mitigation strategy for metoclopramide-containing drugs and warns against chronic use of these products to treat gastrointestinal disorders.[67] Metoclopramide is a dopamine receptor antagonist (D2) that also activates 5-hydroxytryptamine (5HT-4) receptors for the combined effect of increased peristalsis of the duodenum and jejunum, increased tone and amplitude of gastric contractions, and relaxation of the pyloric sphincter and duodenal bulb, while simultaneously increasing lower esophageal sphincter tone.[66] It is a commonly used prokinetic, but may lead to significant neurologic side effects, such as tardive dyskinesia. Domperidone is another D2 antagonist with a better side-effect profile related to less penetration through the blood-brain barrier. Its main adverse side effect is hyperprolactinemia. However, domperidone is not as available in the United States. Although the effect of this drug on gastric motility has been studied in diabetic gastroparesis,[68] its use in SSc requires further research.

Cisapride is another 5HT-4 agonist that has been studied in reflux esophagitis in SSc, but has since been withdrawn from the market because of concern for cardiac arrhythmias.[68] Cisapride increases acetylcholine release from the myenteric plexus and is thought to increase lower esophageal sphincter pressure and gastric emptying through increases in esophageal contracting amplitudes and in the number of gastric contractions.[69] Another high-affinity 5HT-4, prucalopride, is still being studied for promotility for chronic intestinal pseudoobstruction,[66] but is not yet approved by the FDA.

Histamine blockers reduce acid production but, based on animal studies, may also stimulate gastric motility through an inhibitory effect on acetylcholinesterase, which in turn increases cholinergic tone. Ranitidine demonstrates this effect to a greater extent, compared with cimetidine and famotidine. However, the degree to which this phenomenon is operative in humans is unclear. Interestingly, a study of SSc patients revealed that the lower esophageal sphincter pressure was increased significantly by both intravenous cimetidine and famotidine. However, only famotidine caused a significant esophageal pressure increase in patients without an increase of gastric motility. These findings suggest that the inhibition of lower esophageal acetylcholinesterase activity and gastric acid secretion may be involved in the mechanisms of action of cimetidine and famotidine.[69]

Buspirone, which is usually prescribed as an anxiolytic, binds the endogenous neurotransmitter serotonin (5-hydroxytryptamine). Because 5HT1A receptors have been found to have a strong impact on esophageal peristalsis and lower esophageal sphincter (LES) function, buspirone's ability to augment esophageal motility was studied in a 4-week open-label trial of a small group of SSc patients. This medication was found to increase LES pressure and improve GERD symptoms, but not dysphagia or chest pain.[67]

Erythromycin in lower doses than those required for antibiotic effectiveness is thought to act as a motilin agonist as well as motilin mimic, thus stimulating gastric peristalsis. Accordingly, erythromycin was found to be beneficial in a case where food stasis resulted in esophagitis.[70] However, it appears to have little effect on the small intestine. Moreover, tachyphylaxis can occur with prolonged administration of erythromycin. Newer motilin agonists are in development for gastroparesis[71]

In a case study of 3 patients with connective tissue disorders and chronic intestinal pseudo-obstruction refractory to metoclopramide, domperidone, and cisapride, octreotide and antibiotics were found to be beneficial in improving intestinal motility.[72] Although stimulation of phase III migrating motor complexes in the intestines by octreotide was the purported mechanism of action, the concurrent treatment of SIBO for improved motility must be considered when approaching functional motility disorders in SSc patients. Similarly, a recent study found that ghrelin, which works through increasing postprandial gastric motility, stimulated increased gastric emptying in 10 SSc patients.[73] Of note, postprandial satiety was not improved with treatment, suggesting that there may be other factors involved with the patients' symptoms, which again highlights the importance of comanagement of other GIT issues such as SIBO.

Small Intestinal Bacterial Overgrowth Treatment

Treatment of SIBO involves treating the underlying disease. Dysmotility is thought to be a predisposing factor so treatment as described earlier may offer some relief. Nutritional modifications can also provide some benefit through elimination of simple sugars and lactose.[74] Antibiotics appear to be more effective than placebo for breath test normalization in patients with symptoms attributable to SIBO, and breath test normalization may correlate with clinical response. Specific antibiotic dosing and cycling recommendations are limited by evidence based on weak and heterogeneous study designs as well as small sample sizes.[75] Several broad-spectrum systemic antibiotics, such as fluoroquinolones, metronidazole, tetracycline, amoxicillin-clavulanic acid, and chloramphenicol, have been used to manage SIBO, but adverse effects are commonly reported.[76,77] Rifaximin, which is a nonabsorbable antibiotic, is effective and safe for the treatment of SIBO. However, it may not be available to certain patients because of its cost and formulary restrictions.[76] Of note, probiotics supplementation may effectively decontaminate SIBO and relieve abdominal pain, but has been ineffective in preventing SIBO.[78] Furthermore, the association of proton pump inhibitors with SIBO warrants consideration in SSc patients.[79]

Fecal Incontinence Management

Fecal incontinence in SSc may be related to neurogenic factors as well as fibrotic weakening of the muscle walls. Consequently, management may include a combination of antidiarrheal medications and dietary interventions in order to improve stool consistency. As discussed earlier, consideration of concurrent SIBO is important.[77] In small studies of fecal incontinence, sacral stimulation was shown to be beneficial through both temporal[80] and permanent sacral nerve stimulation[81]; however, further studies are needed in SSc to define the role of these procedures.

Surgical Intervention

Surgical options for fecal incontinence in SSc are often associated with both poor results and complications.[80] Endoscopic intervention is necessary for management of stricture, GAVE, and feeding tube placement for nutritional support. Surgical interventions, such as venting gastrostomy, gastrectomy, or gastric stimulators, have a high risk of associated complications and are not recommended.[48]

Liver Disease

Liver disease comprises approximately 1.1% of GIT involvement in SSc, which includes autoimmune hepatitis and PBC.[82] Important considerations in the management of liver disease include hepatic dosing of medications metabolized by the liver and cautious use of prednisone. In SSc patients, prednisone use increases the risk of scleroderma renal crisis. A case series of 5 patients with autoimmune hepatitis and SSc patients suggested that prednisone use was not associated with adverse effects.[82] It is unclear what conclusions may be drawn from this small sample size, although most would agree that blood pressure education and monitoring are imperative. In patients with concurrent autoimmune hepatitis and PBC, consultation with hepatology is indicated. For patients with PBC, treatment with medications, such as ursodeoxycholic acid, is indicated for therapeutic relief of clinical symptoms, such as itch, as well as cirrhosis prevention.

Adverse Effects of Medications

Medical therapeutics for SSc have several important considerations. Long-term consequences of acid suppression in SSc patients have not been assessed, and risks of enteric infection and effects on absorption of vitamins and minerals have not been clarified in this patient population. Adverse drug reactions, such as reflux exacerbation associated with calcium channel blockers and the constipating effect of pain medications, should be considered. Adverse drug reactions related to prokinetic agents include development of medication tolerance with prolonged use, and as these agents may prolong the QT interval resulting in serious arrhythmias, a baseline electrocardiogram should be obtained. Of note, although erythromycin can treat gastroparesis through its effects on motilin, it can also decrease small intestinal motility. Immunosuppressive medications, particularly those which target fibrotic cytokines and intravenous immunoglobulin, are potentially promising for treatment of SSc and warrant further study.[8] However, their effects on the GIT in particular are largely unknown.

SUMMARY

GIT involvement in SSc is associated with significant morbidity and mortality. An improved understanding of the pathogenesis and treatment of GIT involvement in SSc will require longitudinal, multicenter investigations that incorporate noninvasive testing as well as detailed histopathological studies and identification of biomarkers. Initiation of medical therapeutics in SSc patients requires a stepwise approach that incorporates diagnostic testing, and patient education and nutritional support are imperative in all patients with the diagnosis of SSc.

REFERENCES

1. Morrisroe K, Frech T, Schniering J, et al. Systemic sclerosis: the need for structured care. Best Pract Res Clin Rheumatol 2016;30(1):3–21.
2. van den Hoogen F, Khanna D, Fransen J, et al. 2013 classification criteria for systemic sclerosis: an American College of Rheumatology/European League against Rheumatism collaborative initiative. Arthritis Rheum 2013;65(11):2737–47.
3. Khanna D, Nagaraja V, Gladue H, et al. Measuring response in the gastrointestinal tract in systemic sclerosis. Curr Opin Rheumatol 2013;25(6):700–6.
4. Forbes A, Marie I. Gastrointestinal complications: the most frequent internal complications of systemic sclerosis. Rheumatology (Oxford) 2009;48(Suppl 3):iii36–9.
5. Chifflot H, Fautrel B, Sordet C, et al. Incidence and prevalence of systemic sclerosis: a systematic literature review. Semin Arthritis Rheum 2008;37(4):223–35.
6. Malcarne VL, Hansdottir I, McKinney A, et al. Medical signs and symptoms associated with disability, pain, and psychosocial adjustment in systemic sclerosis. J Rheumatol 2007;34(2):359–67.
7. Steen VD, Medsger TA Jr. Severe organ involvement in systemic sclerosis with diffuse scleroderma. Arthritis Rheum 2000;43(11):2437–44.
8. Kumar S, Singh J, Rattan S, et al. Review article: pathogenesis and clinical manifestations of gastrointestinal involvement in systemic sclerosis. Aliment Pharmacol Ther 2017;45(7):883–98.
9. Jimenez SA, Derk CT. Following the molecular pathways toward an understanding of the pathogenesis of systemic sclerosis. Ann Intern Med 2004;140(1): 37–50.
10. Pattanaik D, Brown M, Postlethwaite BC, et al. Pathogenesis of systemic sclerosis. Front Immunol 2015;6:272.
11. Bocchieri MH, Jimenez SA. Animal models of fibrosis. Rheum Dis Clin North Am 1990;16(1):153–67.
12. Thoua NM, Derrett-Smith EC, Khan K, et al. Gut fibrosis with altered colonic contractility in a mouse model of scleroderma. Rheumatology (Oxford) 2012; 51(11):1989–98.
13. Manetti M, Neumann E, Muller A, et al. Endothelial/lymphocyte activation leads to prominent CD4+ T cell infiltration in the gastric mucosa of patients with systemic sclerosis. Arthritis Rheum 2008;58(9):2866–73.
14. Raja J, Denton CP. Cytokines in the immunopathology of systemic sclerosis. Semin Immunopathol 2015;37(5):543–57.
15. Goldblatt F, Gordon TP, Waterman SA. Antibody-mediated gastrointestinal dysmotility in scleroderma. Gastroenterology 2002;123(4):1144–50.
16. Singh J, Mehendiratta V, Del Galdo F, et al. Immunoglobulins from scleroderma patients inhibit the muscarinic receptor activation in internal anal sphincter smooth muscle cells. Am J Physiol Gastrointest Liver Physiol 2009;297(6): G1206–13.
17. Kumar S, Singh J, Kedika R, et al. Role of muscarinic-3 receptor antibody in systemic sclerosis: correlation with disease duration and effects of IVIG. Am J Physiol Gastrointest Liver Physiol 2016;310(11):G1052–60.
18. Veale BJ, Jablonski RY, Frech TM, et al. Orofacial manifestations of systemic sclerosis. Br Dent J 2016;221(6):305–10.
19. Frech TM, Pauling JD, Murtaugh MA, et al. Sublingual abnormalities in systemic sclerosis. J Clin Rheumatol 2016;22(1):19–21.
20. Jung S, Martin T, Schmittbuhl M, et al. The spectrum of orofacial manifestations in systemic sclerosis: a challenging management. Oral Dis 2017;23(4):424–39.

21. Hansi N, Thoua N, Carulli M, et al. Consensus best practice pathway of the UK scleroderma study group: gastrointestinal manifestations of systemic sclerosis. Clin Exp Rheumatol 2014;32(6 Suppl 86):S-214–21.

22. Thonhofer R, Siegel C, Trummer M, et al. Early endoscopy in systemic sclerosis without gastrointestinal symptoms. Rheumatol Int 2012;32(1):165–8.

23. Carlson DA, Crowell MD, Kimmel JN, et al. Loss of peristaltic reserve, determined by multiple rapid swallows, is the most frequent esophageal motility abnormality in patients with systemic sclerosis. Clin Gastroenterol Hepatol 2016;14(10): 1502–6.

24. Richardson C, Agrawal R, Lee J, et al. Esophageal dilatation and interstitial lung disease in systemic sclerosis: a cross-sectional study. Semin Arthritis Rheum 2016;46(1):109–14.

25. Marie I, Ducrotte P, Antonietti M, et al. Watermelon stomach in systemic sclerosis: its incidence and management. Aliment Pharmacol Ther 2008;28(4):412–21.

26. Ingraham KM, O'Brien MS, Shenin M, et al. Gastric antral vascular ectasia in systemic sclerosis: demographics and disease predictors. J Rheumatol 2010;37(3): 603–7.

27. Sallam H, McNearney TA, Chen JD. Systematic review: pathophysiology and management of gastrointestinal dysmotility in systemic sclerosis (scleroderma). Aliment Pharmacol Ther 2006;23(6):691–712.

28. Marie I, Ducrotte P, Denis P, et al. Small intestinal bacterial overgrowth in systemic sclerosis. Rheumatology (Oxford) 2009;48(10):1314–9.

29. Marie I, Ducrotte P, Denis P, et al. Outcome of small-bowel motor impairment in systemic sclerosis–a prospective manometric 5-yr follow-up. Rheumatology (Oxford) 2007;46(1):150–3.

30. Kaneko M, Sasaki S, Teruya S, et al. Pneumatosis cystoides intestinalis in patients with systemic sclerosis: a case report and review of 39 Japanese cases. Case Rep Gastrointest Med 2016;2016:2474515.

31. Assassi S, Fritzler MJ, Arnett FC, et al. Primary biliary cirrhosis (PBC), PBC autoantibodies, and hepatic parameter abnormalities in a large population of systemic sclerosis patients. J Rheumatol 2009;36(10):2250–6.

32. Rigamonti C, Shand LM, Feudjo M, et al. Clinical features and prognosis of primary biliary cirrhosis associated with systemic sclerosis. Gut 2006;55(3):388–94.

33. Kaburaki J, Kuramochi S, Fujii T, et al. Nodular regenerative hyperplasia of the liver in a patient with systemic sclerosis. Clin Rheumatol 1996;15(6):613–6.

34. Assandri R, Monari M, Montanelli A. Development of systemic sclerosis in patients with autoimmune hepatitis: an emerging overlap syndrome. Gastroenterol Hepatol Bed Bench 2016;9(3):211–9.

35. Skare TL, Nisihara RM, Haider O, et al. Liver autoantibodies in patients with scleroderma. Clin Rheumatol 2011;30(1):129–32.

36. Ebert EC. Gastric and enteric involvement in progressive systemic sclerosis. J Clin Gastroenterol 2008;42(1):5–12.

37. Basilisco G, Barbera R, Vanoli M, et al. Anorectal dysfunction and delayed colonic transit in patients with progressive systemic sclerosis. Dig Dis Sci 1993;38(8):1525–9.

38. Fynne L, Worsoe J, Gregersen T, et al. Gastrointestinal transit in patients with systemic sclerosis. Scand J Gastroenterol 2011;46(10):1187–93.

39. D'Angelo G, Stern HS, Myers E. Rectal prolapse in scleroderma: case report and review of the colonic complications of scleroderma. Can J Surg 1985;28(1):62–3.

40. Richard N, Hudson M, Gyger G, et al. Clinical correlates of faecal incontinence in systemic sclerosis: identifying therapeutic avenues. Rheumatology (Oxford) 2017;56(4):581–8.

41. Thoua NM, Abdel-Halim M, Forbes A, et al. Fecal incontinence in systemic sclerosis is secondary to neuropathy. Am J Gastroenterol 2012;107(4):597–603.

42. Koh CE, Young CJ, Wright CM, et al. The internal anal sphincter in systemic sclerosis. Dis Colon Rectum 2009;52(2):315–8.

43. Heyt GJ, Oh MK, Alemzadeh N, et al. Impaired rectoanal inhibitory response in scleroderma (systemic sclerosis): an association with fecal incontinence. Dig Dis Sci 2004;49(6):1040–5.

44. Auluck A, Pai KM, Shetty C, et al. Mandibular resorption in progressive systemic sclerosis: a report of three cases. Dentomaxillofac Radiol 2005;34(6):384–6.

45. Derk CT, Rasheed M, Spiegel JR, et al. Increased incidence of carcinoma of the tongue in patients with systemic sclerosis. J Rheumatol 2005;32(4):637–41.

46. Rajapakse CN, Bancewicz J, Jones CJ, et al. Pharyngo-oesophageal dysphagia in systemic sclerosis. Ann Rheum Dis 1981;40(6):612–4.

47. Rajapakse C. Pharyngoesophageal dysphagia: an under recognised, potentially fatal, but very treatable feature of systemic sclerosis. Intern Med J 2016;46(11): 1340–4.

48. Nagaraja V, McMahan ZH, Getzug T, et al. Management of gastrointestinal involvement in scleroderma. Curr Treatm Opt Rheumatol 2015;1(1):82–105.

49. Shawis TN, Chaloner C, Herrick AL, et al. Pancreatic function in systemic sclerosis. Br J Rheumatol 1996;35(3):298–9.

50. Fynne L, Worsoe J, Laurberg S, et al. Faecal incontinence in patients with systemic sclerosis: is an impaired internal anal sphincter the only cause? Scand J Rheumatol 2011;40(6):462–6.

51. Baron M, Hudson M, Steele R, Canadian Scleroderma Research Group. Malnutrition is common in systemic sclerosis: results from the Canadian Scleroderma Research Group database. J Rheumatol 2009;36(12):2737–43.

52. Krause L, Becker MO, Brueckner CS, et al. Nutritional status as marker for disease activity and severity predicting mortality in patients with systemic sclerosis. Ann Rheum Dis 2010;69(11):1951–7.

53. Baron M, Bernier P, Cote LF, et al. Screening and therapy for malnutrition and related gastro-intestinal disorders in systemic sclerosis: recommendations of a North American expert panel. Clin Exp Rheumatol 2010;28(2 Suppl 58):S42–6.

54. Murtaugh MA, Frech TM. Nutritional status and gastrointestinal symptoms in systemic sclerosis patients. Clin Nutr 2013;32(1):130–5.

55. Baron M, Hudson M, Steele R, Canadian Scleroderma Research Group (CSRG). Is serum albumin a marker of malnutrition in chronic disease? The scleroderma paradigm. J Am Coll Nutr 2010;29(2):144–51.

56. Raja J, Ng CT, Sujau I, et al. High-resolution oesophageal manometry and 24-hour impedance-pH study in systemic sclerosis patients: association with clinical features, symptoms and severity. Clin Exp Rheumatol 2016;34 Suppl 100(5): 115–21.

57. Shah AA, Wigley FM, Hummers LK. Telangiectases in scleroderma: a potential clinical marker of pulmonary arterial hypertension. J Rheumatol 2010;37(1): 98–104.

58. Valenzuela A, Li S, Becker L, et al. Intestinal pseudo-obstruction in patients with systemic sclerosis: an analysis of the Nationwide Inpatient Sample. Rheumatology (Oxford) 2016;55(4):654–8.

59. Frech TM. Understanding empirical therapeutics in systemic sclerosis gastrointestinal tract disease. Rheumatology (Oxford) 2017;56(2):176–7.
60. Spiegel BM, Hays RD, Bolus R, et al. Development of the NIH patient-reported outcomes measurement information system (PROMIS) gastrointestinal symptom scales. Am J Gastroenterol 2014;109(11):1804–14.
61. Alantar A, Cabane J, Hachulla E, et al. Recommendations for the care of oral involvement in patients with systemic sclerosis. Arthritis Care Res (Hoboken) 2011;63(8):1126–33.
62. Yuen HK, Marlow NM, Reed SG, et al. Effect of orofacial exercises on oral aperture in adults with systemic sclerosis. Disabil Rehabil 2012;34(1):84–9.
63. Yuen HK, Weng Y, Bandyopadhyay D, et al. Effect of a multi-faceted intervention on gingival health among adults with systemic sclerosis. Clin Exp Rheumatol 2011;29(2 Suppl 65):S26–32.
64. Katz PO, Gerson LB, Vela MF. Guidelines for the diagnosis and management of gastroesophageal reflux disease. Am J Gastroenterol 2013;108(3):308–28 [quiz: 29].
65. Halmos EP, Power VA, Shepherd SJ, et al. A diet low in FODMAPs reduces symptoms of irritable bowel syndrome. Gastroenterology 2014;146(1):67–75.e5.
66. Paine P, McLaughlin J, Lal S. Review article: the assessment and management of chronic severe gastrointestinal dysmotility in adults. Aliment Pharmacol Ther 2013;38(10):1209–29.
67. Camilleri M. Functional dyspepsia and gastroparesis. Dig Dis 2016;34(5):491–9.
68. Sugumar A, Singh A, Pasricha PJ. A systematic review of the efficacy of domperidone for the treatment of diabetic gastroparesis. Clin Gastroenterol Hepatol 2008;6(7):726–33.
69. Horikoshi T, Matsuzaki T, Sekiguchi T. Effect of H2-receptor antagonists cimetidine and famotidine on interdigestive gastric motor activity and lower esophageal sphincter pressure in progressive systemic sclerosis. Intern Med 1994;33(7): 407–12.
70. Hara T, Ogoshi K, Yamamoto S, et al. Successful treatment of severe reflux esophagitis with erythromycin in a patient with progressive systemic sclerosis and proximal gastrectomy. Tokai J Exp Clin Med 2006;31(2):70–2.
71. Acosta A, Camilleri M. Prokinetics in gastroparesis. Gastroenterol Clin North Am 2015;44(1):97–111.
72. Perlemuter G, Cacoub P, Chaussade S, et al. Octreotide treatment of chronic intestinal pseudoobstruction secondary to connective tissue diseases. Arthritis Rheum 1999;42(7):1545–9.
73. Ariyasu H, Iwakura H, Yukawa N, et al. Clinical effects of ghrelin on gastrointestinal involvement in patients with systemic sclerosis. Endocr J 2014;61(7):735–42.
74. Bures J, Cyrany J, Kohoutova D, et al. Small intestinal bacterial overgrowth syndrome. World J Gastroenterol 2010;16(24):2978–90.
75. Shah SC, Day LW, Somsouk M, et al. Meta-analysis: antibiotic therapy for small intestinal bacterial overgrowth. Aliment Pharmacol Ther 2013;38(8):925–34.
76. Gatta L, Scarpignato C. Systematic review with meta-analysis: rifaximin is effective and safe for the treatment of small intestine bacterial overgrowth. Aliment Pharmacol Ther 2017;45(5):604–16.
77. Gyger G, Baron M. Gastrointestinal manifestations of scleroderma: recent progress in evaluation, pathogenesis, and management. Curr Rheumatol Rep 2012; 14(1):22–9.
78. Zhong C, Qu C, Wang B, et al. Probiotics for preventing and treating small intestinal bacterial overgrowth: a meta-analysis and systematic review of current evidence. J Clin Gastroenterol 2017;51(4):300–11.

79. Lo WK, Chan WW. Proton pump inhibitor use and the risk of small intestinal bacterial overgrowth: a meta-analysis. Clin Gastroenterol Hepatol 2013;11(5):483–90.
80. Kenefick NJ, Vaizey CJ, Nicholls RJ, et al. Sacral nerve stimulation for faecal incontinence due to systemic sclerosis. Gut 2002;51(6):881–3.
81. Malouf AJ, Vaizey CJ, Nicholls RJ, et al. Permanent sacral nerve stimulation for fecal incontinence. Ann Surg 2000;232(1):143–8.
82. You BC, Jeong SW, Jang JY, et al. Liver cirrhosis due to autoimmune hepatitis combined with systemic sclerosis. Korean J Gastroenterol 2012;59(1):48–52.

Drug-Induced Gastrointestinal and Hepatic Disease Associated with Biologics and Nonbiologic Disease-Modifying Antirheumatic Drugs

Patrick R. Wood, MD*, Liron Caplan, MD, PhD

KEYWORDS

- Drug-related ADRs and adverse reactions • Immunosuppressive agents
- Antirheumatic agents • Gastrointestinal diseases • Liver diseases • Mouth diseases
- Pancreatic diseases • Chemical and drug-induced liver injury

KEY POINTS

- Long-term methotrexate use is associated with hepatotoxicity and fibrosis.
- Azathioprine and other nonbiologic disease-modifying antirheumatic drug use is associated with a variety of unique hepatic, biliary, and pancreatic complications.
- Rituximab use is strongly associated with an increased risk of viral hepatitis B virus reactivation, although tumor necrosis factor-alpha inhibitors and other treatments also confer reactivation risk to lesser degrees.
- Tofacitinib and interleukin-6 inhibition use may increase the risk of gastrointestinal perforation events.
- Anti-interleukin-17 therapies have been associated with incident or worsening inflammatory bowel disease, although data are ambiguous.

Disclosure Statement: All authors declare no conflicts of interest in this article, including financial, consultant, institutional, and other relationships that might lead to bias or a conflict of interest. Financial Support: There was no financial or grant support for this article. Dr L. Caplan is supported by VA HSR&D IIR 14-048-3 and the Michelson Fund at the University of Colorado Foundation. Author Contributions: P. Wood and L. Caplan were responsible for drafting, critical revision, and approval of the final article. All authors were involved in the final approval of the version of the article submitted and have agreed to be accountable for all aspects of the work. The views expressed in this article are those of the authors and do not necessarily reflect the position or policy of the Department of Veterans Affairs.
Division of Rheumatology, University of Colorado, Anschutz Medical Campus Barbara Davis Center, 1775 Aurora Court, PO Box 6511, Mail Stop B-115, Aurora, CO 80045, USA
* Corresponding author. Anschutz Medical Campus Barbara Davis Center, 1775 Aurora Court, PO Box 6511, Mail Stop B-115, Aurora, CO 80045.
E-mail address: patrick.wood@ucdenver.edu

Rheum Dis Clin N Am 44 (2018) 29–43
https://doi.org/10.1016/j.rdc.2017.09.003
0889-857X/18/© 2017 Elsevier Inc. All rights reserved.

rheumatic.theclinics.com

INTRODUCTION

The invention and discovery of various nonbiologic and biologic disease-modifying therapies have revolutionized the care of rheumatic and other autoimmune disease. Although the strides made in therapy are remarkable, the use of these agents, as with all therapies, confers risks in the form of adverse drug reactions (ADRs) **(Table 1)**. These ADRs, defined by the World Health Organization as "a response to a drug which is noxious and unintended, and which occurs at doses normally used,"[1] include significant gastrointestinal ADRs, that is, "side effects." The authors briefly introduce and review the mechanism of action of disease-modifying therapies commonly used in the care of rheumatic disease. Frequently encountered and drug-specific gastrointestinal ADRs are discussed, including reviews of the primary literature describing these reactions. Guidelines and standard of care practices, where they exist, for screening, monitoring, and management of these reactions, are summarized.

CONVENTIONAL DISEASE-MODIFYING ANTI-RHEUMATIC DRUGS
Methotrexate

High-dose intravenous formulations of methotrexate (MTX) were first used at as a chemotherapeutic in cancer treatment in the 1940s. Lower dosing regimens via oral and subcutaneous routes were later pioneered and approved for use in psoriasis and rheumatoid arthritis (RA) in the 1960s and 1980s, respectively.[2] MTX is now one of the most widely used antirheumatic medications, used in a variety of inflammatory diseases. It is a folate antimetabolite, and mechanisms of action include inhibition of DNA synthesis, repair, and replication. Specifically, its antimetabolite effects are mediated via inhibition of dihydrofolate reductase and, therefore, purine synthesis. At lower doses typically used in the treatment of rheumatic diseases, this mechanism of action is less important; however, at these doses, MTX and its metabolite MTX-polyglutamate dephosphorylate extracellular adenine nucleotides. Through this effect, it is hypothesized that extracellular adenosine levels are increased, with downstream reductions in lymphocyte proliferation and production of cytokines, including tumor necrosis factor-alpha, interleukin-1 (IL-1), and IL-12.[3–5]

Hepatotoxicity
Hepatotoxicity associated with long-term oral MTX use in psoriasis was initially described in the 1960s. Early reports suggested rates of fibrosis of up to 14% to 50%, and 11% to 26% for clinical cirrhosis following several years of use.[6] At the time of early studies, cumulative MTX exposure was significantly higher than is typically used today, and daily dosing (rather than weekly) was common. In addition, folic acid supplementation (demonstrated to reduce hepatotoxicity[7]) was not commonly used at the time of early landmark studies. Concurrent alcohol use, viral hepatitis, and other uncontrolled factors may also have contributed to the very high rates of toxicity.

Pathologic changes to the liver seen with long-term MTX exposure include steatosis, stellate cell hypertrophy, and fibrosis. The mechanism of action of this toxicity is incompletely understood. Theories include prolonged accumulation of MTX polyglutamate and folate depletion.

Of note, later studies in the setting of RA suggest the incidence of advanced hepatocellular changes at much lower rates, approximately 5%.[8,9] In addition to the uncontrolled factors noted above in early studies, liver function monitoring protocols varied in this population when compared with the early psoriasis literature. It should also be

Table 1
Summary of select adverse drug reactions associated with conventional and biologic disease-modifying therapies

Risk of Select Gastrointestinal ADRs in Conventional and Biologic Disease-Modifying Anti-Rheumatic Drugs (by Agent):

Medication	Nausea/Vomiting	HBV Reactivation	Hepatotoxicity	GIP	HSTCL	Other
Methotrexate	High	Low risk	Moderate(fibrosis)	Low risk	Low risk	Stomatitis, ulcerations
Azathioprine	High	Low risk	Moderate (multiple types)	Possibly associated	Low risk	Pancreatitis, endothelial pathology
Tofacitinib	Moderate	Low risk	Moderate	Moderate	Low risk	
Sulfasalazine	High	Low risk	Moderate (multiple types)	Low risk	Low risk	Acute hypersensitivity, granulomatous hepatitis
Leflunomide	High	Low risk	Moderate (acute injury)	Low risk	Low risk	Enterohepatic recirculation
Hydroxychloroquine	Low risk	Low risk	Low risk	Low risk	Low risk	
Tocilizumab	Low risk	Unclear, probably moderate	Yes	Moderate	Low risk	
Interleukin-17 inhibitors	Low risk	Unclear, probably moderate	Low risk	Low risk	Low risk	Inflammatory bowel disease
B-cell targeted therapies	Moderate[a]	Very high[b]	Low risk	Low risk	Low risk	Lower gastrointestinal obstruction (in cancer patients)
Tumor necrosis factor-alpha inhibitors	Low risk	Moderate	Yes[c]	Possibly associated	Possibly associated	
Ustekinumab	Moderate	Unclear, probably moderate	Low risk	Low risk	Low risk	Appendicitis
Interleukin-1 inhibitors	Low risk	Unclear, probably moderate	Low risk	Low risk	Low risk	
Abatacept	Low risk	Unclear, probably moderate	Yes	Low risk	Low risk	

Note. See text for references and further details.
Abbreviations: GIP, Gastrointestinal Perforation; HSTCL, Hepatosplenic T-cell Lymphoma.
[a] Belimumab.
[b] Rituximab.
[c] Infliximab/adalimumab.

noted that although up to 15% of patients develop intermittent transaminase elevations over the course of long-term use, these events are typically self-limited.

Risk factors for cirrhosis and fibrosis with long-term MTX use include concurrent alcohol use, history of nonalcoholic fatty liver disease, chronic viral hepatitis or other concurrent primary liver disease (including viral hepatitis and nonalcoholic fatty liver disease), diabetes, obesity, hyperlipidemia (metabolic syndrome), concurrent hepatotoxic medication use, absence of folate supplementation, and cumulative MTX dose.[10]

Monitoring and assessment for MTX hepatotoxicity include an ongoing assessment of cumulative dose exposure. Frequent liver function test (LFT) monitoring (including transaminases, alkaline phosphatase, protein, and bilirubin) every 4 to 12 weeks (depending on duration and stability of dose) is standard of care and is included in treatment guidelines. Notably, in older psoriasis literature, LFT abnormalities did not correlate well with biopsy results,[6] although later RA literature in the setting of more regular monitoring suggested LFT abnormalities do correlate well with biopsy abnormalities.[8,9] American College of Rheumatology management guidelines in RA recommend liver biopsy in the event that greater than 6 in 12 LFTs are abnormal over the course of 1 year. In psoriasis patients receiving long-term MTX therapy, serial liver biopsy, regardless of LFT monitoring, was previously recommended once the patient reaches 1.5 g, 3.5 g, and 4.0 g of cumulative MTX exposure. More recent guidelines have suggested liver biopsies may not be required in the absence of other risk factors. Serial monitoring biopsies are not recommended in current RA guidelines.[11–14]

Liver biopsy interpretation in the setting of long-term MTX use for psoriasis is standardized and based on the Roenigk classification. This framework divides hepatocellular changes into 5 grades, with grades above IIIA representing fibrosis. Grades 1 to 2 are commonly seen and do not require any changes to therapy. Grade IIIA suggests a need for repeat/close monitoring by serial biopsy, whereas any changes graded above IIIB preclude further MTX use.[15]

The biomarker procollagen type III amino-terminal peptide is an extension cleavage peptide and marker of collagen turnover used in Europe for MTX monitoring. Levels of this biomarker correlate with hepatic fibrosis. This assay is highly sensitive, but poorly specific, and is not useful in pediatric disease, RA, psoriatic arthritis, or clinical situations with elevated connective tissue turnover. As such, its use is primarily limited to psoriasis, and various European dermatologic management guidelines promote it as an option for MTX monitoring.[16]

In addition to periodic laboratory and biopsy monitoring, avoidance of significant alcohol intake is advised among patients taking MTX. Alcohol intake conveys a 2.5 to 5 times relative risk increase for hepatocellular disease in some studies. Additional caution and attention should be given to other modifiable or nonmodifiable risk factors, such as type II diabetes, obesity, and concurrent hepatotoxic medication use. Finally, a review of high-quality literature examining folic and folinic acid supplementation for the prevention of ADRs of low-dose MTX strongly supports the use of these agents in the prevention of hepatotoxicity as well as discontinuation from MTX for any reason. This review suggested a 77% relative risk reduction in LFT abnormalities with concurrent Folic Acid use, and a 61% relative risk reduction in withdrawal from MTX for any reason.[7,17–21]

Stomatitis, mucositis, upper gastrointestinal distress, and other adverse drug reactions

In addition to hepatotoxicity, a variety of less serious oral and gastrointestinal ADRs are commonly encountered with low-dose MTX use. A *Cochrane Review*[18] incorporating the seminal studies of MTX use in RA identified statistically significant differences in gastrointestinal distress (9% vs 4%) and stomatitis/oral ulcers (9% vs 4%) in MTX users compared with placebo. Nonsignificant differences were also identified in other clinically recognized side effects, such as diarrhea and abdominal pain. Notably, folic or folinic acid supplementation appears to be effective in preventing some of these ADRs and discontinuation from MTX for any reason. A review of controlled trial data of folic acid supplementation showed statistically significant risk reductions for gastrointestinal ADRs, including nausea, vomiting, and abdominal pain. Although a trend was seen supporting its use in the prevention of stomatitis, this trend was not statistically significant based on this review.[7]

Azathioprine

Azathioprine (AZA) is a widely used immunosuppressant first synthesized and used in the late 1950s. It is a thiopurine and prodrug of 6-mercaptopurine, which through enzymatic pathways is converted to 6-thioguanine nucleotides methylthioinosine monophosphate, thioguanine triphosphate, and thio-deoxyguanosine triphosphate. These compounds act as purine analogues and are selectively incorporated into the DNA of rapidly replicating cells, particularly lymphocytes, leading to broad downstream inhibitory effects on the immune system.[22] AZA is widely used in the treatment of systemic lupus erythematosus, RA, inflammatory bowel and muscle disease, autoimmune hepatitis, as well as in post–organ transplant antirejection regimens. As the agent is a prodrug, toxicities vary with genetic polymorphisms of critical enzymes in its metabolic pathways, particularly thiopurine methyltransferase. In addition, concurrent use of agents that affect purine synthesis and salvage pathways (particularly xanthine oxidase inhibitors) may heighten AZA toxicity. Common ADRs include nausea and upper gastrointestinal upset in up to 23% of patients.[23] In addition, a variety of unique hepatobiliary ADRs are seen with AZA use, which should be noted.

Acute cholestatic hepatitis/hypersensitivity syndrome

Both acute hepatocellular and cholestatic reactions are seen in new AZA users. Some studies suggest nearly 8% of users develop LFTs that are at least 1 to 2 times the upper limit of normal (ULN) on a yearly basis, although this appears most commonly in the first year of therapy.[24] US Food and Drug Administration (FDA) guidelines suggest close LFT monitoring (weekly in the first 3 months) as a result of these data, with monitoring reduced to monthly for 3 months and then quarterly thereafter. Older American College of Rheumatology guidelines[25] suggested only obtaining baseline transaminase levels for monitoring AZA in RA, without subsequent testing. Newer guidelines do not make recommendations for AZA.[12] Few formal guidelines exist on dose alterations or protocols for abnormal results, although it is common for dose reductions by one-third to one-half to be made until normalization of LFTs, and for the drug to be discontinued if normalization is not achieved with these changes or with severe LFT anomalies.

Peliosis hepatis, nodular regenerative hyperplasia, sinusoidal obstruction syndrome

A variety of unique and otherwise rare hepatotoxicities have been observed in association with long-term AZA use. These ADRs' include peliosis hepatis (peliosis hepatitis), a syndrome manifesting as multiple blood-filled hepatic cavities; nodular regenerative hyperplasia, a widespread parenchymal nodulosis along septal tracts; and the sinusoidal obstruction syndrome and veno-occlusive disease. The pathophysiologic changes of these rare entities are incompletely understood, but are thought to relate to endothelial injury in the sinusoids and terminal venules, rather than a parenchymal or hepatocyte injury. Unlike acute hepatotoxic reactions or hypersensitivity, these reactions are typically seen years after initiation of therapy, appear to be cumulative dose-dependent, and should be considered in otherwise unexplained laboratory anomalies or portal hypertension in long-term AZA users.[26–29]

Acute pancreatitis

So-called drug-induced pancreatitis has been linked to a variety of agents, including commonly used drug classes such as ACE inhibitors, thiazide diuretics, oral contraceptive pills, and statins. This entity is relatively rare, but has been described in association with AZA. Danish case control data[30] suggest a significantly elevated relative risk for pancreatitis in AZA users, although the absolute risk rate was 1 in 659 patient-years, and the population-attributable risk (the proportion of all cases attributable to AZA) was less than 0.5%. Despite this relatively low absolute risk, AZA is generally acknowledged as a potential culprit for otherwise unexplained pancreatitis, and patients and prescribing physicians should be aware of this risk.

Hepatobiliary malignancy

Hepatosplenic T-cell lymphoma (HSTCL) is a very rare and highly fatal malignancy of unclear incidence that was initially described in the early 1990s. It is a form of peripheral T-cell, non-Hodgkin lymphoma that presents with systemic symptoms and hepatosplenomegaly without lymphadenopathy. Some investigators have associated this malignancy with autoimmune disease (particularly inflammatory bowel disease) but also possibly with treatment with AZA (in addition to mercaptopurine and tumor necrosis factor inhibitor, TNFi). The basis for this potential association is a series of 43 FDA-reported cases in the 2010s among users of these agents. Of note, most patients in this series were exposed to AZA and had inflammatory bowel disease, although 3 cases were using TNFi therapy without AZA for RA or psoriasis. Based on these reports, a large-scale observational study was performed in the Netherlands[31] that showed an extremely low incidence of HSTCL overall, and no association with either immune-mediated disease or treatments, including AZA. This controversy reflects the broader topic of risk for hematologic and other malignancies ascribed to these agents. Hepatobiliary carcinoma (or cholangiocarcinoma) has been reported in association with AZA use; however, this risk is confounded by the underlying inflammatory disease process in many AZA users, particularly primary sclerosing cholangitis (PSC), which has a well-described and widely accepted risk association with this malignancy. A retrospective study in Germany and Norway in 2016 showed no additional risk for cholangiocarcinoma attributable to AZA use in patients with PSC.[32]

Tofacitinib

Tofacitinib is an oral, small molecule inhibitor of Janus kinases (primarily JAK 1 and 3). Downstream effects of its use include reduction in activation in the JAK-STAT pathway, which ultimately leads to reduced cytokine expression, proliferation, and activation of $CD4^+$ T cells. Tofacitinib has been FDA approved for the treatment of RA since 2012. Gastrointestinal ADRs reported in conjunction with tofacitinib use include hepatotoxicity (up to 1% with LFT elevations >3× ULN), hepatic steatosis, diarrhea (4%), gastritis, nausea, and vomiting. As a result of sporadic transaminase elevations reported in clinical trials, routine LFT monitoring is recommended during use, although unlike traditional oral disease-modifying anti-rheumatic drugs (DMARDs), this is not typically recommended on a long-term basis.[33]

Gastrointestinal perforation

Gastrointestinal perforations (GIP) were reported in clinical trials for tofacitinib, and as a result, product labels include a warning regarding this ADR, particularly in those with a history of diverticulitis. GIPs were relatively rare events in the clinical trials; however, subsequent large-scale observational work by Xie and colleagues[34] confirmed that the risk of perforation with tofacitinib use may indeed be significantly elevated compared with users of other immunosuppressive agents (TNFi), with an adjusted hazard ratio of 3.24 (1.05–10.04). A history of gastrointestinal comorbidities (particularly diverticulitis), moderate or greater dose of glucocorticoid use, and age were additional risk factors for GIP while taking this agent.

The mechanism of these risks is still unclear, although data from translational experiments[35] suggest a potentially important role for IL-6 in the maintenance, integrity, and turnover of gastrointestinal mucosal barriers, as well as in the pathogenesis of inflammatory bowel disease and colon cancer. Therefore, a plausible mechanism for these adverse ADRs includes downstream inhibition of IL-6, leading to reduced gastrointestinal barrier turnover and subsequent perforation risks. This proposed mechanism is consistent with similar risks seen in association with the IL-6 receptor inhibitor tocilizumab (see later discussion).

Sulfasalazine

Sulfasalazine (SSZ) was initially investigated as early as the 1940s for use as an RA treatment and was resurrected following positive study results in the late 1970s to early 1980s. The drug is a compound of 2 potentially active agents, 5-aminosalicylic acid (5-ASA) and sulfa-pyridine. Its mechanism of action is incompletely understood.[36] In inflammatory bowel disease, 5-ASA, which is primarily excreted intact without absorption, is likely the active metabolite, whereas sulfa-pyridine, which is absorbed systemically, is likely the primary active component in RA treatment. The mechanism of action for sulfa-pyridine is also incompletely understood, although it may reduce production of certain cytokines, including IL-8. In addition, a small proportion of the compound molecule is absorbed systemically, and SSZ may possess inhibitory effects on nuclear factor kappa-light-chain-enhancer of activated B cells (NF-κB) independent of the 2 component molecules. The most common gastrointestinal effects of SSZ include dose-dependent gastrointestinal distress.

Acute hypersensitivity with hepatic injury

Idiosyncratic acute hepatitis events have been described with SSZ use, and the drug may cause a unique syndrome of fever, rash, eosinophilia, and severely elevated LFTs (even including fulminant hepatic necrosis), occurring in up to 1 in 200 patients. Hepatotoxicity is more common with a history of viral hepatitis and concomitant use of isoniazid. Because of these risks, most expert opinion suggests close LFT monitoring at 2- to 4-week intervals initially, and no less frequent than every 12 weeks even on longstanding therapy.[29,37–39]

Granulomatous hepatitis

In addition, case reports have described a unique presentation of cholestatic LFT anomalies in conjunction with granulomas on liver biopsy for patients taking SSZ. These anomalies were described initially in patients with Crohn disease, but have been seen in patients taking SSZ for other indications. The pathologic and laboratory changes resolved with discontinuation of the agent, suggesting this is indeed a rare idiosyncratic reaction to the medication itself.[29,40]

Leflunomide

Leflunomide (LEF) is structurally unrelated to MTX, although it has a similar mechanism of action as an antimetabolite. Its primary mechanism of action is via inhibiting synthesis of a pyrimidine ribonucleotide (uridine, monophosphate) by the primary metabolite teriflunomide. This inhibition inhibits cell-cycle progression. In addition, LEF inhibits leukocyte adhesion, dendritic cell function, reduction in NF-κB activation, and reduction of T-cell activation via Janus kinase inhibition.[41] The agent is widely used in the treatment of RA.

Common and significant adverse effects for LEF are primarily gastrointestinal, including nausea and diarrhea in up to 15% of patients, although this is rarely severe enough to warrant drug discontinuation.[42] Loading doses (no longer recommended) were also associated with greater numbers of gastrointestinal ADRs.[43] In addition, severe aminotransferase abnormalities have been noted (as well as fatal liver failure), although these risks are probably similar to MTX.[44] As a result, present guidelines recommend periodic monitoring of LFTs occurring on a weekly basis at initiation and quarterly with stable long-term use. FDA guidelines suggest particularly close monitoring for those using MTX and LEF concurrently, and those with preexisting liver disease; patients with a history of LFTs >2× ULN should not take LEF. Special note should be made regarding the enterohepatic recirculation of LEF and extremely long effective half-life. In instances with severe LFT abnormalities (greater than 2× ULN) or unplanned pregnancy while on LEF (which has an unacceptable antenatal/prenatal risk profile), a "cholestyramine washout" may be used to eliminate the drug rapidly. This protocol calls for 8 g oral cholestyramine 3 times daily for 11+ days until LFTs have normalized. In the instance of a planned pregnancy within 3 months or an unplanned pregnancy, cholestyramine is continued until drug levels are confirmed less than 0.02 mg/L on 2 separate tests separated by at least 2 weeks.

Hydroxychloroquine and Other Antimalarials

The mechanism of anti-inflammatory action for hydroxychloroquine (HCQ) and other antimalarials remains incompletely understood. The most widely accepted proposed mechanisms include alteration of vacuolar and lysosomal pH, thereby altering processes such as protein degradation and macromolecule assembly. In addition, antimalarials likely inhibit the stimulation of, and downregulate, toll-like receptors, leading to downstream inhibitory effects on a variety of innate immune responses. HCQ and other antimalarial agents are widely used in the treatment of systemic lupus erythematosus, RA, and other inflammatory conditions.

Long-term antimalarial use is typically well tolerated, with the most feared complication of retinal toxicity well known and described elsewhere. Although much time and effort are spent on these rare but potentially irreversible ADRs, the most common adverse events with antimalarial use are gastrointestinal, and include anorexia, diarrhea, nausea, and vomiting. These adverse events occur commonly, although they are rarely severe enough to prompt therapeutic changes. HCQ-based disease management has been subject to recent tumult as a result of drug manufacturing issues. Formulary and drug patent changes are relevant because recent preliminary data suggest some gastrointestinal ADRs may be formulation or brand dependent.[45]

BIOLOGIC AGENTS
Tocilizumab

Tocilizumab is a humanized monoclonal antibody directed against the IL-6 receptor. The binding of soluble and membrane-bound receptors to IL-6 results in widespread downstream anti-inflammatory effects. The agent was developed in the late 1990s and early 2000s, approved for use in RA in the early 2010, and recently approved for use in giant cell arteritis in 2017. Tocilizumab has been associated with a variety of gastrointestinal adverse events. Most common among these include significant transaminase elevations in up to 36% of users. These perturbations in LFTs are reversible and as yet have not been strongly associated with clinically meaningful long-term hepatic injury such as cirrhosis.[46]

Gastrointestinal perforation
In addition, tocilizumab use has been strongly associated with an increased risk of lower GIP events. In Xie and colleagues,[34] the relative risk of lower GIP among tocilizumab users was 2.55 (1.33–4.88) relative to TNFi users. As noted above, recent basic and translational science has implicated IL-6 as important in the maintenance of gastrointestinal mucosal integrity and turnover. Presumably, loss of this protection underlies the mechanism for GIPs.[47–49]

Interleukin-17 Inhibitors

Secukinumab is a humanized monoclonal antibody against IL-17, a cytokine produced by Th17 T cells that has been implicated in the disease pathways of psoriasis, psoriatic arthritis, spondyloarthritis, and other diseases. It is approved by the FDA for treatment of psoriasis, psoriatic arthritis, and ankylosing spondylitis.[49] Ixekizumab is a related agent approved for the treatment of psoriasis. Typical gastrointestinal ADRs to agents in this class include diarrhea and candidiasis.

Inflammatory bowel disease
Postmarketing reports have raised concern for incident cases and worsening of ulcerative colitis and Crohn disease among secukinumab users.[50] Interpretation of these data has been controversial, however, because Crohn and ulcerative colitis are pathophysiologically linked with spondyloarthritides, separate from any drug effect. The risks of developing inflammatory bowel disease are up to 2-to 4-fold higher in spondyloarthritis than in the general population. In addition, subclinical gut inflammation may occur in up to 50% of ankylosing spondylitis patients. Of note, more recent data[51] suggest the elevated risk of inflammatory bowel disease among secukinumab users may be no different than those receiving other treatments. Nonetheless, patients should be counseled on the potential risk for incident or worsening inflammatory bowel disease with anti-IL-17 treatments.[49,52]

B-Cell–Directed Therapies

Rituximab (RXN) is a chimeric monoclonal antibody directed at CD20-positive B cells, which induces apoptosis and complement-mediated cytotoxicity of these cells. It is widely used in the treatment of a variety of neoplastic and inflammatory conditions, including RA, dermatomyositis, and vasculitis, among others. Nausea, vomiting, and diarrhea are commonly seen with its administration, present in up to 10% to 20% of users. Bowel obstruction and perforation have been reported in association with RXN use, although this severe ADR has been primarily been seen primarily in posttransplant lymphoproliferative disease, non-Hodgkin lymphoma, and other oncologic applications of the medication.[53]

Viral hepatitis reactivation and rituximab
Hepatitis B virus (HBV) reactivation has occurred with RXN, including cases of fulminant liver failure and death. As such, FDA labeling for the agent includes a "black box" warning that recommends screening for HBV before treatment to reduce this risk. Screening typically includes serologic testing for HBV surface antigen (HBVsAg) and

core antibodies (HBVcAb).[54] Those who are sAg positive are at very high risk of RXN-induced reactivation; those with only core antibody positivity are at a more moderate risk, possibly similar to antigen-positive patients receiving TNFi. Of note, even antigen-positive patients receiving nonbiologic antirheumatic agents under most circumstances will be at low risk for viral reactivation. Moderate- to high-risk patients, on the other hand, should be treated with prophylactic antiviral therapy during and 6 to 12 months following treatment with RXN. These patients should also be monitored closely for reactivation, with serial liver function testing on a quarterly basis; HBV serum polymerase chain reaction testing should also be obtained serially, because PCR serologic recurrence may precede transaminase elevations. Data have shown that institution of prophylactic treatments in the setting of high reactivation risk medications reduces the risk of HBV reactivation.[54–57] In contrast to HBV, hepatitis C virus (HCV) reactivation with RXN is relatively uncommon, and RXN may be used in many cases of HCV infection. Although case reports have described rare examples of viral reactivation in this setting,[58] RXN is used as a therapy in HCV-associated mixed cryoglobulinemia. Recent guidelines suggest caution with RXN use in HCV in high-risk situations, including acute infection and high-grade cirrhosis, even under antiviral treatment.[12]

Belimumab

Belimumab is a humanized monoclonal antibody against B-cell activating factor (BAFF) also known as B-lymphocyte stimulator. BAFF is a required factor for B-cell stimulation and survival. Belimumab may primarily bind to circulating soluble BAFF, as the agent does not produce the cellular cytotoxicity and reduction in circulating CD-20 positive B cells seen with RXN. Although belimumab, an FDA-approved treatment for systemic lupus erythematosus, has been associated with some ADRs and risks similar to RXN (including catastrophic progressive multifocal leukoencephalopathy, and other infections), there has been no association with HBV reactivation. Common mild gastrointestinal ADRs seen in clinical trials and postmarketing data have included nausea and vomiting.

Tumor Necrosis Factor-Alpha Inhibitors

The tumor necrosis factor-alpha inhibitors (TNFis) include the monoclonal antibodies, infliximab, adalimumab, and golimumab, as well as the related PEGylated protein, certolizumab pegol, and receptor fusion protein, etanercept. These agents are widely used in the treatment of RA, spondyloarthritis, inflammatory bowel disease, and other inflammatory diseases. Although these therapeutics have a variety of systemic and organ-specific potential adverse effects, their use has been associated with relatively few adverse gastrointestinal manifestations. Postmarketing reports of rare hepatotoxic events, including fatal drug-induced liver injury, as well as well as drug-related autoimmune hepatitis, have been reported. Most of these reports were associated with infliximab or adalimumab. Although these were sporadic and rare events, recommended routine monitoring includes semiannual LFTs while taking any of these agents. As discussed above, HSTCL has been reported in association with infliximab, adalimumab, and etanercept use. Most of these cases have been in the setting of concurrent AZA and in the setting of inflammatory bowel disease treatment; it is unclear if this is an epidemiologically/statistically significant association. Of note, large-scale retrospective population studies have not confirmed a statistical association between any immunosuppressive treatment and this rare malignancy.[29]

Viral hepatitis reactivation

It has been hypothesized that inhibition of tumor necrosis factor-alpha may alter T-cell activation and interferon production, potentially leading to reactivation of latent viral infections. HBV reactivation, in particular, has occurred with TNFi therapy, although this has not been as frequent or strongly associated as in RXN use.[59,60] Like RXN, TNFi should be avoided in the setting of untreated chronic HBV or HBV with significant liver injury. Viral hepatitis screening should be performed before therapy, similar to that recommended for RXN. The risk of reactivation is lower in TNFi users than in RXN. As such, antigen-negative patients with HBVcAb positivity may be monitored closely with treatment, typically including serial HBV DNA and LFTs on a quarterly basis, but do not universally require treatment or prophylaxis.[54] Surface antigen (HBVsAg) -positive patients should be treated for HBV before initiation of the TNFi. In addition to HBV reactivation concerns, HCV progression has also been observed in some patients receiving TNFis, although investigations have also investigated etanercept as a potential adjunctive *treatment* therapy for HCV, with positive results. As such, etanercept may, in fact, be the most appropriate TNFi for individuals requiring these treatments with active or prior exposure to HCV.[56,61,62]

Other Biologic Agents

Ustekinumab

Ustekinumab is a monoclonal antibody that binds the shared p40 subunit of IL-12 and IL-23. It is FDA approved for the treatment of psoriasis and psoriatic arthritis, as well as Crohn disease as of 2016. IL-12 and IL-23 are important cytokines in the pathways of natural killer and CD4[+] T-cell activation. Downstream effects include downregulation of other cytokines, including TNF-alpha and IL-8. Appendicitis events were reported rarely in initial trials, although no subsequent large-scale data have determined the significance of this risk; common ADRs of nausea and vomiting were noted in trials in up to 4% of users.[63]

Interleukin-1 inhibitors

The IL-1 receptor antagonist anakinra, the related protein rilonacept, and monoclonal antibody canakinumab all target the IL-1 cytokine pathway, leading to a downstream reduction in a variety of innate immune pathways. These agents are used in the treatment of a variety of familial periodic fever and other autoinflammatory disorders as well as Still disease, Behcet disease, and other inflammatory diseases. Aside from elevated infection risk, cytopenias are the most common serious ADR relatively specific to IL-1 blockade. A variety of gastrointestinal anomalies have been reported in clinical trials at rates greater than 5% of users, including nausea, diarrhea, and elevated aminotransferases.[64]

Abatacept

Abatacept is a fusion protein of an immunoglobulin G1 fragment crystallizable region and the extracellular domain of Cytotoxic T-Lymphocyte Associated Protein 4. For the treatment of RA and other inflammatory diseases, its primary mechanism of action is the competitive binding of CD80/CD86, blocking costimulatory signal by antigen-presenting cells, and, thus, the downstream activation of T cells. The primary serious gastrointestinal events seen in abatacept use have been HBV reactivation (see earlier discussion). In addition, GIPs have been reported, although these risks are probably no higher than in TNFi users based on large cohort data.[34]

SUMMARY

A variety of gastrointestinal ADRs are seen for nearly all conventional antirheumatic medications, ranging from nausea to potentially life-threatening drug-induced liver injury. Rheumatologists should be particularly familiar with hepatotoxicity associated with long-term MTX use, and the range of unique hepatopancreatic manifestations associated with AZA. HBV reactivation is the most serious gastrointestinal disease risk associated with many biological therapies, particularly RXN. Finally, GIP may be an additional and relatively specific risk for agents directed at IL-6 pathways or T cells, whereas the relationship of IL-17 inhibition to incident or worsening inflammatory bowel disease remains uncertain.

REFERENCES

1. International drug monitoring: the role of national centres. Report of a WHO meeting. World Health Organ Tech Rep Ser 1972;498:1–25.
2. Thompson RN, Watts C, Edelman J, et al. A controlled two-centre trial of parenteral methotrexate therapy for refractory rheumatoid arthritis. J Rheumatol 1984; 11:760–3.
3. Morabito L, Montesinos MC, Schreibman DM, et al. Methotrexate and sulfasalazine promote adenosine release by a mechanism that requires ecto-5′-nucleotidase-mediated conversion of adenine nucleotides. J Clin Invest 1998;101: 295–300.
4. Furst DE, Kremer JM. Methotrexate in rheumatoid arthritis. Arthritis Rheum 1988; 31:305–14.
5. Cronstein BN. Molecular therapeutics. Methotrexate and its mechanism of action. Arthritis Rheum 1996;39:1951–60.
6. Nyfors A. Liver biopsies from psoriatics related to methotrexate therapy. 3. Findings in post-methotrexate liver biopsies from 160 psoriatics. Acta Pathol Microbiol Scand A 1977;85:511–8.
7. Shea B, Swinden MV, Tanjong GE, et al. Folic acid and folinic acid for reducing side effects in patients receiving methotrexate for rheumatoid arthritis. Cochrane Database Syst Rev 2013;(5):CD000951.
8. Kremer JM, Kaye GI, Kaye NW, et al. Light and electron microscopic analysis of sequential liver biopsy samples from rheumatoid arthritis patients receiving long-term methotrexate therapy. Followup over long treatment intervals and correlation with clinical and laboratory variables. Arthritis Rheum 1995;38:1194–203.
9. Kremer JM, Furst DE, Weinblatt ME, et al. Significant changes in serum AST across hepatic histological biopsy grades: prospective analysis of 3 cohorts receiving methotrexate therapy for rheumatoid arthritis. J Rheumatol 1996;23: 459–61.
10. Kalb RE, Strober B, Weinstein G, et al. Methotrexate and psoriasis: 2009 National Psoriasis Foundation Consensus Conference. J Am Acad Dermatol 2009;60: 824–37.
11. Menter A, Korman NJ, Elmets CA, et al. Guidelines of care for the management of psoriasis and psoriatic arthritis: section 4. Guidelines of care for the management and treatment of psoriasis with traditional systemic agents. J Am Acad Dermatol 2009;61:451–85.
12. Saag KG, Teng GG, Patkar NM, et al. American College of Rheumatology 2008 recommendations for the use of nonbiologic and biologic disease-modifying antirheumatic drugs in rheumatoid arthritis. Arthritis Rheum 2008;59:762–84.
13. Singh JA, Furst DE, Bharat A, et al. 2012 update of the 2008 American College of Rheumatology recommendations for the use of disease-modifying antirheumatic drugs and biologic agents in the treatment of rheumatoid arthritis. Arthritis Care Res (Hoboken) 2012;64:625–39.

14. Aithal GP, Haugk B, Das S, et al. Monitoring methotrexate-induced hepatic fibrosis in patients with psoriasis: are serial liver biopsies justified? Aliment Pharmacol Ther 2004;19:391–9.

15. Roenigk HH Jr, Auerbach R, Maibach H, et al. Methotrexate in psoriasis: consensus conference. J Am Acad Dermatol 1998;38:478–85.

16. Pathirana D, Ormerod AD, Saiag P, et al. European S3-guidelines on the systemic treatment of psoriasis vulgaris. J Eur Acad Dermatol Venereol 2009;23(Suppl 2): 1–70.

17. van Ede AE, Laan RF, Rood MJ, et al. Effect of folic or folinic acid supplementation on the toxicity and efficacy of methotrexate in rheumatoid arthritis: a forty-eight week, multicenter, randomized, double-blind, placebo-controlled study. Arthritis Rheum 2001;44:1515–24.

18. Lopez-Olivo MA, Siddhanamatha HR, Shea B, et al. Methotrexate for treating rheumatoid arthritis. Cochrane Database Syst Rev 2014;(6):CD000957.

19. Prey S, Paul C. Effect of folic or folinic acid supplementation on methotrexate-associated safety and efficacy in inflammatory disease: a systematic review. Br J Dermatol 2009;160:622–8.

20. King PD, Perry MC. Hepatotoxicity of chemotherapy. Oncologist 2001;6:162–76.

21. Bath RK, Brar NK, Forouhar FA, et al. A review of methotrexate-associated hepatotoxicity. J Dig Dis 2014;15:517–24.

22. Elion GB. The purine path to chemotherapy. Science 1989;244:41–7.

23. Weinshilboum RM, Sladek SL. Mercaptopurine pharmacogenetics: monogenic inheritance of erythrocyte thiopurine methyltransferase activity. Am J Hum Genet 1980;32:651–62.

24. Bjornsson ES, Gu J, Kleiner DE, et al. Azathioprine and 6-mercaptopurine-induced liver injury: clinical features and outcomes. J Clin Gastroenterol 2017; 51:63–9.

25. Guidelines for monitoring drug therapy in rheumatoid arthritis. American College of Rheumatology Ad Hoc Committee on Clinical Guidelines. Arthritis Rheum 1996;39:723–31.

26. Daniel F, Cadranel JF, Seksik P, et al. Azathioprine induced nodular regenerative hyperplasia in IBD patients. Gastroenterol Clin Biol 2005;29:600–3.

27. Musumba CO. Review article: the association between nodular regenerative hyperplasia, inflammatory bowel disease and thiopurine therapy. Aliment Pharmacol Ther 2013;38:1025–37.

28. Gisbert JP, Gonzalez-Lama Y, Mate J. Thiopurine-induced liver injury in patients with inflammatory bowel disease: a systematic review. Am J Gastroenterol 2007; 102:1518–27.

29. Hirten R, Sultan K, Thomas A, et al. Hepatic manifestations of non-steroidal inflammatory bowel disease therapy. World J Hepatol 2015;7:2716–28.

30. Floyd A, Pedersen L, Nielsen GL, et al. Risk of acute pancreatitis in users of azathioprine: a population-based case-control study. Am J Gastroenterol 2003; 98:1305–8.

31. Montgomery M, van Santen MM, Biemond BJ, et al. Hepatosplenic T-cell lymphoma: a population-based study assessing incidence and association with immune-mediated disease. Gastroenterol Hepatol (N Y) 2015;11:160–3.

32. Zenouzi R, Weismuller TJ, Jorgensen KK, et al. No evidence that azathioprine increases risk of cholangiocarcinoma in patients with primary sclerosing cholangitis. Clin Gastroenterol Hepatol 2016;14:1806–12.

33. Wollenhaupt J, Silverfield J, Lee EB, et al. Safety and efficacy of tofacitinib, an oral janus kinase inhibitor, for the treatment of rheumatoid arthritis in open-label, longterm extension studies. J Rheumatol 2014;41:837–52.

34. Xie F, Yun H, Bernatsky S, et al. Brief report: risk of gastrointestinal perforation among rheumatoid arthritis patients receiving tofacitinib, tocilizumab, or other biologic treatments. Arthritis Rheumatol 2016;68:2612–7.

35. Kuhn KA, Manieri NA, Liu TC, et al. IL-6 stimulates intestinal epithelial proliferation and repair after injury. PLoS One 2014;9:e114195.

36. Smedegard G, Bjork J. Sulphasalazine: mechanism of action in rheumatoid arthritis. Br J Rheumatol 1995;34(Suppl 2):7–15.

37. Singh JA, Saag KG, Bridges SL Jr, et al. 2015 American College of Rheumatology guideline for the treatment of rheumatoid arthritis. Arthritis Rheumatol 2016;68:1–26.

38. Fuchs HA. Use of sulfasalazine in rheumatic diseases. Bull Rheum Dis 1997;46:3–4.

39. Marinos G, Riley J, Painter DM, et al. Sulfasalazine-induced fulminant hepatic failure. J Clin Gastroenterol 1992;14:132–5.

40. Fich A, Schwartz J, Braverman D, et al. Sulfasalazine hepatotoxicity. Am J Gastroenterol 1984;79:401–2.

41. Fox RI. Mechanism of action of leflunomide in rheumatoid arthritis. J Rheumatol Suppl 1998;53:20–6.

42. Strand V, Cohen S, Schiff M, et al. Treatment of active rheumatoid arthritis with leflunomide compared with placebo and methotrexate. Leflunomide Rheumatoid Arthritis Investigators Group. Arch Intern Med 1999;159:2542–50.

43. Siva C, Eisen SA, Shepherd R, et al. Leflunomide use during the first 33 months after Food and Drug Administration approval: experience with a national cohort of 3,325 patients. Arthritis Rheum 2003;49:745–51.

44. van Roon EN, Jansen TL, Houtman NM, et al. Leflunomide for the treatment of rheumatoid arthritis in clinical practice: incidence and severity of hepatotoxicity. Drug Saf 2004;27:345–52.

45. Srinivasa A, Tosounidou S, Gordon C. Increased incidence of gastrointestinal side effects in patients taking hydroxychloroquine: a brand-related issue? J Rheumatol 2017;44:398.

46. Singh JA, Beg S, Lopez-Olivo MA. Tocilizumab for rheumatoid arthritis: a Cochrane systematic review. J Rheumatol 2011;38:10–20.

47. Schiff MH, Kremer JM, Jahreis A, et al. Integrated safety in tocilizumab clinical trials. Arthritis Res Ther 2011;13:R141.

48. Gout T, Ostor AJ, Nisar MK. Lower gastrointestinal perforation in rheumatoid arthritis patients treated with conventional DMARDs or tocilizumab: a systematic literature review. Clin Rheumatol 2011;30:1471–4.

49. Patel DD, Lee DM, Kolbinger F, et al. Effect of IL-17A blockade with secukinumab in autoimmune diseases. Ann Rheum Dis 2013;72(Suppl 2):ii116–23.

50. Hueber W, Sands BE, Lewitzky S, et al. Secukinumab, a human anti-IL-17A monoclonal antibody, for moderate to severe Crohn's disease: unexpected results of a randomised, double-blind placebo-controlled trial. Gut 2012;61:1693–700.

51. Deodhar AA, Schreiber S, Gandhi K, et al. No increased risk of inflammatory bowel disease among secukinumab-treated patients with moderate to severe psoriasis, psoriatic arthritis, or ankylosing spondylitis: data from 14 phase 2 and phase 3 clinical studies [Abstract]. Suppl 10. Arthritis Rheumatol. 68. 9–28-2016. Ref Type: Proceedings. Available at: http://acrabstracts.org/abstract/no-increased-risk-of-

inflammatory-bowel-disease-among-secukinumab-treated-patients-with-moderate-to-severe-psoriasis-psoriatic-arthritis-or-ankylosing-spondylitis-data-from-14-phase-2-and-phase-3-c/. Accessed October 28, 2017.

52. Langley RG, Elewski BE, Lebwohl M, et al. Secukinumab in plaque psoriasis–results of two phase 3 trials. N Engl J Med 2014;371:326–38.
53. Cornejo A, Bohnenblust M, Harris C, et al. Intestinal perforation associated with rituximab therapy for post-transplant lymphoproliferative disorder after liver transplantation. Cancer Chemother Pharmacol 2009;64:857–60.
54. Di Bisceglie AM, Lok AS, Martin P, et al. Recent US Food and Drug Administration warnings on hepatitis B reactivation with immune-suppressing and anticancer drugs: just the tip of the iceberg? Hepatology 2015;61:703–11.
55. Mozessohn L, Chan KK, Feld JJ, et al. Hepatitis B reactivation in HBsAg-negative/HBcAb-positive patients receiving rituximab for lymphoma: a meta-analysis. J Viral Hepat 2015;22:842–9.
56. Li S, Kaur PP, Chan V, et al. Use of tumor necrosis factor-alpha (TNF-alpha) antagonists infliximab, etanercept, and adalimumab in patients with concurrent rheumatoid arthritis and hepatitis B or hepatitis C: a retrospective record review of 11 patients. Clin Rheumatol 2009;28:787–91.
57. Loomba R, Rowley A, Wesley R, et al. Systematic review: the effect of preventive lamivudine on hepatitis B reactivation during chemotherapy. Ann Intern Med 2008;148:519–28.
58. Lin KM, Lin JC, Tseng WY, et al. Rituximab-induced hepatitis C virus reactivation in rheumatoid arthritis. J Microbiol Immunol Infect 2013;46:65–7.
59. Lee YH, Bae SC, Song GG. Hepatitis B virus reactivation in HBsAg-positive patients with rheumatic diseases undergoing anti-tumor necrosis factor therapy or DMARDs. Int J Rheum Dis 2013;16:527–31.
60. Perez-Alvarez R, Diaz-Lagares C, Garcia-Hernandez F, et al. Hepatitis B virus (HBV) reactivation in patients receiving tumor necrosis factor (TNF)-targeted therapy: analysis of 257 cases. Medicine (Baltimore) 2011;90:359–71.
61. Pompili M, Biolato M, Miele L, et al. Tumor necrosis factor-alpha inhibitors and chronic hepatitis C: a comprehensive literature review. World J Gastroenterol 2013;19:7867–73.
62. Carroll MB, Bond MI. Use of tumor necrosis factor-alpha inhibitors in patients with chronic hepatitis B infection. Semin Arthritis Rheum 2008;38:208–17.
63. Sandborn WJ, Gasink C, Gao LL, et al. Ustekinumab induction and maintenance therapy in refractory Crohn's disease. N Engl J Med 2012;367:1519–28.
64. Bresnihan B, Alvaro-Gracia JM, Cobby M, et al. Treatment of rheumatoid arthritis with recombinant human interleukin-1 receptor antagonist. Arthritis Rheum 1998; 41:2196–204.

Gastrointestinal Involvement in Behçet Disease

Ibrahim Hatemi, MD[a], Gulen Hatemi, MD[b],
Aykut Ferhat Çelik, MD[a],*

KEYWORDS

- Behçet syndrome • Mouth diseases • Intestinal diseases • Gastrointestinal diseases
- Epidemiology • Colonoscopy • Antirheumatic agents • TNF inhibitors

KEY POINTS

- There is a wide variation across countries in the reported frequency of gastrointestinal involvement among Behçet disease patients. Frequencies of less than or equal to 50% were reported from the Far East, whereas it is approximately 1% in Turkey.
- The scope of gastrointestinal involvement in Behçet disease includes ulcers in the ileocolonic region, which is the most commonly involved area; ulcers in other parts of the intestines; and Budd-Chiari syndrome due to hepatic vein and/or inferior vena cava thrombosis.
- The most common symptoms are abdominal pain of variable intensity, usually in the right lower quadrant; diarrhea, with or without bleeding; and fever.
- Presence of typical ulcers on colonoscopy is essential for the diagnosis. Histopathologic examination of surgical samples show neutrophilic infiltration of the vessel wall, perivascular area, and intravascular area with more frequent involvement of venules compared with arteries.
- Management consists of 5-aminosalicylate derivatives in mild cases, azathioprine in moderate to severe cases, and glucocorticoids during acute exacerbations.

INTRODUCTION

Behçet disease (BD) was first described by a Turkish dermatologist as a triple-symptom complex that consists of oral aphthous ulcers, genital ulcers, and uveitis. It is now considered a unique vasculitic condition that causes inflammation of vessels of all size with involvement of several organs and organ systems.[1,2] Nodular lesions,

[a] Division of Gastroenterology, Department of Internal Medicine, Cerrahpasa Medical School, Istanbul University, Koca Mustafa Pasa Mahallesi, Cerrahpaşa Caddesi No:53, 34096 Fatih/Istanbul, Turkey; [b] Division of Rheumatology, Department of Internal Medicine, Cerrahpasa Medical School, Istanbul University, Koca Mustafa Paşa Mahallesi, Cerrahpaşa Caddesi No:53, 34096 Fatih/Istanbul, Turkey
* Corresponding author. Department of Internal Medicine, Cerrahpasa Medical School, Istanbul University, Fatih, Istanbul, Turkey.
E-mail address: afcelik@superonline.com

Rheum Dis Clin N Am 44 (2018) 45–64
https://doi.org/10.1016/j.rdc.2017.09.007
0889-857X/18/© 2017 Elsevier Inc. All rights reserved.

papulopustular lesions, arterial and venous involvement, central nervous system, and gastrointestinal (GI) involvement are other manifestations. GI involvement causes both macroscopic and histopathologic inflammatory changes that resemble inflammatory bowel diseases (IBDs), creating a diagnostic challenge, as well as vasculitis-driven relapsing ischemic features that result in higher perforation and major GI bleeding rates compared with IBD.[3]

EPIDEMIOLOGY
Epidemiology of Behçet Disease

The prevalence of BD shows a wide geographic variation.[4] It is known to be higher in countries along the ancient Silk Route starting from the Mediterranean and reaching the Far East.[4] The highest prevalence was reported from Turkey, with equal to or less than 421 cases per 100,000 (95% CI 340–510) in a population-based survey.[5] In the Far East, the prevalence has been reported as 14 per 100,000 in China and 13.5 per 100,000 in Japan.[6,7] Differences between ethnic populations within the same country have also been reported. A study from Israel reported that the overall BD prevalence was 15.2 per 100,000 but 146.4 among Druze, 26.2 among Arabs, and 8.6 among the Jews living in Israel.[8] The prevalence in Europe decreases from South to North and was reported as 15.9 per 100,000 in Southern Italy, 6.4 per 100,000 in Spain, 0.64 per 100,000 in the United Kingdom and 0.3 per 100,000 in Scotland; rates thus decrease as distance from the Silk Route increases.[9–12] BD prevalence among immigrants from a high-prevalence country who move to a low-prevalence country has been estimated to belong between the 2 extremes, suggesting a role for both genetics and environment in the pathogenesis.[13] Moreover, BD seems to run a less severe course in nonendemic countries, providing another clue for the role of environmental factors.[14] Finally, a recent metaanalysis of 45 prevalence studies showed that, although there was clearly a wide variation across countries, methodologic issues (ie, registry-based studies vs direct population sampling) may be responsible for some of the variation.[15]

Epidemiology of Gastrointestinal Involvement of Behçet Disease

The frequency of GI involvement among patients with BD also shows a wide variation across geographies, being much more common in the Far East compared with the Middle East and Europe[4] (**Table 1**). The frequency was as high as 50% in a Japanese cohort[16] and 1% in a formal study in Turkey.[17]

Caution is required when interpreting the frequencies reported in different studies. Some sources of bias in reporting the frequency of GI involvement may be:

- Mode of diagnosis, such as symptom-based compared with endoscopy. Earlier symptom-based studies report a higher frequency compared with endoscopy or imaging-based reports in Japan, where BD is endemic, and other inflammatory bowel conditions, such as Crohn disease (CD), are rare. Moreover, a recent Korean study showed that only half of the subjects with upper GI symptoms did actually have esophageal involvement confirmed by endoscopy.[18]
- Use of highly sensitive techniques such as capsule enteroscopy or double-balloon enteroscopy. Such methods can pick up incidental nonspecific lesions even in healthy individuals and may cause an overestimation for the frequency of GI involvement.[19]
- Differences in criteria used for diagnosis. GI involvement is 1 of the items in Japanese criteria, whereas it does not appear in the International Study Group (ISG) criteria.[20,21] Consequently, use of Japanese criteria may result in a higher proportion of patients with GI involvement in the total pool.

Table 1
Frequency of gastrointestinal involvement in Behçet disease cohorts from different countries

Author	Country	Year	Total Number of Subjects with BD	GI Involvement (%)
Shimizu[93]	Japan	1971	Not provided	50
O'Duffy[94]	USA	1971	10	30
Yamamato[95]	Japan	1974	2031	25
Chamberlain[96]	UK	1977	32	6
Eun[97]	Korea	1984	32	5.3
Jankowski[98]	UK	1992	114	40
Dilsen[99]	Turkey	1993	15	5
Yurdakul[100]	Turkey	1996	496	0.7
Gurler[101]	Turkey	1997	2147	2.8
Bang[102]	Korea	1997	1155	4
Bang[103]	Korea	2003	1901	3.2
Tursen[104]	Turkey	2003	2313	1.4
Seyahi[105]	Turkey	2003	121	0.8
Yi[106]	Korea	2008	842	8
Alli[107]	Turkey	2009	213	2.8
Neves[108]	Brazil	2009	106	6.6
El Menyawi[109]	Egypt	2009	35	19
Davatchi[110]	Iran	2010	6500	7.4
Oliveira[111]	Brazil	2011	60	3.3
Zhang[112]	China	2012	334	17
Kobayashi[113]	Japan	2012	135	37
Kobayashi[113]	USA	2012	634	34
Singal[114]	India	2013	29	3.4
Olivieri[115]	Italy	2013	11	18
Mohammad[116]	Sweden	2013	40	0
Sibley[117]	Turkey	2014	107	0
Sibley[117]	USA	2014	112	37.5
Kim[118]	Korea	2014	3674	8
Rodriguez-Carballeira[119]	Spain	2014	496	1.4
Khabbazi[120]	Iran (Azeri population)	2014	166	0.6
Hamzaoui[121]	Tunis	2014	430	1.6
Ndiaye[122]	Senegal	2015	50	2
Lennikov[123]	Russia	2015	250	25.2
Ajose[124]	Nigeria	2015	15	20
Bonitsis[125]	Germany	2015	747	11.5
Kirino[126]	Japan	2016	578	12.3
Nanthapisal[127]	UK (pediatric)	2016	46	58.7
Uskudar-Cansu[128]	Turkey	2016	329	0
Ryu[129]	Korea	2016	193	11.4
Hatemi[130]	Turkey	2016	8763	0.8

- Misdiagnosis of nonsteroidal antiinflammatory drug (NSAID) ulcers or intestinal infections (eg, tuberculosis) as BD with GI involvement.
- Differences in study methodology. Retrospective chart reviews are typically less reliable compared with formal cross-sectional or prospective screening for GI involvement.
- In low-prevalence countries, the preferential diagnosis of patients with more severe disease, including GI involvement, compared with patients with only mild symptoms. A surprisingly high frequency of GI disease has been reported from countries with very low BD prevalence, such as the United Kingdom and the United States.[11,22] This may be attributed to the failure to identify milder (skin or mucosa-limited) BD in low-prevalence countries, where clinicians are not as familiar with BD. This may lead to a biased reporting that favors severe disease, which is more likely to include GI manifestations.

Overall, BD prevalence seems to be similar among men and women (male/female ratio 1:1), but the disease follows a more severe course with more major organ involvement among men.[23] However, GI involvement has similar frequency among men and women.[3] The mean age of onset of GI involvement is around the late thirties, but there may be a bimodal distribution because a high frequency has been reported in children.[3,24]

Pathogenesis and Pathophysiology

Genetic and environmental factors are thought to play role in the development of BD, but the exact pathogenesis is unknown. HLAB51 is the best known genetic factor, and infectious agents, especially streptococci, have been proposed as environmental factors.[2] Disease clusters have long been identified in BD. It is hypothesized that different pathogenic mechanisms may be responsible for these clusters, mainly because they show differences in drug response and disease course.[25] There have been few studies that specifically explored the pathogenesis of GI involvement of BD and even fewer studies that included BD subjects without GI involvement, CD subjects, and healthy individuals as controls.

Although HLAB51 is the most closely associated genetic factor, a metaanalysis of 78 studies showed that only around half of BD subjects are HLAB51-positive in several reports and the population-attributable risks for BD in relationship with HLAB51 or HLAB52 is between 32% and 52% in different geographies.[26] Moreover, another metaanalysis of studies looking at HLAB51 frequency according to type of involvement showed that HLAB51 is negatively associated with GI involvement (odds ratio 0.70, 95% CI 0.52–0.94).[27]

Additional candidate loci that play role in the pathogenesis of BD had been identified in genome-wide association studies, but none of these studies looked at the association of these loci with specific types of involvement, including GI involvement. The interleukin (IL)-23R and IL-12RB2 locus has been shown to carry genome-wide significance in 2 studies in Japanese and Turkish BD subjects, but not in Korean, Middle Eastern, Greek, and British subjects.[28,29] Whether this differed according to the types of organ involvement was not presented. Interestingly, a Korean study showed that specific single nucleotide polymorphisms (SNPs) in IL-17A, IL-23R, and signal transducer and activator of transcription 4 protein may modulate susceptibility to intestinal BD.[30] However, this study was limited because no BD subjects without GI involvement were included as controls.

Another study suggested a role for innate immunity in the pathogenesis of both BD and CD through sharing of IL-23R and IL-10 susceptibility. The role of TLR8, which mediates innate inflammatory response, was also implied through a trend toward the association of rs2407992 with BD and rs5744067 with CD (reaching significance only among women).[31] The investigators considered Toll Like Receptor 8 as a candidate genetic susceptibility locus for both conditions, but this could not be demonstrated definitively. It should be noted that only 19% of BD subjects in this study had GI involvement and their results were not separately analyzed.

In a study that explored 3 common Caspase Activation and Recruitment Domain 15 variants predisposing to CD (R702W, G908R, and L1007fsinsC), none of these loci were associated with BD among Turkish subjects, including 2 with GI involvement.[32]

Intestinal macrophages up-regulate triggering receptor expressed on myeloid cells-1 (TREM-1) in the intestine for patients with CD and ulcerative colitis (UC); this expression is correlated with disease activity.[33] Based on this finding, a more recent study explored 3 TREM-1 SNPs (rs9471535, rs2234237, and rs3789205) in intestinal BD, CD, and UC subjects, and healthy controls.[34] Interestingly, TREM-1 SNPs were significantly associated with intestinal BD, but not CD or UC.

The T helper (Th)-1 dominance, which is well described in BD, has been confirmed in intestinal tissues of BD subjects with GI involvement in 2 small studies.[35,36] More recently, the IL-17–IL-23 axis was evaluated in parallel with Th1 in the serum and ileal biopsy specimens of BD subjects with GI symptoms, ankylosing spondylitis (AS), and CD subjects.[37] A Th1, but not a Th17, response has been observed in BD subjects with GI involvement, in contrast to AS and CD subjects. It has been suggested that, although the clinical phenotypes are similar, differing immunologic alterations and pathogenic mechanisms may be operative in BD compared with AS and CD.

Further studies with adequate sample size and appropriate diseased and healthy controls are needed to elucidate the pathogenesis of GI involvement in BD.

Histopathology

BD can show vasculitic involvement of large, medium, and small arteries, as well as veins. The most common histologic finding in intestinal resection material is phlebitis, which is defined as neutrophilic infiltration of the vein wall.[38] It has been reported that the venules are involved more frequently than the arteries. Of note, the neutrophilic inflammation affects both the perivascular area and the intravascular area. Some investigators have reported that intestinal ulcers in BD originate from Peyer patches, explaining, in part, the pattern of skip lesions.[39]

The involved vessel type, duration, and severity determine the clinical manifestations. An acute transmural ischemia can cause bowel infarction and perforation, whereas chronic ischemia can result in strictures. Transient mild or moderate ischemia can cause an acute transient ischemic enteritis and/or colitis that can resolve spontaneously.[40]

This acute exacerbating course with ischemia is typically a result of vasculitis as the underlying pathologic condition in BD. This is in contrast to CD, in which the disease course is generally chronic and progressive, and perforations or massive bleeding are relatively uncommon.

Anatomic Distribution of Gastrointestinal Involvement and Symptoms

The most frequently involved anatomic GI location for BD is the ileocolonic region, but the whole GI tract can be involved. Furthermore, venous thrombosis as a manifestation of BD can affect the hepatic veins, causing Budd-Chiari syndrome[41–49] (**Table 2**).

Ileocolonic involvement

Similar to the presentation in CD and intestinal tuberculosis, the ileocolonic site is the most commonly involved GI location in BD; it occurs in equal to or less than 96% of BD patients with GI involvement.[50] Ileocolonic involvement typically causes single or few,

Table 2
Anatomic distribution

Location	Involvement	Evidence	Reference
Mouth or pharynx	Ulcer 92.4%–100%	Case series	3,41
Esophagus	Ulcer 4.7% Esophagitis 5%	Prospective cohort	18,42
Stomach	Ulcer 8%–9.2%	Prospective cohort	18,43
Duodenum	Ulcer 4.7%–8%	Prospective cohort	18,43
Pancreas	Pancreatitis	Case report	44
Liver	Hepatic vein thrombosis	Case series	45,46
Gall bladder	Not available	—	—
Small intestine	Ulcer 2.5%	Case series	41
Colon	Ulcer 18.4%–32%	Case series	3,41
Rectum	Ulcer 2.4% Rectovaginal fistula	Case series Case report	41,47–49

oval or round, deep ulcers, most commonly in the ileocecal area but also in the ileum, ileocecal valve, or in different segments of the colon.[3,50] The area of involvement can be focal, segmental, or diffuse.[3,50–52] (**Fig. 1**). GI involvement in BD shows a relapsing character and nearly 29% of the subjects followed for 5 years have chronic symptoms or relapses.[53] The symptoms of ileocolonic involvement depend on the severity of vasculitis and whether the patient presents during an acute or a chronic phase. Abdominal pain is the most common symptom, followed by diarrhea with or without bleeding, and fever.[50] Patients with acute severe involvement may present with perforations and/or massive bleeding.

Perforation and bleeding About 30% of the patients present with acute abdomen findings such as perforation or with GI bleeding.[3] Closed perforation with abscess formation can also be seen in chronic cases.

The prevalence of acute lower GI bleeding is reported as 11.2% to 25% in BD patients with GI involvement.[50,54] In a retrospective cohort, bleeding was the first manifestation of GI involvement in 36% of these subjects. The rate of rebleeding was high (35%), even with medical and/or surgical treatment.[54] Age older than 52 years and nodular ulcer margins were associated with bleeding risk.

Abdominal pain The most common symptom of GI involvement in BD is abdominal pain (87%–92%).[50,55] Most patients with GI involvement present with chronic abdominal pain with or without mild to moderate diarrhea.[3,55] The severity of abdominal pain ranges from mild abdominal discomfort to severe intractable pain.[51] Ileocecal involvement commonly causes right lower quadrant pain, but pain can be over the whole abdomen.[55]

Diarrhea Chronic diarrhea was reported in 12.7% to 29% of patients with GI involvement.[3,41] Diarrhea is less severe and frequent in BD than CD, due to a more focal or segmental involvement rather than extensive inflammation.[41]

Fever Fever can be seen in approximately 25% of patients with GI involvement.[3] An interesting association of trisomy 8–positive myelodysplastic syndrome (MDS) and GI involvement of BD has been reported.[56] These are generally seen in patients with more severe GI involvement whose disease tends to be resistant to immunosuppressives.[56–58] Fever may be especially common in such patients and is suggested that this is related to trisomy

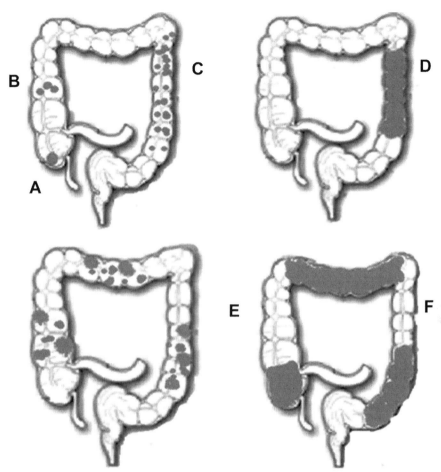

Fig. 1. Patterns of GI involvement in BD. (*A*) Focal single ulcer. (*B*) Focal multiple ulcers. (*C*) Segmental multiple ulcers. (*D*) Segmental diffuse ulceration. (*E*) Multisegmental multiple ulcers. (*F*) Multisegmental diffuse ulceration.

8, rather than MDS.[56] Fever also requires the clinician to exercise caution because it may represent thromboembolic disease and acute or chronic infections (eg, tuberculosis) in BD patients.

Fistulas Enteroabdominal fistulas are relatively less frequent in BD (7.6%) and may occur when there is ongoing inflammation following bowel resection.[41,59]

Esophageal involvement
Esophageal involvement is uncommon, reported as 4.7% in symptomatic BD patients, and usually manifests as nonspecific ulceration.[18] Bleeding, perforation, or stricture of the esophagus are rarely described in BD.[60] Pill-induced or infectious (cytomegalovirus or herpetic) esophagitis should be ruled out.

Hepatic vein thrombosis
Hepatic vein thrombosis in BD may have a rapid progression and poor prognosis. Mortality was reported as 47% during the 10 months after diagnosis.[45] Most patients

have vena cava inferior thrombosis along with hepatic vein involvement.[45] BD should be kept in mind as an important cause of mesenteric vascular thrombosis or Budd-Chiari syndrome in endemic countries because this may be the presenting manifestation before the diagnosis of BD in some patients.[61]

Diagnostic Evaluation

The diagnosis of GI involvement is straightforward in a patient with typical GI ulcers who already has a diagnosis of BD, provided that NSAID ulcers and infections such as GI tuberculosis are excluded. The difficulty arises when GI manifestations precede other systemic manifestations of BD or when the presenting signs and symptoms are fairly nonspecific, such as oral ulcers or skin lesions that may be seen in CD or UC.[52] It has been reported that only around 30% of BD patients with ileocolonic ulcers fulfill BD criteria after a mean follow-up of 33 months following the discovery of ileocolonic ulcers.[62]

Another diagnostic challenge is the appearance of a GI ulcer that is coincidentally discovered in an asymptomatic patient. In a study from China, colonoscopy was performed in 148 consecutive BD subjects and ileocolonic ulcers were observed in 13.5%.[63] Among the subjects with ulcers, 20% did not have any GI symptoms. Such subjects should be scrutinized for other ulcer causes before being labeled as having GI involvement of BD. The morphology of the ulcer may be helpful in this case. For subjects with typical Behçet ulcers (defined as single oval or round ulcers with discrete margins), the frequency of fulfilling ISG criteria increases from 19% to 53.2% after a mean follow-up of 63.9 plus or minus 50.9 months.[64]

The Korean IBD study group has proposed an algorithm that combines endoscopic findings with clinical manifestations to facilitate the diagnosis of BD-related GI involvement[65] (**Table 3**). This tool categorizes BD patients with ileocecal ulcers as definite, probable, suspected, and nondiagnostic.

Diagnostic Modalities

Colonoscopy

- Colonoscopic appearance of ulcers located in the intestines or the colon are usually well demarcated, oval or round (77%), and deep[3,51] (**Fig. 2**). They can be single or multiple and can be seen at the ileum, ileocecal area, on the ileocecal valve, or at different segments of the colon. The area of involvement can be segmental or diffuse.[51,52]

Table 3
Diagnosis of gastrointestinal involvement of Behçet disease according to the Korean Inflammatory Bowel Disease study group

Endoscopic Findings (Ileocecal Area)	Clinical Findings[b]	Diagnosis of Intestinal BD
Typical intestinal ulcer[a]	Systemic BD	Definite
	Oral ulcer only	Probable
	None	Suspected
Atypical intestinal ulcer	Systemic BD	Probable
	Oral ulcer only	Suspected
	None	Nondiagnostic

[a] ≤5 ulcers, oval, deep, discrete borders.
[b] According to the Japanese criteria.
Data from Cheon JH, Kim ES, Shin SJ, et al. Development and validation of novel diagnostic criteria for intestinal Behçet's disease in Korean patients with ileocolonic ulcers. Am J Gastroenterol 2009;104:2492–9.

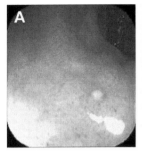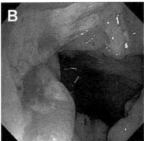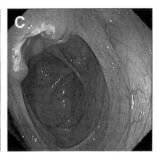

Fig. 2. Ulcers in GI BD. (*A*) Aphthous ulcer. (*B*) Large, deep geographic ulcer. (*C*) Large, deep volcano-type ulcer.

- The most common type of ulcer is the focal single ulceration reported in 45% to 67% and the most common location is the ileocecal region reported in 61% to 96% of the cases.[3,50,66]
- In some cases, aphtoid lesions, geographic or star-shaped ulcers can also be seen.[3]
- Ulcer shape may have a prognostic value, notably a volcano-type ulcer defined as a well demarcated, deep ulcer with nodular margins that forms a pseudopolyp appearance is associated with poor prognosis.[67,68] Persistence of GI ulcers during clinical remission is predictive for clinical relapse.[69]

Capsule endoscopy

- A retrospective study with capsule endoscopy showed intestinal ulcers in 47.4% of BD subjects with GI involvement compared with none of the controls with other diseases. Among these subjects, 26.3% did not have ileal or colonic lesions on colonoscopy.[70]
- Two studies including 10 subjects each with GI symptoms and no ulcers on colonoscopy showed that capsule endoscopy detected ulcers in 8 and 9 of these subjects.[71,72] Capsule endoscopy can be useful in symptomatic BD subjects in whom conventional endoscopic investigations are negative.

Laboratory findings and biomarkers

- Elevated C-reactive protein levels can predict reactivation and postsurgical relapse of GI involvement in BD.[73,74]
- Fecal calprotectin may be elevated during active GI involvement in BD and may be helpful in the decision to perform colonoscopy in patients with mild GI symptoms.[75,76] Further data are needed to show whether it can replace colonoscopy for predicting active disease and relapses in patients with already known GI involvement.

Serologic markers

- There are currently no reliable serologic markers for the diagnosis or follow-up of GI involvement of BD.
- Anti-*Saccharomyces cerevisiae* antibodies (ASCA), which is a well-known serologic marker for CD, was evaluated in BD and was positive in 44.3% of BD subjects with GI involvement, 3.3% in those without GI involvement, and 8.8% in healthy controls. ASCA positivity was more frequent in subjects who required operations but did not predict postsurgical relapses.[77]

- In 1 study, immunoglobulin-M anti-alpha-enolase antibody was found in 67.5% of BD subjects with GI involvement.[78]
- IL-12 B was also reported as a potential marker in GI involvement of BD because it was associated with clinical and endoscopic activity.[79]

Histopathology

Histopathology is usually not helpful in the diagnosis, because the histopathologic findings indicating vasculitis are seldom seen in endoscopic biopsy samples because these samples are usually too superficial to include the vessels necessary to document vasculitis.[3,40] Moreover even bulky surgical samples may be insufficient because acute vasculitic features may disappear soon after the flare. Occasionally, thrombotic occlusive vessels reported as vasculopathy are seen, but whether this represents a late stage of vasculitis or is a distinct pathologic condition is not clear.[3,40] The inflammatory findings that are usually observed in mucosal biopsies are similar to those seen in other chronic inflammatory conditions.[40]

Differential Diagnosis

The ileocecal region can be involved in many inflammatory conditions other than BD, such as CD or GI tuberculosis. Navigating the differential diagnosis is made even more difficult because these conditions have similar endoscopic features. Diagnosis can only be made by combining clinical, laboratory, endoscopic, radiologic, histologic, microbiologic, and serologic findings.

Inflammatory bowel diseases

- Some manifestations that are common in BD, such as oral ulcers, nodular lesions, or arthritis, can also occur in CD and UC (**Table 4**). This can make the differential diagnosis even more difficult. However, a formal study of 93 CD and 130 UC subjects showed that only 1.3% of UC and none of the CD subjects fulfilled ISG criteria for BD.[80] The presence of scarring genital ulcers, posterior uveitis, and vascular involvement are especially helpful in diagnosing BD.
- Ulcer morphology and distribution detected by endoscopy can help to differentiate CD and BD. Comparative studies showed that oval, deep penetrating, 5 or fewer ulcers with discrete borders located in the ileocecal region, absence of cobblestone appearance, and aphtoid lesions and the presence of focal involvement would typically suggest BD.[65,81]
- An algorithm has been described for differentiating BD from CD.[81] According to this algorithm, round ulcers indicate BD and longitudinal ulcers indicate CD. If the ulcers are irregular, geographic, or diffuse with segmental involvement, CD should be favored; focal involvement suggests BD.[81]
- Chronic fistulizing perianal disease would strongly suggest CD, but this finding has a low sensitivity.[41,66]
- Strictures are more common in CD.[41]

Tuberculosis

The possibility of GI tuberculosis should never be underestimated, especially in a patient who has weight loss and fever. Chest imaging, Purified Protein Derivative of Tuberculin, and/or quantiferon test should be performed. Culture and polymerase chain reaction testing of endoscopically obtained tissues for tuberculosis and acid-fast staining with a careful histopathological examination for granuloma are crucial.[82]

In conclusion, endoscopic morphology and clinical findings are integral to the diagnosis of GI involvement in BD. Before labeling a patient with BD-associated GI

Table 4
Frequency of Behçet manifestations in patients with gastrointestinal involvement of Behçet disease and Crohn disease

	GI Involvement of BD	CD	Reference
Oral ulcers	92.4%–100%	9.9%–21.3%	3,41,64
Genital ulcers	42.4%–85%	0.9%	3,41,64
Papulopustular lesions	43.1%–70%	16.6%- 23.6%	41,64
Nodular lesions	48%	2.1%	3,64
Positive pathergy test	49%	10.7%	3,64
Arthritis or arthralgia	30%–31.9%	19%	3,41
Venous thrombosis	18%	0	3,64
Eye involvement	19.6%–28%	0%–7.5%	3,41,64
Nervous system involvement	%5	0	3,64
Features of GI involvement			
Ileal or ileocecal	83%–94.6%	83.1%–90%	41,80
Rectal	2%–2.4%	25%–37%	41,80
Upper GI involvement	3.3%	2.4%	41
Stricture	7.2%–13%	24%	41,80
Abdominal or internal fistula	7.6%–10%	27.4%	3,41
Perianal fistula	2.5%–5%	39.2%	3,41
Perforation	12.7%–18.3%	8.7%	3,41
ASCA positivity	41.7%–44.3%	49.4%	3,76
Ulcer type and location	A few round or oval ulcers, focal involvement	Longitudinal ulcers, diffuse segmental involvement	65,80
Granuloma in mucosal biopsy	2%	14%	3,60

involvement, ulcers caused by NSAIDs or other drugs should be excluded with a detailed history. Sometimes, a conservative approach (stopping the suspected drug and repeat endoscopy in 3 months) can clarify the cause. Exclusion of GI tuberculosis is crucial to avoid prescribing immunosuppressives to a patient with tuberculosis. On the other hand, an initial misdiagnosis of CD as BD or vice versa may not be clinically important because the management is similar. It is important to carefully follow these patients over time because of their high rate of complication, as previously described.

Management

Medical treatment
Management of BD ideally involves (1) suppression of the exacerbation rapidly and effectively in patients with active disease and (2) prevention of new exacerbations after remission is obtained.[83] In BD patients presenting with an acute exacerbation of GI involvement, the choice of treatment depends on the severity of the involvement. Glucocorticoids may be used for a short duration to induce remission. Patients with small and relatively superficial ulcers that carry a low risk of bleeding and perforation can be managed with systemic and/or local 5-aminosalicylate (5-ASA) derivatives.[84] Patients with moderate or severe disease can be managed with immunosuppressives such as azathioprine. In a retrospective study, 37 subjects with moderate or severe involvement started on azathioprine and 16 subjects with mild lesions started on 5-ASA

produced positive results; almost two-thirds of the subjects achieved complete clinical and endoscopic remission using these agents without withdrawal due to adverse events.[3] A Korean retrospective study showed a similar initial remission rate of 66.7% at week 8 among their 93 subjects who were started on medical treatment of GI involvement.[85] Their initial treatment modalities consisted of mesalamine 2 to 4 g, oral, or intravenous prednisolone 0.5 to 1 mg/kg, and azathioprine in cases of inadequate response. Total parenteral nutrition and bowel rest was also applied during the acute periods.

Prevention of new exacerbations after remission with these agents has also been studied. The relapse rates were 8.1%, 22.6%, 31.2%, and 46.7% at 1, 3, 5, and 10 years among the 143 subjects who achieved remission with 5-ASA and 5.8%, 28.7%, 43.7%, and 51.7% at 1, 2, 3, and 5 years among the 39 subjects treated with azathioprine.[73,86]

In subjects who do not obtain remission with these agents or who relapsed during treatment, thalidomide and/or tumor necrosis factor inhibitor (TNFi) may be preferred. Although there are no controlled studies with these agents for GI involvement, a systematic review of uncontrolled studies and case reports showed that 84% of 19 subjects who were prescribed thalidomide and 58% of 86 subjects who were prescribed infliximab for refractory GI involvement achieved clinical remission.[87] Infliximab was stopped due to an adverse event in 1 of the 49 subjects according to available safety data. A recent open-label 52-week phase III Japanese trial with adalimumab in 20 BD subjects with GI involvement who had an ileocecal ulcer of at least 1 cm in diameter and a global GI symptom score of at least 3 showed marked improvement in 12 out of 20 (60%) and complete remission in 4 out of 20 (20%) subjects.[88] Fifteen of these subjects continued an extension trial that lasted equal to or less than 100 weeks with 40% achieving marked improvement and 15% achieving complete remission at the end of this period. Monoclonal TNFi is usually preferred in the management of GI involvement, mainly based on the adverse experience with etanercept in CD. However, a small open-label study showed a higher clinical remission rate (Relative risk 1.74, 95% CI 1.22–2.49) and healing of intestinal ulcers (Relative risk 1.66, 95% CI 1.22–2.25) with etanercept compared with conventional treatment with methotrexate or prednisolone.[89]

An alternative approach for the management of GI involvement may be use of TNFi as a first-line agent in severe cases. Japanese Consensus Statements recommend 0.5 to 1 mg/kg prednisolone for 1 to 2 weeks, followed by slow tapering in patients with severe symptoms and deep ulcers. They also suggest that adalimumab or infliximab should be considered for induction therapy in such patients.[90] The decision to start TNFi as induction or in refractory cases should take into account an individual's disease severity, risk of adverse events such as tuberculosis, and economic considerations.

Surgery

Surgery may be life-saving in emergency situations such as perforations or major bleeding that cannot be controlled with glucocorticoids and immunosuppressives. In a retrospective cohort, almost a third of the subjects required emergency surgery due to perforation, major bleeding, or obstruction.[3] Postoperative use of immunosuppressives may be beneficial for decreasing the risk of postoperative complications and recurrences, which usually occur at or close to the anastomosis site.[3] A retrospective study comparing the outcomes of laparoscopic surgery with open surgery showed that operation duration and blood loss was less profound with laparoscopy, and the rate of postoperative complications, reoperation, mortality, and hospital stay were similar between the 2 groups.[91]

Disease assessment and follow-up

Follow-up of patients who achieve remission is challenging. As is the case with all other manifestations of BD, GI involvement is subject to acute exacerbations rather than following a chronic, indolent course. Further research is needed to determine the ideal time for surveillance colonoscopy in patients who achieve clinical remission, the role of acute phase reactants or fecal calprotectin in predicting relapse in such patients, and the decision to treat asymptomatic patients who are shown to have ulcers on endoscopy.

Disease assessment during follow-up in clinical trials is also challenging. The Disease Activity Index for Intestinal BD (DAIBD), a modified version of the CD activity index, was developed specifically for GI involvement of BD.[92] However, 3 of the 8 items (general well-being, fever, and extraintestinal manifestations) can be positive in BD patients due to conditions unrelated to the GI tract. Thus, patients with mucosal or skin lesions, uveitis, and arterial or venous involvement can have high scores even if their GI involvement is in remission. This may explain the weak correlation between DAIBD scores and endoscopic activity.[68]

SUMMARY

GI involvement of BD presents as a combination of both vasculitis and IBD-type characteristics. Therefore, clinical presentation and complications are consistent with a vasculitic picture, but IBD-type features may also be prominent enough to complicate the diagnosis. Due to the lack of controlled studies, reflecting the rarity of GI involvement in BD even in endemic geographies, management relies on uncontrolled data and extrapolation from IBD treatment strategies.

REFERENCES

1. Behçet H. [Über rezidivierende, aphtöse, durch ein Virus verursachte Geschwüre am Mund, am Auge und an den Genitalien]. Dermatol Wochenschr 1937;105:1152–63.
2. Hatemi G, Seyahi E, Fresko I, et al. Behçet's syndrome: a critical digest of the 2012-2013 literature. Clin Exp Rheumatol 2013;31:108–17.
3. Hatemi I, Esatoglu SN, Hatemi G, et al. Characteristics, treatment, and long-term outcome of gastrointestinal involvement in Behcet's Syndrome: a strobe-compliant observational study from a dedicated multidisciplinary center. Medicine (Baltimore) 2016;95:e3348.
4. Yurdakul S, Yazıcı Y. Epidemiology of Behçet's syndrome and regional differences in disease expression. In: Yazıcı Y, Yazıcı H, editors. Behçet's syndrome. New York: Springer NY; 2010. p. 35–52.
5. Azizlerli G, Köse AA, Sarica R, et al. Prevalence of Behçet's disease in Istanbul, Turkey. Int J Dermatol 2003;42:803–6.
6. Zhang Z, He F, Shi Y. Behcet's disease seen in China: analysis of 334 cases. Rheumatol Int 2013;33:645–8.
7. Nakae K, Masaki F, Hashimoto T, et al. Recent epidemiological features of Behçet's disease in Japan. In: Wechsler B, Godeau P, editors. Behçet's disease. Amsterdam: Excerpta Medica; 1993. p. 145–51.
8. Krause I, Yankevich A, Fraser A, et al. Prevalence and clinical aspects of Behcet's disease in the north of Israel. Clin Rheumatol 2007;26:555–60.
9. Olivieri I, Leccese P, Padula A, et al. High prevalence of Behçet's disease in southern Italy. Clin Exp Rheumatol 2013;31:28–31.

10. González-Gay MA, García-Porrúa C, Brañas F, et al. Epidemiologic and clinical aspects of Behçet's disease in a defined area of Northwestern Spain, 1988-1997. J Rheumatol 2000;27:703–7.

11. Chamberlain MA. Behcet's syndrome in 32 patients in Yorkshire. Ann Rheum Dis 1977;36:491–9.

12. Jankowski J, Crombie I, Jankowski R. Behçet's syndrome in Scotland. Postgrad Med J 1992;68:566–70.

13. Papoutsis NG, Abdel-Naser MB, Altenburg A, et al. Prevalence of Adamantiades-Behçet's disease in Germany and the municipality of Berlin: results of a nationwide survey. Clin Exp Rheumatol 2006;24:S125.

14. Leccese P, Yazici Y, Olivieri I. Behcet's syndrome in nonendemic regions. Curr Opin Rheumatol 2017;29:12–6.

15. Maldini C, Druce K, Basu N, et al. Exploring the variability in Behçet's disease prevalence: a meta-analytical approach. Rheumatology (Oxford) 2017. https://doi.org/10.1093/rheumatology/kew486.

16. Oshima Y, Shimizu T, Yokohari R, et al. Clinical studies on Behcet's syndrome, with special reference to 100 personal cases. Naika 1962;9:701–14 [in Japanese].

17. Yurdakul S, Tuzuner N, Yurdakul I, et al. Gastrointestinal involvement in Behçet's syndrome: a controlled study. Ann Rheum Dis 1996;55:208–10.

18. Yi SW, Cheon JH, Kim JH, et al. The prevalence and clinical characteristics of esophageal involvement in patients with Behçet's disease: a single center experience in Korea. J Korean Med Sci 2009;24:52–6.

19. Goldstein JL, Eisen GM, Lewis B, et al. Video capsule endoscopy to prospectively assess small bowel injury with celecoxib, naproxen plus omeprazole, and placebo. Clin Gastroenterol Hepatol 2005;3:133.

20. Kobayashi K, Ueno F, Bito S, et al. Development of consensus statements for the diagnosis and management of intestinal Behçet's disease using a modified Delphi approach. J Gastroenterol 2007;42:737–45.

21. Criteria for diagnosis of Behçet's disease. International Study Group for Behçet's disease. Lancet 1990;335:1078–80.

22. Ward EM, Woodward TA, Mazlumzadeh M, et al. Gastrointestinal disease in Behçet's disease. Adv Exp Med Biol 2003;528:459–64.

23. Yazici H, Tüzün Y, Pazarli H, et al. Influence of age of onset and patient's sex on the prevalence and severity of manifestations of Behçet's syndrome. Ann Rheum Dis 1984;43:783–9.

24. Hung CH, Lee JH, Chen ST, et al. Young children with Behçet disease have more intestinal involvement. J Pediatr Gastroenterol Nutr 2013;57:225–9.

25. Hatemi G, Yazici Y, Yazici H. Behçet's syndrome. Rheum Dis Clin North Am 2013;39:245–61.

26. de Menthon M, Lavalley MP, Maldini C, et al. HLA-B51/B5 and the risk of Behçet's disease: a systematic review and meta-analysis of case-control genetic association studies. Arthritis Rheum 2009;61:1287–96.

27. Maldini C, Lavalley MP, Cheminant M, et al. Relationships of HLA-B51 or B5 genotype with Behçet's disease clinical characteristics: systematic review and meta-analyses of observational studies. Rheumatology (Oxford) 2012;51:887–900.

28. Mizuki N, Meguro A, Ota M, et al. Genome-wide association studies identify IL23R–IL12RB2 and IL10 as Behçet's disease susceptibility loci. Nat Genet 2010;42:703–6.

29. Remmers EF, Cosan F, Kirino Y, et al. Genome-wide association study identifies variants in the MHC class I, IL10, and IL23R–IL12RB2 regions associated with Behcet's disease. Nat Genet 2010;42:698–702.

30. Kim ES, Kim SW, Moon CM, et al. Interactions between IL17A, IL23R, and STAT4 polymorphisms confer susceptibility to intestinal Behcet's disease in Korean population. Life Sci 2012;22(90):740–6.

31. Ortiz-Fernández L, García-Lozano JR, Montes-Cano MA, et al. Association of haplotypes of the TLR8 locus with susceptibility to Crohn's and Behçet's diseases. Clin Exp Rheumatol 2015;33:S117–22.

32. Uyar FA, Saruhan-Direskeneli G, Gül A. Common Crohn's disease-predisposing variants of the CARD15/NOD2 gene are not associated with Behçet's disease in Turkey. Clin Exp Rheumatol 2004;22:S50–2.

33. Schenk M, Bouchon A, Seibold F, et al. TREM-1-expressing intestinal macrophages crucially amplify chronic inflammation in experimental colitis and inflammatory bowel diseases. J Clin Invest 2007;117:3097–106.

34. Jung YS, Kim SW, Yoon JY, et al. Expression of a soluble triggering receptor expressed on myeloid cells-1 (sTREM-1) correlates with clinical disease activity in intestinal Behcet's disease. Inflamm Bowel Dis 2011;17:2130–7.

35. Nara K, Kurokawa MS, Chiba S, et al. Involvement of innate immunity in the pathogenesis of intestinal Behçet's disease. Clin Exp Immunol 2008;152:245–51.

36. Imamura Y, Kurokawa MS, Yoshikawa H, et al. Involvement of Th1 cells and heat shock protein 60 in the pathogenesis of intestinal Behcet's disease. Clin Exp Immunol 2005;139:371–8.

37. Ferrante A, Ciccia F, Principato A, et al. A Th1 but not a Th17 response is present in the gastrointestinal involvement of Behçet's disease. Clin Exp Rheumatol 2010;28:S27–30.

38. Hayasaki N, Ito M, Suzuki T, et al. Neutrophilic phlebitis is characteristic of intestinal Behçet's disease and simple ulcer syndrome. Histopathology 2004;45:377–83.

39. Isomoto H, Shikuwa S, Suematsu T, et al. Ileal lesions in Behçet's disease originate in Peyer's patches: findings on magnifying endoscopy. Scand J Gastroenterol 2008;43:249–50.

40. Demirkesen C, Oz B, Göksal S. Behçet's disease: pathology. In: Yazici Y, Yazici H, editors. Behçet's syndrome. New York: Springer; 2010. p. 215–43.

41. Jung YS, Cheon JH, Park SJ, et al. Long-term clinical outcomes of Crohn's disease and intestinal Behcet's disease. Inflamm Bowel Dis 2013;19:99–105.

42. Houman MH, Ben Ghorbel I, Lamloum M, et al. Esophageal involvement in Behcet's disease. Yonsei Med J 2002;43:457–60.

43. Cakmak SK, Cakmak A, Gul U, et al. Upper gastrointestinal abnormalities and Helicobacter pylori in Behçet's disease. Int J Dermatol 2009;48:1174–6.

44. Ben Yaghlène L, Hammel P, Palazzo L, et al. Acute pancreatitis revealing Behçet disease. Gastroenterol Clin Biol 2005;29:294–6.

45. Seyahi E, Caglar E, Ugurlu S, et al. An outcome survey of 43 patients with Budd-Chiari syndrome due to Behçet's syndrome followed up at a single, dedicated center. Semin Arthritis Rheum 2015;44:602–9.

46. Desbois AC, Rautou PE, Biard L, et al. Behçet's disease in Budd-Chiari syndrome. Orphanet J Rare Dis 2014;9:104.

47. Adiamah A, Wong LS. Behçet's disease: a rare cause of rectovaginal fistula. BMJ Case Rep 2010;2010 [pii:bcr0620103130].

48. Chawla S, Smart CJ, Moots RJ. Recto-vaginal fistula: a refractory complication of Behcet's disease. Colorectal Dis 2007;9:667–8.

49. Teh LS, Green KA, O'Sullivan MM, et al. Behçet's syndrome: severe proctitis with rectovaginal fistula formation. Ann Rheum Dis 1989;48:779–80.

50. Lee CR, Kim WH, Cho YS, et al. Colonoscopic findings in intestinal Behçet's disease. Inflamm Bowel Dis 2001;7:243–9.

51. Cheon JH, Kim WH. An update on the diagnosis, treatment, and prognosis of intestinal Behçet's disease. Curr Opin Rheumatol 2015;27:24–31.

52. Kim DH, Cheon JH. Intestinal Behçet's disease: a true inflammatory bowel disease or merely an intestinal complication of systemic vasculitis? Yonsei Med J 2016;57:22–32.

53. Jung YS, Cheon JH, Park SJ, et al. Clinical course of intestinal Behcet's disease during the first five years. Dig Dis Sci 2013;58:496–503.

54. Park J, Cheon JH, Park YE, et al. Risk factors and outcomes of acute lower gastrointestinal bleeding in intestinal Behcet's disease. Int J Colorectal Dis 2017;32:745–51.

55. Bayraktar Y, Ozaslan E, Van Thiel DH. Gastrointestinal manifestations of Behcet's disease. J Clin Gastroenterol 2000;30:144–54.

56. Esatoglu SN, Hatemi G, Salihoglu A, et al. A reappraisal of the association between Behçet's disease, myelodysplastic syndrome and the presence of trisomy 8: a systematic literature review. Clin Exp Rheumatol 2015;33:145–51.

57. Toyonaga T, Nakase H, Matsuura M, et al. Refractoriness of intestinal Behçet's disease with myelodysplastic syndrome involving trisomy 8 to medical therapies - our case experience and review of the literature. Digestion 2013;88:217–21.

58. Soysal T, Salihoglu A, Esatoglu SN, et al. Bone marrow transplantation for Behçet's disease: a case report and systematic review of the literature. Rheumatology (Oxford) 2014;53:1136–41.

59. Kasahara Y, Tanaka S, Nishino M, et al. Intestinal involvement in Behçet's disease: review of 136 surgical cases in the Japanese literature. Dis Colon Rectum 1981;24:103–6.

60. Morimoto Y, Tanaka Y, Itoh T, et al. Esophagobronchial fistula in a patient with Behcet's disease: report of a case. Surg Today 2005;35:671–6.

61. Melikoğlu M, Uğurlu S, Tascilar K, et al. Large vessel involvement in Behçet's syndrome: a retrospective survey. Ann Rheum Dis 2008;67(Suppl II):67.

62. Jung HC, Rhee PL, Song IS, et al. Temporal changes in the clinical type or diagnosis of Behcet's colitis in patients with aphthoid or punched-out colonic ulcerations. J Korean Med Sci 1991;6:313–8.

63. Zou J, Shen Y, Ji DN, et al. Endoscopic findings of gastrointestinal involvement in Chinese patients with Behcet's disease. World J Gastroenterol 2014;20: 17171–8.

64. Shin SJ, Lee SK, Kim TI, et al. Chronological changes in the systemic manifestations of intestinal Behçet's disease and their significance in diagnosis. Int J Colorectal Dis 2010;25:1371–6.

65. Cheon JH, Kim ES, Shin SJ, et al. Development and validation of novel diagnostic criteria for intestinal Behçet's disease in Korean patients with ileocolonic ulcers. Am J Gastroenterol 2009;104:2492–9.

66. Zhang T, Hong L, Wang Z, et al. Comparison between intestinal Behçet's disease and Crohn's disease in characteristics of symptom, endoscopy, and radiology. Gastroenterol Res Pract 2017;2017:3918746.

67. Kim JS, Lim SH, Choi IJ, et al. Prediction of the clinical course of Behcet's colitis according to macroscopic classification by colonoscopy. Endoscopy 2000;32: 635–40.

68. Lee HJ, Kim YN, Jang HW, et al. Correlations between endoscopic and clinical disease activity indices in intestinal Behcet's disease. World J Gastroenterol 2012;18:5771–8.

69. Yim SM, Kim DH, Lee HJ, et al. Mucosal healing predicts the long-term prognosis of intestinal Behcet's disease. Dig Dis Sci 2014;59:2529–35.

70. Arimoto J, Endo H, Kato T, et al. A.Clinical value of capsule endoscopy for detecting small bowel lesions in patients with intestinal Behçet's disease. Dig Endosc 2016;28:179–85.

71. Hamdulay SS, Cheent K, Ghosh C, et al. Wireless capsule endoscopy in the investigation of intestinal Behçet's syndrome. Rheumatology (Oxford) 2008;47: 1231–4.

72. Neves FS, Fylyk SN, Lage LV, et al. Behçet's disease: clinical value of the video capsule endoscopy for small intestine examination. Rheumatol Int 2009;29: 601–3.

73. Jung YS, Hong SP, Kim TI, et al. Long-term clinical outcomes and factors predictive of relapse after 5-aminosalicylate or sulfasalazine therapy in patients with intestinal Behcet disease. J Clin Gastroenterol 2012;46:e38–45.

74. Jung YS, Yoon JY, Lee JH, et al. Prognostic factors and long-term clinical outcomes for surgical patients with intestinal Behcet's disease. Inflamm Bowel Dis 2011;17:1594–602.

75. Kim DH, Park Y, Kim B, et al. Fecal calprotectin as a non-invasive biomarker for intestinal involvement of Behçet's disease. J Gastroenterol Hepatol 2017;32: 595–601.

76. Esatoglu SN, Hatemi I, Ozguler Y, et al. Fecal calprotectin level is useful in identifying active disease in Behçet's syndrome patients with gastrointestinal involvement: a controlled Study [abstract]. Arthritis Rheumatol 2016;68:3993–4.

77. Choi CH, Kim TI, Kim BC, et al. Anti-*Saccharomyces cerevisiae* antibody in intestinal Behçet's disease patients: relation to clinical course. Dis Colon Rectum 2006;49:1849–59.

78. Shin SJ, Kim BC, Kim TI, et al. Anti-alpha-enolase antibody as a serologic marker and its correlation with disease severity in intestinal Behçet's disease. Dig Dis Sci 2011;56:812–8.

79. Lee HW, Chung SH, Moon CM, et al. The correlation of serum IL-12B expression with disease activity in patients with inflammatory bowel disease. Medicine (Baltimore) 2016;95:e3772.

80. Hatemi I, Hatemi G, Celik AF, et al. Frequency of pathergy phenomenon and other features of Behçet's syndrome among patients with inflammatory bowel disease. Clin Exp Rheumatol 2008;26:S91–5.

81. Lee SK, Kim BK, Kim TI, et al. Differential diagnosis of intestinal Behcet's disease and Crohn's disease by colonoscopic findings. Endoscopy 2009;41:9–16.

82. Erzin Y, Esatoglu SN, Hatemi I, et al. P259 Comparative retrospective assessment of prospectively recorded endoscopic and histological findings between CD and GI-TB; the first Eastern European registry data. J Crohns Colitis 2014; 8:S171.

83. Ozguler Y, Hatemi G, Yazici H. Management of Behçet's syndrome. Curr Opin Rheumatol 2014;26:285–91.

84. Hatemi G, Silman A, Bang D, et al, EULAR Expert Committee. EULAR recommendations for the management of Behçet disease. Ann Rheum Dis 2008;67:1656–62.

85. Chung MJ, Cheon JH, Kim SU, et al. Response rates to medical treatments and long-term clinical outcomes of nonsurgical patients with intestinal Behçet disease. J Clin Gastroenterol 2010;44:e116–22.

86. Jung YS, Cheon JH, Hong SP, et al. Clinical outcomes and prognostic factors for thiopurine maintenance therapy in patients with intestinal Behcet's disease. Inflamm Bowel Dis 2012;18:750–7.

87. Hatemi I, Hatemi G, Pamuk ON, et al. TNF-alpha antagonists and thalidomide for the management of gastrointestinal Behcet's syndrome refractory to the conventional treatment modalities: a case series and review of the literature. Clin Exp Rheumatol 2015;33:S129–37.

88. Inoue N, Kobayashi K, Naganuma M, et al. Long-term safety and efficacy of adalimumab for intestinal Behçet's disease in the open label study following a phase 3 clinical trial. Intest Res 2017;15:395–401.

89. Ma D, Zhang CJ, Wang RP, et al. Etanercept in the treatment of intestinal Behcet's disease. Cell Biochem Biophys 2014;69:735–9.

90. Hisamatsu T, Ueno F, Matsumoto T, et al. The 2nd edition of consensus statements for the diagnosis and management of intestinal Behçet's disease: indication of anti-TNFα monoclonal antibodies. J Gastroenterol 2014;49:156–62.

91. Baek SJ, Baik SH, Kim CW, et al. Short- and long-term outcomes of laparoscopic surgery for intestinal Behcet's disease: a comparative study with open surgery. Surg Endosc 2016;30:99–105.

92. Cheon JH, Han DS, Park JY, et al, Korean IBD Study Group. Development, validation, and responsiveness of a novel disease activity index for intestinal Behçet's disease. Inflamm Bowel Dis 2011;17:605–13.

93. Shimizu T, Ehrlich GE, Inaba G, et al. Behçet disease (Behçet syndrome). Semin Arthritis Rheum 1979;8:223–60.

94. O'Duffy JD, Carney JA, Deodhar S. Behçet's disease. Report of 10 cases, 3 with new manifestations. Ann Intern Med 1971;75:561–70.

95. Yamamato T, Toyokkawa H, Matsubara JT, et al. Anation-wide surwey of Behçet's disease in Japon. Jpn J opthalmol 1974;18:282–90.

96. Chamberlain MA. Behcet's syndrome in 32 patients in Yorkshire. Ann Rheum Dis 1977;36:491–9.

97. Eun HC, Chung H, Choi SJ. Clinical analysis of 114 patients with behçet's disease. J Korean Med Assoc 27:933–939.

98. Jankowski J, Crombie I, Jankowski R. Behçet's syndrome in Scotland. Postgrad Med J 1992;68:566–70.

99. Dilsen N, Konice M, Aral O, et al. Risk factors of vital organ involvement in Behçet's disease. In: Weschle B, Godeau F, editors. Behçet's disease. Proceedings of the sixty International confereance on Behçet's disease. Excrepta Medica. Amsterdam, sayda 165–169.

100. Yurdakul S, Tüzüner N, Yurdakul I, et al. Gastrointestinal involvement in Behçet's syndrome: a controlled study. Ann Rheum Dis 1996;55:208–10.

101. Gürler A, Boyvat A, Türsen U. Clinical manifestations of Behçet's disease: an analysis of 2147 patients. Yonsei Med J 1997;38:423–7.

102. Bang D, Yoon KH, Chung HG, et al. Epidemiological and clinical features of Behçet's disease in Korea. Yonsei Med J 1997;38:428–36.

103. Bang DS, Oh SH, Lee KH, et al. Influence of sex on patients with Behçet's disease in Korea. J Korean Med Sci 2003;18:231–5.

104. Tursen U, Gurler A, Boyvat A. Evaluation of clinical findings according to sex in 2313 Turkish patients with Behçet's disease. Int J Dermatol 2003;42:346–51.
105. Kural-Seyahi E, Fresko I, Seyahi N, et al. The long-term mortality and morbidity of Behçet syndrome: a 2-decade outcome survey of 387 patients followed at a dedicated center. Medicine (Baltimore) 2003;82:60–76.
106. Yi SW, Kim JH, Lim KY, et al. The Behcet's disease quality of life: reliability and validity of the Korean version. Yonsei Med J 2008;49:698–704.
107. Alli N, Gur G, Yalcin B, et al. Patient characteristics in Behçet disease: a retrospective analysis of 213 Turkish patients during 2001-4. Am J Clin Dermatol 2009;10:411–8.
108. Neves FS, Caldas CA, Lage LV, et al. Faraway from the silk route: demographic and clinical features of Behçet's disease in 106 Brazilian patients. Clin Rheumatol 2009;28:543–6.
109. El Menyawi MM, Raslan HM, Edrees A. Clinical features of Behcet's disease in Egypt. Rheumatol Int 2009;29:641–6.
110. Davatchi F, Shahram F, Chams-Davatchi C, et al. Behcet's disease in Iran: analysis of 6500 cases. Int J Rheum Dis 2010;13:367–73.
111. Oliveira AC, Buosi AL, Dutra LA, et al. Behçet disease: clinical features and management in a Brazilian tertiary hospital. J Clin Rheumatol 2011;17:416–20.
112. Zhang Z, He F, Shi Y. Behcet's disease seen in China: analysis of 334 cases. Rheumatol Int 2013;33:645–8.
113. Kobayashi T, Kishimoto M, Swearingen CJ, et al. Differences in clinical manifestations, treatment, and concordance rates with two major sets of criteria for Behçet's syndrome for patients in the US and Japan: data from a large, three-center cohort study. Mod Rheumatol 2013;23:547–53.
114. Singal A, Chhabra N, Pandhi D, et al. Behçet's disease in India: a dermatological perspective. Indian J Dermatol Venereol Leprol 2013;79:199–204.
115. Olivieri I, Leccese P, Padula A, et al. High prevalence of Behçet's disease in southern Italy. Clin Exp Rheumatol 2013;31:28–31.
116. Mohammad A, Mandl T, Sturfelt G, et al. Incidence, prevalence and clinical characteristics of Behçet's disease in southern Sweden. Rheumatology (Oxford) 2013;52:304–10.
117. Sibley C, Yazici Y, Tascilar K, et al. Behçet syndrome manifestations and activity in the United States versus Turkey a cross-sectional cohort comparison. J Rheumatol 2014;41:1379–84.
118. Kim DY, Choi MJ, Cho S, et al. Changing clinical expression of Behçet disease in Korea during three decades (1983-2012): chronological analysis of 3674 hospital-based patients. Br J Dermatol 2014;170:458–61.
119. Rodríguez-Carballeira M, Alba MA, Solans-Laqué R, et al. Registry of the Spanish network of Behçet's disease: a descriptive analysis of 496 patients. Clin Exp Rheumatol 2014;32:S33–9.
120. Khabbazi A, Noshad H, Shayan FK, et al. Demographic and clinical features of Behçet's disease in Azerbaijan. Int J Rheum Dis 2014.
121. Hamzaoui A, Jaziri F, Ben Salem T, et al. Comparison of clinical features of Behcet disease according to age in a Tunisian cohort. Acta Med Iran 2014;52:748–51.
122. Ndiaye M, Sow AS, Valiollah A, et al. Behçet's disease in black skin. A retrospective study of 50 cases in Dakar. J Dermatol Case Rep 2015;9:98–102.
123. Lennikov A, Alekberova Z, Goloeva R, et al. Single center study on ethnic and clinical features of Behcet's disease in Moscow, Russia. Clin Rheumatol 2015;34:321–7.

124. Ajose FO, Adelowo O, Oderinlo O. Clinical presentations of Behçet's disease among Nigerians: a 4-year prospective study. Int J Dermatol 2015;54(8):888–97.

125. Bonitsis NG, Luong Nguyen LB, LaValley MP, et al. Gender-specific differences in Adamantiades-Behçet's disease manifestations: an analysis of the German registry and meta-analysis of data from the literature. Rheumatology (Oxford) 2015;54:121–33.

126. Kirino Y, Ideguchi H, Takeno M, et al. Continuous evolution of clinical phenotype in 578 Japanese patients with Behçet's disease: a retrospective observational study. Arthritis Res Ther 2016;18:217.

127. Nanthapisal S, Klein NJ, Ambrose N, et al. Paediatric Behçet's disease: a UK tertiary centre experience. Clin Rheumatol 2016;35:2509–16.

128. Cansu DÜ, Kaşifoğlu T, Korkmaz C. Do clinical findings of Behçet's disease vary by gender?: A single-center experience from 329 patients. Eur J Rheumatol 2016;3:157–60.

129. Ryu HJ, Seo MR, Choi HJ, et al. Clinical phenotypes of Korean patients with Behcet disease according to gender, age at onset, and HLA-B51. Korean J Intern Med 2017. https://doi.org/10.3904/kjim.2016.202.

130. Hatemi I, Esatoglu SN, Hatemi G, et al. Characteristics,treatment, and long-term outcome of gastrointestinal involvement in Behcet's syndrome: a strobe-compliant observational study from a Dedicated Multidisciplinary Center. Medicine (Baltimore) 2016;95:e3348.

Rheumatic Manifestations in Autoimmune Liver Disease

 CrossMark

Carlo Selmi, MD, PhD[a,b,]*, Elena Generali, MD[a],
Merrill Eric Gershwin, MD[c]

KEYWORDS

- Immune tolerance • Personalized medicine • Autoimmune comorbidity • Cholangitis
- Hepatitis • Osteoporosis • Methotrexate • Autoantibody

KEY POINTS

- Autoimmune hepatitis (AIH) is a rare disease that is the result of an autoimmune destruction of the hepatocytes, manifesting with high liver aminotransferase and serum autoantibody levels that may be specific for the disease.
- Primary biliary cholangitis (PBC) and primary sclerosing cholangitis (PSC) are chronic autoimmune cholestatic diseases that affect the biliary tree. PBC is characterized by antimitochondrial antibody positivity in almost all cases, whereas, conversely, PSC has no association with autoantibodies, suggesting a different pathogenesis.
- Rheumatic diseases are found in nearly 20% of patients with autoimmune liver diseases and may be associated with different prognoses for the patients. For this reason, the identification of the co-occurring disease at an early stage or even preclinically (using autoantibodies) is of pivotal importance.
- Bone density is reduced in patients with AIH because of prolonged steroid use and in PBC/PSC because of chronic cholestasis; therefore, osteoporosis management is an important issue in the care of these patients.
- Treatment options should be personalized to address coexisting conditions, especially if overlapping with specific rheumatic or autoimmune diseases.

INTRODUCTION

The link between autoimmune liver diseases and rheumatologic disease traces back to the first report in the mid-1950s, when findings of active chronic hepatic disease were described in the setting of systemic lupus erythematosus (SLE). These findings

Conflicts of Interest: The authors have no conflicts of interest.
[a] Division of Rheumatology and Clinical Immunology, Humanitas Research Hospital, Via A. Manzoni 56, Rozzano, Milan 20089, Italy; [b] BIOMETRA Department, University of Milan, Via Luigi Vanvitelli, 32, 20129 Milano, MI, Italy; [c] Division of Rheumatology, Allergy, and Clinical Immunology, University of California, Davis, 4860 Y Street, Suite 2500, Sacramento, CA 95817, USA
* Corresponding author. Division of Rheumatology and Clinical Immunology, Humanitas Research Hospital, via A. Manzoni 56, Rozzano, Milan 20089, Italy.
E-mail address: carlo.selmi@unimi.it

Rheum Dis Clin N Am 44 (2018) 65–87
https://doi.org/10.1016/j.rdc.2017.09.008
0889-857X/18/© 2017 Elsevier Inc. All rights reserved.
rheumatic.theclinics.com

led to the concept of lupoid hepatitis with positive LE cell tests and mild signs of rheumatic disease.[1,2] When discussing autoimmune liver disease, it is possible to distinguish autoimmune hepatitis (AIH; affecting hepatocytes) from primary biliary cholangitis (PBC, until recently known as primary biliary cirrhosis), and primary sclerosing cholangitis (PSC) based on the target tissue.[3,4] Cirrhosis and liver failure are potential complications shared by inflammatory hepatobiliary diseases, regardless of the target tissue, whereas the pathogenesis and therapeutics may vary within the clinical spectrum.[5] The epidemiology of autoimmune liver diseases is similar to that of other rare autoimmune or inflammatory disorders.[6–8] Similarly, serum autoantibodies represent the hallmark for AIH and PBC, but not PSC, and are usually positive years before the diagnosis (**Table 1**).[9–11]

Since the earliest reports, several others have shown the associations between PBC and systemic sclerosis (SSc),[12,13] as well as Sjögren syndrome (SjS).[14] Moreover, the epidemiologic links between these liver diseases and systemic rheumatic manifestations are also reflected in shared pathogenic mechanisms. These links are elegantly represented by the concept of autoimmune epithelitis, coined as a descriptor for PBC and SjS.[15] Serologic profiles are also similar with regard to antinuclear antibody (ANA) positivity[16] and common laboratory abnormalities are present, as is the case for hypergammaglobulinemia.[17] Most importantly, therapeutic strategies may also overlap, because steroids represent the first-line therapy in most cases,[18] whereas new targeted approaches are emerging.[19,20] Nonclassic associations have been also reported between spondyloarthritis and PSC with regard to inflammatory bowel diseases (IBD).[21] In addition, because corticosteroids and chronic liver diseases are associated with bone density loss, osteoporosis and bone fractures demand the attention of rheumatologists managing such patients.[22–24]

This article (1) provides an overview of the characteristics of the 3 major autoimmune liver diseases, namely AIH, PBS, and PSC; and (2) elucidates the existing associations between these conditions and rheumatic diseases. Particular attention is paid to both the shared and unique epidemiology, serum autoantibodies, and treatments, as well as the approach to bone density loss. The term lupoid hepatitis was introduced by our unit in 195CiL to describe cases of active chronic hepatitis associated with a positive LE cell test and occasionally minor manifestations of SLE.

AUTOIMMUNE HEPATITIS

AIH is a chronic inflammatory disease of unknown cause resulting from the immune-mediated destruction of hepatocytes with autoimmune features.[25,26] AIH is characterized by the presence of typical but nonspecific findings on liver biopsy, serum autoantibodies, and increased serum aminotransferase and gamma-globulin levels.[27] The incidence, although not precise, is estimated at approximately 1 per 100,000 person-years, with higher possible incidence in Scandinavia.[28] AIH most commonly affects women, with a male/female ratio of 1:4,[28] and manifests a 2-peak incidence during adolescence and at 30 to 45 years of age.[25,29] The onset of AIH is most frequently insidious, with 20% to 30% of patients presenting with an acute icteric hepatitis, consistently associated with hypergammaglobulinemia. Clinical manifestations are nonspecific and include hepatosplenomegaly, jaundice, anorexia, and fatigue.[27,30] The most common extrahepatic manifestations are arthralgia and rash.

Clinical Features

Two types of AIH are distinguished, primarily based on autoantibody patterns: AIH type 1 with ANA and/or anti–smooth muscle antibodies (anti-SMA), and AIH type 2

Table 1
Serum autoantibodies in autoimmune liver diseases

Antibody	Liver Disease	Prevalence (%)
ANA	AIH	Homogeneous pattern 34–58, speckled 21–34
	PBC	Nuclear pore complex targeting gp210 and nucleoporin p62, multiple nuclear dots targeting Sp100: 50–70
	PSC	20
SMA	AIH	81
	PSC	0–73
LKM1	Type 2 AIH	—
LC1	Type 2 AIH	50, only autoantibody in 10 of cases
pANCA	AIH	—
	PSC	33
SLA/LP	AIH	10–30
LKM3	Type 2 AIH	—
ASGPR	AIH	90
	PBC	—
AMA	AIH	9
	PBC	90–95
ACA	AIH	0–25
	PBC	9–30
Anti-dsDNA	AIH	23–34
	PBC	0–22
Rheumatoid factor	AIH	21
Antihistones	AIH	35
Anti-Ro/SSA	AIH	26
	PBC	10–28
Anti-La/SSB	AIH	4.3
Anti-CCP	AIH	9
Anticardiolipin IgG/IgM	AIH	40
	PBC	IgM 75
Antinucleosome	AIH	21.7
	PBC	14.2
	PSC	20
Anti-RNP	AIH	8.6
	PSC	5
Anti-Sm	AIH	4.3
Antiribosomal P	AIH	4.3
	PSC	5

Abbreviations: ANA, antinuclear antibodies; ASGPR: Asialoglycoprotein receptor antibodies; CCP, cyclic citrullinated peptides; dsDNA, downstream DNA; IgG, immunoglobulin G; IgM, immunoglobulin M; LC1, liver cytosol type 1; LKM1, liver kidney microsomal type 1; LKM3, liver kidney microsomal type 3; pANCA, perinuclear antineutrophil cytoplasmic antibodies; RNP: Ribonucleoprotein; SMA, smooth muscle antibodies .

with anti–liver kidney microsomal type 1 antibody (anti-LKM1) and/or anti–liver cytosol type 1 antibody (anti-LC1). Type I AIH (AIH-1) can affect individuals of any age and sex. Patients with human leukocyte antigen (HLA) DRB1*0301 AIH-1 are more likely to be male, present with high immunoglobulin (Ig) G levels, be ANA/anti-SMA positive, deteriorate despite glucocorticoid treatment, and progress more frequently to liver transplant. Type II AIH (AIH-2) primarily affects girls and young women, and has been linked to alleles encoding the DR3 (DRB1*0301) and DR7 (DRB1*0701) molecules.[26] It also associates with anti-LKM antibodies.[27,31,32] The diagnosis of AIH is defined as definite or probable, based on the diagnostic criteria of the International Autoimmune Hepatitis Group (IAIH-G; **Table 2**).[33,34] The clinical criteria for the diagnosis are sufficient to establish or rule out a definite or probable AIH in most patients. The revised scoring system was developed as a research tool to ensure the comparability of study populations in clinical trials, and can be used to assess treatment response (**Table 3**), similar to classification criteria used in rheumatology.[34] A pretreatment score of 10 points or higher, or a posttreatment score of 12 points or higher, indicate probable AIH at presentation, with a sensitivity of 100%, a specificity of 73%, and diagnostic accuracy of 67%. A pretreatment score of 15 points indicates definite AIH and has a sensitivity of 95%, a specificity of 97%, and a diagnostic accuracy of 94%.[35]

The clinical course of untreated AIH results in significant mortality, with 5-year and 10-year survival rates of 50% and 10% respectively. The use of glucocorticoids has dramatically improved the disease course, with a 10-year survival rate now exceeding 90%.[25] The complications associated with AIH are similar to those of other progressive liver diseases, because chronic hepatitis can evolve to cirrhosis and ultimately to hepatocellular carcinoma (HCC), despite the use of immunosuppressives. At the time of diagnosis, approximately 30% of adults have histologic evidence of cirrhosis; however, when appropriately treated, only a small number develop cirrhosis during follow-up if biochemical and histology inflammation resolves. The occurrence of HCC in patients with AIH is rare and only develops in long-standing cirrhosis. In the absence of definitive data, primary liver neoplasia incidence is assumed to be similar to that of other nonviral cases of cirrhosis.[25]

Association with Rheumatic Diseases

AIH was originally described in association with SLE and currently extrahepatic autoimmune manifestations are found in 20% to 50% of patients,[36] with the most common being autoimmune thyroiditis, diabetes, rheumatoid arthritis (RA), and ulcerative colitis (UC). Up to 43% of AIH cases have a family history of autoimmune diseases, in particular thyroid diseases and type 1 diabetes.[37] The occurrence of other autoimmune diseases in AIH is included in the original and revised International Autoimmune Hepatitis Scoring System (see **Table 3**).[33] Concurrent autoimmune disorders tend to cluster in women with AIH type 1, particularly if positive for HLA-DR4.[38] Moreover, elderly patients with AIH have higher frequency of concurrent rheumatic conditions than young adults.[39] SjS has been reported in up to 7% of patients with AIH, whereas RA has been reported in 2% to 4%. Although liver dysfunction has been reported in up to 60% of patients with SLE, overlapping with AIH is rare.[36]

An AIH-like entity linked to anti–tumor necrosis factor (TNF) treatment has recently been described in case reports.[40] Although these result in significant liver injury, the pathogenesis remains clear.[41] Liver biopsy seems to be useful; however, differentiation between drug-induced liver injury is not an easy task. Most cases respond well to corticosteroids.[42]

Autoantibodies

Autoantibodies represent a critical feature of AIH and may guide the diagnosis (see **Table 2**). In 2004, the IAIH-G established procedures and reference guidelines for more reliable serum autoantibody testing to overcome the lack of standardization.[43] In addition to serum ANA, anti-SM, and anti-LKM,[44] other autoantibodies should also be sought in suspected cases, including anti-LC1, perinuclear antineutrophil

Table 2
Revised original scoring system of the International Autoimmune Hepatitis Group

Criteria	Points
Sex	
Male	0
Female	+2
Ratio of ALP vs AST/ALT	
>2.0	+3
1.5–2.0	+2
1.0–1.5	+1
<1.0	0
Autoantibodies (ANA, SMA, LKM1) titer	
>1:80	+3
1:80	+2
1:40	+1
<1:40	0
AMA	
Positive	−4
Negative	0
Seropositivity for other autoantibodies	+2
Viral Hepatitis Markers	
Negative	+3
Positive	−3
History of Drug Use	
Yes	−4
No	+1
Average Alcohol Consumption (g/d)	
<25	+2
>60	−2
Presence of genetic factors (HLA, DR3, or DR4)	+1
Presence of other autoimmune disorders (thyroiditis, colitis, others)	+2
Liver Histology	
Interface hepatitis	+3
Predominant lymphocytic infiltrate	+1
Rosetting of liver cells	+1
None of the above	−5
Biliary changes	−3
Other changes	−3
Response to Therapy	
Complete	+2
Relapse	+3

A score greater than 15 or greater than 17 indicates a definite diagnosis of AIH before or after treatment, respectively. In contrast, scores between 10 and 15 and between 12 and 17 indicate a probable diagnosis, before or after therapy, respectively.

Abbreviations: ALP, alkaline phosphatase; ALT, alanine transaminase; AST, aspartate transaminase; AMA, antimitochondrial autoantibodies.

Adapted from Manns MP, Czaja AJ, Gorham JD, et al. Diagnosis and management of autoimmune hepatitis. Hepatology 2010;51(6):2195–6; with permission.

Table 3		
Codified diagnostic criteria of the International Autoimmune Hepatitis Group		
Features	**Definite**	**Probable**
Liver histology	Interface hepatitis of moderate or severe activity with or without lobular hepatitis or central portal bridging necrosis, but without biliary lesions or well-defined granulomas or other prominent changes suggestive of a different cause	Same as for definite
Serum biochemistry	Any abnormality in serum aminotransferase levels, especially if the serum alkaline phosphatase level is not markedly increased. Normal serum concentrations of alpha-antitrypsin, copper and ceruloplasmin	Same as for definite but patients with abnormal serum concentrations of copper or ceruloplasmin may be included, provided that Wilson disease has been excluded by appropriate investigations
Serum immunoglobulins	Total serum globulin or gamma globulin or IgG concentrations >1.5 times the upper normal limit	Any increase of serum globulin or gamma globulin or IgG concentrations above the upper normal limit
Serum autoantibodies	Seropositivity for ANA, SMA or anti-LKM1 antibodies at titers >1:80. Lower titers (particularly of anti-LKM1) may be significant in children. Seronegativity for AMA	Same as for definite but at titers of 1:40 or greater. Patients who are seronegative for these antibodies but who are seropositive for other antibodies may be included
Viral markers	Seronegativity for markers of current infection with hepatitis A, B, and C viruses	Same as for definite
Other causal factors	Average alcohol consumption <25 g/d No history of recent use of known hepatotoxic drugs	Alcohol consumption <50 g/d and no recent use of known hepatotoxic drugs Patients who have consumed larger amounts of alcohol or who have recently taken potentially hepatotoxic drugs may be included if there is clear evidence of continuing liver damage after abstinence from alcohol or withdrawal of the drug

From Manns MP, Czaja AJ, Gorham JD, et al. Diagnosis and management of autoimmune hepatitis. Hepatology 2010;51(6):2195; with permission.

cytoplasmic antibodies (pANCA), SLA/LP, and the antiasialoglycoprotein receptor antibodies.[45] In addition, less specific autoantibodies may be detected in a subset of patients, including anticardiolipin, antichromatin, anti–double-stranded DNA (dsDNA), rheumatoid factor, antihistones, anti-Ro/SSA, and anticyclic citrullinated peptides (anti-CCP) antibodies. Serum ANA were the first autoantibodies observed in AIH sera more than 50 years ago and remain the most sensitive marker of AIH.[46] These most frequently produce a homogeneous or speckled pattern. However, the test is not specific for AIH, because ANA positivity is common in viral diseases, other auto-immune liver diseases, as well as in up to 15% of healthy individuals, especially in older age groups.[47] Serum SMA are autoantibodies reacting with different proteins (actin, tubulin, vimentin, desmin, cytokeratins) of the cytoskeletal components (micro-filaments, microtubules, intermediate filaments). Their presence characterizes both autoimmune (AIH-1, celiac disease) and viral diseases (chronic hepatitis C, infectious mononucleosis). When detected at high titers (>1:80), they are considered a sensitive marker for AIH-1, being found in up to 80% of cases. A recent study showed that anti–SMA-T/G–positive subjects with normal liver function were at low risk of progression to AIH, whereas subjects with positive SMA and increased alanine transaminase (ALT) levels (>55IU/L) were at higher risk, although the positive predictive value is only 22%.[48] Serum autoantibodies against LKM-1 are the main serologic markers of AIH-2, recognizing the proximal renal tubule and hepatocellular cytoplasm. Serum anti-SLA/LP antibodies are occasionally found in patients with AIH who are negative for ANA, SMA, or anti-LKM and are cumulatively detected in 10% to 30% of cases of AIH-1 and AIH-2. Anti-SLA/LP antibodies are detectable by radioimmunoassay and enzyme-linked immunosorbent assay (ELISA) but not by immunofluorescence and are directed against different epitopes of a UGA transfer RNA suppressor. Anti-LC1 antibodies are detected by indirect immunofluorescence in sera from up to 50% of patients with type 2 AIH and less frequently in type 1 AIH or chronic hepatitis C. Importantly, ho, anti-LC1 are the only detectable markers in 10% of AIH cases. Note that serum anti-LC1 antibodies correlate with AIH severity and progression. An-tibodies to the asialoglycoprotein receptor are observed in up to 90% of patients with AIH and often coexist with other autoantibodies, although they lack specificity for the disease. However, similar to anti-LC1, antiasialoglycoprotein titers are associated with a more florid inflammatory disease activity and may allow monitoring of treatment response.

With regard to nonspecific antibodies, anti-CCP can be found in 9% of AIH sera, and their detection is independent of concurrent RA but may distinguish early-stage RA from nonspecific arthralgia.[39] Moreover, it has been reported than anti-CCP–pos-itive patients are at higher risk of cirrhosis at diagnosis and die more frequently from hepatic failure.[21] Anticardiolipin antibodies occur in nearly 40% of AIH, which is more frequently than hepatitis C (20%) and B (14%) infections. The presence of anti-cardiolipin IgG/IgM is associated with cirrhosis and inflammatory activity,[49] with the IgM subtype being more frequent in AIH than PBC.[50] Further, pANCA can be detected by indirect immunofluorescence in sera from patients with AIH-1 but also in a sub-group of patients with PSC or chronic viral hepatitis. Antibodies to histones are pre-sent in 35% of ANA-positive patients with AIH, whereas anti-dsDNA is detected in 23% to 34% cases, depending on the nature of the assay and substrate used for their detection.[51] Patients with antihistones are not distinguished by the severity of their disease,[52] whereas anti-dsDNA–positive subjects do not respond, or respond less, to corticosteroid treatment.[53]

Therapy

In contrast with PBC and PSC, immunosuppressants represent the treatment of choice for AIH, based on the good biochemical and histologic response, and survival (**Table 4**).[43,54] Glucocorticoids, in particular prednisone, in monotherapy or in combi-nation with azathioprine are the first-line treatment and induce remission (ie, normal ALT and IgG) in more than 80% of the patients, regardless of the presence of cirrhosis.[31] Once achieved, remission can be maintained with azathioprine alone after steroid tapering. The dosage of azathioprine is typically low compared with rheumatic diseases, usually requiring only 50 mg/d and never exceeding 150 mg/d.[18] Relapses following steroid discontinuation are common, because only 20% of patients remain in sustained remission. However, subgroups of patients manifest disease progression (approximately 10%) or are intolerant to standard therapy (13%). In such patients, other drugs have been anecdotally tried, including methotrexate,[55] cyclophospha-mide, tacrolimus, ursodeoxycholic acid (UDCA), cyclosporine, and mycophenolate mofetil, the last 2 constituting the most frequently reported alternatives.[18,56] Biologic therapies commonly used in rheumatology are of particular interest, because proin-flammatory cytokines (eg, TNF-alpha) are involved in AIH pathogenesis.[18] Infliximab has been used in refractory cases of AIH with reduction of aminotransferases and IgG levels.[57] Rituximab has been tried in a few refractory AIH cases, resulting in improved liver enzyme and IgG levels, no significant side effects, and a reduction in prednisolone dose for some patients.[58] Future developments may include regulatory T-cell therapy, which could allow the avoidance of prolonged, often lifelong, global immunosuppression in patients with AIH.[59] Liver transplant is the most definitive treat-ment of patients with AIH presenting with acute liver failure or end-stage chronic liver disease and for those with HCC who meet the transplant criteria. Although liver trans-plant for these patients is very successful, AIH may recur after transplant. Patients with AIH undergoing liver transplant have overall 5-year and 10-year survival rates of 90% and 75%, respectively, although infectious complications and disease recurrence are common.[60–63]

PRIMARY BILIARY CHOLANGITIS

PBC is a chronic cholestatic disease characterized by high-titer serum antimitochon-drial antibodies (AMA) in nearly 100% of patients when sensitive techniques are used.[64] It results in autoimmune-mediated destruction of the small and medium-sized intrahepatic bile ducts.[17,65] PBC prevalence varies substantially according to geography; the highest rates are in the northern United Stat, with a point prevalence of 402 per million in Minnesota.[66] Similar to other autoimmune diseases, PBC most commonly affects women, with a 1:9 male/female ratio,[17] and the average age at PBC diagnosis is within the fifth and sixth decades of life.[17]

Recently, PBC nomenclature has shifted from the term cirrhosis to cholangitis, which is more precise and removes the stigma associated with cirrhosis. This change reflects the dramatically improved PBC prognosis and treatment, because nowadays 2 out of 3 patients diagnosed with PBC and treated with UDCA have an expected sur-vival comparable with that of the general population and only a minority ever develop cirrhosis.[67,68]

Clinical Features

Early PBC symptoms are classically described as fatigue and pruritus, whereas phys-ical findings may include skin hyperpigmentation, hepatosplenomegaly, and (rarely) xanthelasmas. Fatigue and pruritus are nonspecific symptoms present in 70% of pa-tients with PBC. In contrast, end-stage symptoms are secondary to the complications of liver cirrhosis, including ascites, jaundice, hepatic encephalopathy, and upper digestive bleeding. Portal hypertension is frequently found in patients with PBC and, importantly, does not imply the presence of liver cirrhosis. Metabolic bone disease is increased in PBC compared with sex-matched and age-matched healthy individ-uals (discussed later). Similar to other types of cirrhosis, end-stage PBC can be complicated by the occurrence of HCC. The progression of PBC varies widely, and the factors influencing the severity and progression of the disease are largely

Table 4
Treatment of autoimmune liver diseases with rheumatic disease-modifying antirheumatic drugs and biologic therapy

Drug	Dosage	Safety
AIH		
Prednisone	First-line treatment (1 mg/kg/d, maximum 60 mg/d in monotherapy)	Acute: hyperglycemia, high blood pressure Chronic: diabetes, osteoporosis, glaucoma, cataract
Azathioprine	Induction therapy (1–2 mg/kg/d, maximum 200 mg/d) in combination with prednisone (30 mg/d) Maintenance therapy (50 mg/d or up to 2 mg/kg/d)	Leukopenia, liver toxicity, infections, nausea and vomiting
Mycophenolate mofetil	Second line (1.5–2 g daily)	Infections, nausea and vomiting, cytopenia, contraindicated in pregnancy
Cyclosporine	Refractory cases (2–5 mg/kg daily)	Hypertension, increased serum creatinine level, hirsutism
Methotrexate	Refractory cases: case reports	Liver toxicity, infections, contraindicated in pregnancy
Infliximab	Refractory cases: case reports	Liver toxicity, induction of AIH, contraindicated in pregnancy
Rituximab	Refractory cases: case reports	Contraindicated in pregnancy
PBC		
Azathioprine	Refractory cases (50 mg/d) + prednisone (30 mg/d) + UDCA	Leukopenia, liver toxicity, infections, nausea and vomiting
Cyclosporine	Refractory cases	Hypertension, increased serum creatinine level, hirsutism
Methotrexate	Refractory cases (0.25 mg/kg/wk PO)	Liver toxicity, infections, contraindicated in pregnancy
Mycophenolate mofetil	Refractory cases (1–2 mg/d)	Infections, nausea and vomiting, cytopenia, contraindicated in pregnancy
Colchicine	Refractory cases (1.2 mg/d)	Diarrhea, myelosuppression
Ustekinumab	Under evaluation (90 mg SC weeks 0–4 and then every 8 wk)	Infections, contraindicated in pregnancy
Abatacept	Under evaluation	
PSC		
Cyclosporine	Refractory cases	Hypertension, increased serum creatinine level, hirsutism
Methotrexate	Refractory cases	Liver toxicity, infections, contraindicated in pregnancy

Abbreviations: PO, by mouth; SC, subcutaneously; UDCA, ursodeoxycholic acid.

unknown. However, the presence of symptoms at presentation are a major factor determining PBC survival rates; asymptomatic PBC produces 10-year survival rates lower than those in the general population, but symptomatic PBC produces even lower survival rates.[68]

The diagnosis of PBC is generally based on the presence of 2 of the following 3 criteria: (1) biochemical evidence of cholestasis with increase of alkaline phosphatase activity over 6 months; (2) presence of serum AMA at significant titers; and (3) histologic nonsuppurative cholangitis and destruction of small or medium-sized bile ducts on biopsy specimen. The differential diagnosis includes a cholestatic drug reaction, biliary obstruction, sarcoidosis, AIH, and PSC (see **Table 4**).[69]

Association with Rheumatic Diseases

PBC is commonly associated with several extrahepatic autoimmune conditions. A recent monocentric study identified a co-occurrence in more than 60% of patients, with the most common being SjS in 30% of patients, followed by Raynaud phenomenon in 18%, and Hashimoto thyroiditis. PBC and SSc are associated in 6% of cases,[70] whereas a higher frequency of RA (up to 10%) has been reported since the 1970s.[71,72] PBC has also been reported in the presence of HLA-B27 enthesopathy.[73] Note that 5% of patients with PBC also have autoimmune cutaneous conditions.[74,75] Surprisingly, when extrahepatic autoimmune diseases co-occur with PBC, the cases tend to be less severe; severe SjS occurs in 10.5% of PBC cases, and the PBC disease is usually milder and at early stage (stage I–II at liver histology) in the presence of SjS.[76,77] The same observation has been made with PBC and SSc. PBC most commonly associates with limited cutaneous SSc (lSSc), and patients with PBC/SSc overlap have a slower rate of liver disease progression compared with matched patients with PBC alone.[78] Female sex is the only significant risk factor for having a second autoimmune condition,[70] whereas neither autoantibodies nor liver histology differ.

Autoantibodies

PBC is characterized serologically by the presence of AMA, which are highly specific for the disease. These antibodies are found in 90% to 95% of patients with PBC compared with less than 1% of healthy individuals.[79] Similar to other autoimmune diseases, AMA positivity arises years before the development of PBC,[9] and AMA are included in the internationally accepted criteria for PBC diagnosis (**Box 1**).[80] AMA are directed against components of the 2-oxoacid dehydrogenase (2-OADC) family of enzymes within the mitochondrial respiratory chain, most frequently the E2 and E3-binding protein (E3BP) components of the pyruvate dehydrogenase complex and the E2 components of the 2-oxoglutarate dehydrogenase and branched-chain

---

Box 1
Diagnostic criteria for primary biliary cholangitis. Diagnosis is made in the presence of at least 2 out of 3 of the criteria

Parameters

Increased ALP level greater than 2 times ULN or GGT greater than 5 times ULN

AMA positivity

Chronic granulomatous cholangitis at liver biopsy

Abbreviations: ALP, alkaline phosphatase; AMA, antimitochondrial antibodies; GGT, gamma-glutamyltransferase; ULN, upper limit of normal.

2-oxoacid dehydrogenase complexes.[81] All 3 antigen epitopes contain the motif DKA, with lipoic acid covalently bound to the lysine (K) residue.[78] ANA have been identified in 52% of patients, with the most specific patterns being nuclear rim and multiple nuclear dots, produced by antibodies directed against the nuclear membrane gp120 and nucleoporin 62, and the nuclear body sp100, sp140, and promyelocytic leukemia proteins, respectively (see **Table 1**).[82–85] ANA-positive patients are more frequently AMA negative, possibly because of the lack of a masking effect of these latter antibodies in such sera. Although anticentromere antibodies (ACA) are most specific for lSSc, found in up to 90% of patients, they are also detectable in 9% to 30% of patients with PBC. This prevalence exceeds that of the PBC/SSc overlap syndrome.[86,87] ACA recognize 6 centromere polypeptides belonging to the kinetochore proteins: CENP-A, CENP-B, CENP-C, CENP-D, CENP-E, CENP-F, with the major autoantigen being CENP-B. The clinical significance of ACA in PBC remains ill-defined because it is unclear whether ACA represents a preclinical marker of lSSc or a subclinical form of the disease. Moreover, ACA could simply represent an epiphenomenon of the immune dysregulation present in PBC.[78] Some clinicians have posited that because ACA can predict the development of SSc and because early SSc may be frequent in PBC, these may facilitate timely detection of complications, preventing disability and reducing the probability of liver transplant.[78,88] In any case, patients with PBC and positive ACA with SSc-related symptoms should be assessed for organ involvement and, in particular, assessment of pulmonary arterial hypertension by echocardiography should be considered in all patients with PBC/SSc. However, currently used tools to predict this pulmonary arterial hypertension (eg, the Detection of PAH/SSc score) have not been evaluated in patients with PBC.[89] Furthermore, although PBC/SSc seems to have a milder disease course, ACA-positive patients with PBC have a more severe bile duct injury and more frequently portal hypertension.[78] With regard to other autoantibodies,[90] anti-extractable nuclear antigens are positive in up to 40% of PBC cases, regardless of the extrahepatic autoimmunity,[70] with no effect on disease severity or progression. Anti-Ro/SSA are found in PBC/SjS overlap in 10% of cases[90]; anti-dsDNA in 22% of patients with PBC[90]; whereas anticardiolipin IgM is positive in 75% of PBC, advanced-stage disease.[91]

Therapy

PBC treatment is currently based on UDCA, which is the only approved drug. Its mechanism of action is incompletely understood and possibly dependent on the various phases of the disease.[5,92] During the early disease, short-term glucocorticoids might be effective; however, prolonged use raises safety concerns. Budesonide, because of its high first-pass metabolism, has minimum systemic adverse effects and, at 6 to 9 mg daily, has been shown to be superior to UDCA in terms of both histology and biochemical markers. Other immunosuppressants, such as methotrexate and azathioprine, have also been suggested and there is evidence supporting the use of the latter in PBC with AIH overlap syndrome.[93] The use of biologics targeting TNF-alpha has been reported in few cases of overlap syndromes with rheumatic diseases.[94,95] In the last years, improved understanding of PBC pathogenesis has led to the testing of new targeted therapies, especially those modulating the interleukin-17/23 axis. However, ustekinumab, a monoclonal antibody against the p40 subunit, showed only a very modest decrease in alkaline phosphatase level after 28 weeks of therapy, and was otherwise deemed ineffective.[19] Other therapies targeting T cells,[96] including those that bind Cytotoxic T-Lymphocyte Antigen (CTLA-4) (abatacept) or antagonize cluster differentiation (CD) 40 (FFP104), are under investigation.[69,97,98] Of note, the use CTLA-4 Ig in a PBC murine model prevents cholangitis manifestations (AMA production, intrahepatic T-cell infiltrates, and bile duct damage) and reduces disease severity in established murine disease.[99] When the disease has already progressed and bile has accumulated, obeticholic acid (OCA), an analogue of chenodeoxycholic acid with a much higher affinity to the farnesoid X receptor, has been shown to decrease bile synthesis, promote secretion, and induce liver regeneration in animal models. Furthermore, a recent phase III trial of OCA administered with UDCA or as monotherapy for 12 months showed decreases in alkaline phosphatase and total bilirubin levels compared with placebo.[97] Ultimately, UDCA represents the cornerstone therapy for PBC and doses ranging from 13 to 15 mg/kg lead to optimum bile enrichment, with 50% of patients normalizing their alkaline phosphatase levels. Other immunosuppressive treatments should be started only in combination with UDCA.

Liver transplant may be necessary for end-stage PBC, with survival rates of 92% and 85% at 1 and 5 years after transplant, respectively. Recurrence is common and seems to be influenced by immunosuppressives, whereas the use of UDCA for recurrence is safe and recommended.

PRIMARY SCLEROSING CHOLANGITIS

PSC is a progressive cholestatic liver disease of unknown cause presenting with chronic inflammatory features of the bile ducts of any size and associated with significant morbidity and mortality.[100,101] In contrast with PBC, PSC can affect all tracts of the biliary tree, including the extrahepatic bile ducts, visible with imaging modalities, and the small bile ducts, observed via liver histology. The prevalence of PSC is approximately 10 per 100000 in northern Europe[28] and in the United States, whereas it is far less common in southern Europe and Asia; recent data from Olmstead County, Minnesota, report a prevalence of 20.9 per 100 000 men and 6.3 per 100,000 women.[102] Different from PBC and AIH, PSC more frequently affects men, with a 2:1 male/female ratio.[102]

Clinical Features

PSC symptoms are generally nonspecific and include abdominal pain, jaundice, and fever in the case of bacterial cholangitis, whereas, at more advanced stages, symptoms include those typical of decompensated cirrhosis or neoplasia. Commonly, PSC is complicated by episodic bacterial cholangitis precipitated by biliary strictures. Discrete subgroups of patients manifest the small-duct or overlap syndrome variants. Because of the nonspecific symptoms, PSC is usually diagnosed during routine blood tests in otherwise healthy individuals or patients with IBD.[103] Testing characteristically reveals a biochemical cholestatic pattern, as represented by increased serum alkaline phosphatase and gamma-glutamyltransferase levels, although tests of liver function are normal until late stages. Imaging (particularly bile duct MRI or endoscopy) represents a useful diagnostic tool, because it may identify the classic strictured and dilated intrahepatic or extrahepatic bile ducts.[102] Performing a liver biopsy is generally not necessary for the diagnosis of PSC, except in the case of small-duct PSC, which requires histologic examination. The natural history of this form is fairly benign and only a minority (12%) of patients progress to classic PSC. The median timespan from diagnosis to liver-related death or liver transplant is 18 years, and the prognosis is influenced by the onset of cholangiocarcinoma (CCA). CCA is more common with chronic biliary inflammation and is difficult to distinguish from stricturing PSC.[101]

Association with Rheumatic Diseases

The association of PSC with IBD is well established. Nearly 70% of PSC cases also show findings of IBD,[104] frequently in mild asymptomatic forms, whereas 7% of patients with IBD have PSC.[105] Liver abnormalities are more frequently found in psoriatic patients, and this is typically attributed to nonalcoholic or alcoholic fatty liver.[106] However, in generalized pustular psoriasis, a less common form of psoriasis associated with extracutaneous manifestations, evidence for biliary involvement has been suggested, and neutrophilic cholangitis has been observed on liver biopsy, whereas magnetic resonance cholangiopancreatography showed features similar to those observed in PSC.[107]

Autoantibodies

In contrast with other autoimmune liver diseases, autoantibodies are of limited use in the diagnosis of PSC because of low sensitivity and specificity; for example, only a limited percentage of patients (33%) have positive pANCA.[108,109] Only for PSC forms overlapping with AIH is serum ANA typically detected.

Therapy

The treatment of PSC is largely an unmet need and currently includes medical and endoscopic measures, short of liver transplant.[110,111] UDCA has been investigated in several clinical trials, with conflicting results. Overall, the available evidence suggests that UDCA does not produce a substantial change in the course of PSC, despite remaining the most prescribed drug. However, it seems that high-dose UDCA (20 mg/kg/d) or norUDCA, a side chain–shortened homologue of UDCA, may reduce biochemical indices of cholestasis[112] and the rate of progression, and might prevent the development of colon cancer (particularly in patients with UC/PSC overlap). Based on these inconclusive data, the use of UDCA in PSC varies widely, reflecting regional practice trends rather than science. Endoscopic interventions are indicated to treat complicated PSC through the dilation of short-segment and long-segment stenosis of the common bile duct and short-segment stenosis of the hepatic ducts near to the bifurcation. The treatment can be repeated over time once restenosis ensues and resulting survival rates are higher compared with patients not treated endoscopically. Biologics, mainly anti-TNF, have been used in PSC with concomitant IBD or rheumatic diseases with improvement in laboratory measurements,[113,114] but patients with PSC are generally excluded from IBD clinical trials, thus preventing firm conclusions regarding efficacy. In addition, PSC represents an important indication for liver transplant because patients are younger than their counterparts with PBC. Recurrence of disease occurs in 20% to 40% of transplanted patients during prolonged follow-up. The ability of UDCA to prolong survival after disease recurrence remains a point of contention.

OVERLAP SYNDROMES

Autoimmune liver diseases, similarly to rheumatic disease, may overlap and present with both hepatocellular and cholangiocellular patterns according to biochemical, histologic, and imaging-based analysis. When left without treatment, these patients show a more progressive course toward liver cirrhosis and failure. AIH-PBC overlap syndrome is found in 10% of adults with AIH whereas AIH-PSC overlap syndrome affects 6% to 8% of children, adolescents, and young adults with AIH; PBC-PSC overlap syndrome is exceptionally rare (**Table 5**). Besides overlaps, transitions are also possible in rare cases from PBC to AIH, AIH to PBC, or AIH to PSC.[115]

AIH may have an atypical presentation with increased serum alkaline phosphatase level, AMA positivity, histologic features of bile duct injury/loss, or cholangiographic findings of focal biliary strictures and dilatations. These manifestations characterize

Table 5
Diagnostic features of overlap syndromes

Overlap Syndrome	Laboratory Features	Histologic Findings
AIH/PBC	ANA or SMA Hypergammaglobulinemia Serum IgG level increased Marked serum AST/ALT abnormalities ALP or GGT > ULN AMA positive	Interface hepatitis Lymphocytic portal infiltrate Portal plasma cells Destructive cholangitis

AIH/PBC (Paris criteria)	AIH features (2 of 3):
	  Serum ALT ≥5-fold ULN
	  Serum IgG ≥2-fold ULN or SMA
	   present
	  Interface hepatitis
	PBC features (2 of 3):
	  Serum ALP ≥2-fold ULN or GGT
	   ≥5-fold ULN
	  AMA positive
	  Florid duct lesions
		Interface hepatitis (moderate to
		  severe)
		Destructive cholangitis

AIH/PSC	ANA or SMA
	Hypergammaglobulinemia
	Serum IgG level increased
	Marked serum AST/ALT
	  abnormalities
	Focal biliary strictures and
	  dilatations
		Lymphocytic portal infiltrate
		Ductular proliferation
		Periductular fibrosis
		Portal edema
		Cholate stasis
		Fibrous obliterative cholangitis
		  (rare)
		Ductopenia
		Increased stainable hepatic copper
		  concentration

AIH and undefined cholestatic syndrome	ANA or SMA
	Hypergammaglobulinemia
	Serum IgG level increased
	Marked serum AST/ALT
	  abnormalities
	AMA negative
	No biliary strictures or dilatations
		Interface hepatitis plus at least:
		  Destructive cholangitis
		  Periductular fibrosis
		  Ductopenia
		  Portal edema

Abbreviation: ALP, alkaline phosphatase.

the overlap syndromes. The clues to an overlap syndrome consist of (1) serum alkaline phosphatase level more than 2-fold the upper limit of normal (ULN) at presentation, which is present in only 20% of patients with AIH; (2) serum GGT level greater than ULN unimproved or worsened during therapy; (3) AMA positivity; (4) histologic findings of bile duct injury or loss; (5) concurrent IBD; (6) corticosteroid treatment failure or incomplete response.[115]

Overlap features of PBC usually refer to simultaneous AIH in patients who have a diagnosis of AMA-positive PBC and not to patients with AIH who have coincidental AMA. AMA occur in about 5% of patients with AIH in the absence of other biliary features (serologic overlap), but may disappear or persist for decades without an evolution into PBC. Approximately 4% of PBC cases have simultaneous features of AIH. There are 2 different scoring systems that have been used to evaluate patients with PBC for simultaneous evidence of overlapping AIH: (1) the IAIH-G score; (2) looking for the presence of 2 of (i) ALT activity 5 times ULN, (ii) IgG level 2 times ULN and/or positive anti-SMA antibody, and overlap by (iii) liver biopsy with moderate or severe periportal or periseptal inflammation. A PBC/AIH overlap syndrome may also refer to patients with sequential PBC followed by AIH, a condition occurring in 2.4% of cases. In these cases, the diagnosis of PBC with positive AMA occurs first and initially responds biochemically to UDCA therapy; subsequently, these patients present with clinical features of AIH, lose their AMA seropositivity, show liver histology more typical of AIH, and respond to immunosuppressive therapy.

The term autoimmune cholangitis was first coined to indicate AMA-negative PBC, possibly with serum ANA. More recently, a broader concept has emerged that includes (1) serum ANA and/or SMA positivity and/or hypergammaglobulinemia; (2) serum AMA negativity by immunofluorescence; (3) biochemical and/or histologic features of cholestatic and hepatocellular injury; and (4) exclusion of chronic viral, metabolic, or toxic liver disease. This definition possibly subsumes PBC with atypical presentation, small-duct PSC, idiopathic adulthood ductopenia, AIH with bile duct damage, concurrent AIH and small-duct PSC, and various transitional stages of the classic diseases. Consensus is still wanting on this issue, and standardization of diagnostic criteria for overlap syndromes is impeded by their uncommon occurrence in the setting of rare diseases.

OSTEOMETABOLIC CONSEQUENCES OF CHRONIC AUTOIMMUNE LIVER DISEASE

Advancements in the management of autoimmune liver diseases and cirrhosis complications have increased survival rates. However, longer survival rates, compounded by an aging population, have increased the risk of complications such as osteoporosis. Osteoporosis is associated with increased risk of fracture, which is 2-fold higher in cirrhotic patients regardless of the liver disease cause and persists for years after liver transplant.[116–119] Moreover, patients receiving glucocorticoids for AIH have an additional decrease in their bone mass.

According to the World Health Organization definition, osteoporosis is diagnosed when bone density is less than 2.5 standard deviations less than the peak value obtained from normal adults and adjusted for gender (T score).[120] This definition is limited in that the threshold was established from studies of postmenopausal white women, rather than for patients with liver diseases.[117] Therefore, some investigators favor the term hepatic osteodystrophy, although this term also includes osteomalacia.[121]

The mechanisms of cirrhosis-related osteoporosis are not fully understood, but it is generally recognized that the association between liver and bone diseases occurs because of an imbalance of bone turnover, which depends on the osteoblastic and osteoclastic activity.[122] In PBC, although the exact mechanism is also not completely understood, there is evidence that hormone balance, genetics, and cholestasis may contribute to determine bone structure and density changes. There has been conflicting evidence as to whether PBC-related osteoporosis results from diminished bone formation, which is a low-turnover state, or from increased bone resorption, which is a high-turnover state. However, recent data suggest that bone formation is the cause. Cirrhosis is associated with the reduced levels of specific growth factors, such as insulinlike growth factor 1, which impairs osteoblast function and bone formation; severe cholestasis can allow buildup of lithocholic acid, which inhibits osteoblast activity and can interfere with genetic regulation of bone formation.[23]

The prevalence of osteoporosis in cirrhotic patients ranges from 12% to 70% according to the diagnostic modality and the liver disease cause, with cholestatic diseases having a higher prevalence (20%–44%, even without an established diagnosis of cirrhosis). Moreover, fracture rates are increased in cholestatic diseases, varying from 13% to 22% according to the degree of liver function.[120]

Screening for osteoporosis is an important part of liver diseases management, and the guidelines indicate that patients with cirrhosis and PBC should be screened by an initial dual-energy x-ray absorptiometry (DXA) examination.[121] If initial results are normal, the DXA examination should be repeated every 1 to 3 years to assess significant bone loss, depending on the presence of additional risk factors (body mass index <19 kg/m^2, heavy alcohol use, tobacco use, early menopause [age <45 years], glucocorticoid use >3 months, or family history of bone fragility fractures).[121] In addition, BMD should be measured before liver transplant.

Laboratory test are also helpful for evaluating bone metabolism, and include serum calcium, 25-hydroxyvitamin D, phosphorus, osteocalcin, procollagen I carboxyterminal peptide, and parathyroid hormone (PTH), as well as urinary amino telopeptides of collagen I and urinary calcium. Routine monitoring of calcium, phosphorus, 25-hydroxyvitamin D, and PTH should be performed every 1 to 2 years.[123]

The treatment of osteoporosis is based on results obtained from trials assessing postmenopausal women, and few studies have included patients with liver diseases. Educational strategies include elimination of modifiable risk factors, such as smoking and alcohol consumption. Calcium and vitamin D supplementation is part of osteoporosis treatment. The total calcium intake should achieve a daily ingestion of 1.0 to 1.5 g, preferably from diet to facilitate patients' compliance.[120] Oral cholecalciferol (vitamin D$_3$) can be prescribed at 1000 to 4000 IU/d or ergocalciferol (vitamin D$_2$) at 50,000 IU/mo. Given that calcitriol (1,25-dihydroxycholecalciferol or 1,25-dihydroxyvitamin D$_3$) is the final active vitamin D metabolite, it may represent a better treatment of liver disease. Calcitriol is usually prescribed as a daily oral dose of 800 IU but can also be taken at a weekly dose of 5000 IU.[120] In PBC, calcium and vitamin D supplementation alone was inferior to hormonal replacement therapy in improving BMD.[124,125] However, testing for vitamin D deficiency in cholestatic patients is useful to allow appropriate supplementation, particularly in those taking cholestyramine, because this impairs vitamin D absorption.[116]

Bisphosphonates represent the treatment of choice for osteoporosis in cirrhotic patients, because they attach to the bone surface and prevent resorption.[126] However, the threshold of intervention in patients with liver disease may be lower than in the general population because PBC T scores less than -1.5 are associated with a significant risk for vertebral fractures.[127] A recent randomized controlled trial for osteoporosis therapy in patients with PBC showed that both monthly ibandronic acid and weekly alendronic acid improve bone mass and are comparable in safety, although adherence is higher with the monthly regimen.[128] Moreover, bisphosphonates and teriparatide reduce the risk of vertebral fractures in chronically glucocorticoid-treated patients.[129,130] Hormone replacement therapy does not show any osteoporosis benefit for patients with PBC, but its use is no longer contraindicated in chronic cholestasis.[131] Ultimately, treating PBC with UDCA may also have beneficial effects on the bone, because UDCA may increase osteoblast differentiation and mineralization, and may neutralize the detrimental effects of lithocholic acid, bilirubin, and sera from jaundiced patients on osteoblastic cells.[132]

SUMMARY

The coexistence of liver and rheumatic diseases represents an ideal example of the need for an interdisciplinary approach to individualize treatments. Patients with autoimmune liver diseases may be undertreated with antirheumatic drugs for liver safety concerns (as in the case of methotrexate), whereas liver test changes may raise unnecessary concerns. Furthermore, new biologics may be beneficial for more than

1 condition, although insufficient data exist from the hepatology perspective. In addition, the rapid deterioration of bone health associated with chronic liver diseases is an obvious area of collaboration between gastroenterology and rheumatology. With the current focus on personalized medicine, the coexistence of liver autoimmunity and rheumatic disease is an ideal area to develop and investigate the benefits of shared clinical practice.

REFERENCES

1. Cowling DC, Mackay IR, Taft LI. Lupoid hepatitis. Lancet 1956;271(6957): 1323–6.
2. Adiga A, Nugent K. Lupus hepatitis and autoimmune hepatitis (lupoid hepatitis). Am J Med Sci 2017;353(4):329–35.
3. Doherty DG. Immunity, tolerance and autoimmunity in the liver: a comprehensive review. J Autoimmun 2016;66:60–75.
4. Liberal R, Selmi C, Gershwin ME. Diego and Giorgina Vergani: the two hearts of translational autoimmunity. J Autoimmun 2016;66:1–6.
5. Molinaro A, Marschall HU. Why doesn't primary biliary cholangitis respond to immunosuppressive medications? Curr Hepatol Rep 2017;16(2):119–23.
6. Gatselis NK, Zachou K, Lygoura V, et al. Geoepidemiology, clinical manifestations and outcome of primary biliary cholangitis in Greece. Eur J Intern Med 2017;42:81–8.
7. Kim BH, Choi HY, Ki M, et al. Population-based prevalence, incidence, and disease burden of autoimmune hepatitis in South Korea. PLoS One 2017;12(8): e0182391.
8. Ji J, Sundquist J, Sundquist K. Gender-specific incidence of autoimmune diseases from national registers. J Autoimmun 2016;69:102–6.
9. Ma WT, Chang C, Gershwin ME, et al. Development of autoantibodies precedes clinical manifestations of autoimmune diseases: a comprehensive review. J Autoimmun 2017;83:95–112.
10. Toh BH. Diagnostic autoantibodies for autoimmune liver diseases. Clin Transl Immunology 2017;6(5):e139.
11. Watad A, Azrielant S, Bragazzi NL, et al. Seasonality and autoimmune diseases: the contribution of the four seasons to the mosaic of autoimmunity. J Autoimmun 2017;82:13–30.
12. Murray-Lyon IM, Thompson RP, Ansell ID, et al. Scleroderma and primary biliary cirrhosis. Br Med J 1970;3(5717):258–9.
13. Clarke AK, Galbraith RM, Hamilton EB, et al. Rheumatic disorders in primary biliary cirrhosis. Ann Rheum Dis 1978;37(1):42–7.
14. Morgan MY. Primary biliary cirrhosis, scleroderma and keratoconjunctivitis sicca. Proc R Soc Med 1973;66(11):1112.
15. Selmi C, Meroni PL, Gershwin ME. Primary biliary cirrhosis and Sjogren's syndrome: autoimmune epithelitis. J Autoimmun 2012;39(1–2):34–42.
16. Sirotti S, Generali E, Ceribelli A, et al. Personalized medicine in rheumatology: the paradigm of serum autoantibodies. Auto Immun Highlights 2017;8(1):10.
17. Selmi C, Bowlus CL, Gershwin ME, et al. Primary biliary cirrhosis. Lancet 2011; 377(9777):1600–9.
18. Cropley A, Weltman M. The use of immunosuppression in autoimmune hepatitis: a current literature review. Clin Mol Hepatol 2017;23(1):22–6.

19. Hirschfield GM, Gershwin ME, Strauss R, et al. Ustekinumab for patients with primary biliary cholangitis who have an inadequate response to ursodeoxycholic acid: a proof-of-concept study. Hepatology 2016;64(1):189–99.

20. Chimenti MS, Talamonti M, Novelli L, et al. Long-term ustekinumab therapy of psoriasis in patients with coexisting rheumatoid arthritis and Sjogren syndrome. Report of two cases and review of literature. J Dermatol Case Rep 2015;9(3): 71–5.

21. Card TR, Langan SM, Chu TP. Extra-gastrointestinal manifestations of inflammatory bowel disease may be less common than previously reported. Dig Dis Sci 2016;61(9):2619–26.

22. Whittier X, Saag KG. Glucocorticoid-induced osteoporosis. Rheum Dis Clin North Am 2016;42(1):177–89, x.

23. Glass LM, Su GL. Metabolic bone disease in primary biliary cirrhosis. Gastroenterol Clin North Am 2016;45(2):333–43.

24. Imam MH, Talwalkar JA, Lindor KD. Clinical management of autoimmune biliary diseases. J Autoimmun 2013;46:88–96.

25. Liberal R, Krawitt EL, Vierling JM, et al. Cutting edge issues in autoimmune hepatitis. J Autoimmun 2016;75:6–19.

26. Hardtke-Wolenski M, Dywicki J, Fischer K, et al. The influence of genetic predisposition and autoimmune hepatitis inducing antigens in disease development. J Autoimmun 2017;78:39–45.

27. Krawitt EL. Autoimmune hepatitis. N Engl J Med 2006;354(1):54–66.

28. Jepsen P, Gronbaek L, Vilstrup H. Worldwide incidence of autoimmune liver disease. Dig Dis 2015;33(Suppl 2):2–12.

29. Floreani A, Liberal R, Vergani D, et al. Autoimmune hepatitis: contrasts and comparisons in children and adults - a comprehensive review. J Autoimmun 2013; 46:7–16.

30. Wang Q, Yang F, Miao Q, et al. The clinical phenotypes of autoimmune hepatitis: a comprehensive review. J Autoimmun 2016;66:98–107.

31. Liberal R, Grant CR, Mieli-Vergani G, et al. Autoimmune hepatitis: a comprehensive review. J Autoimmun 2013;41:126–39.

32. Webb GJ, Hirschfield GM. Using GWAS to identify genetic predisposition in hepatic autoimmunity. J Autoimmun 2016;66:25–39.

33. Alvarez F, Berg PA, Bianchi FB, et al. International Autoimmune Hepatitis Group report: review of criteria for diagnosis of autoimmune hepatitis. J Hepatol 1999; 31(5):929–38.

34. Manns MP, Czaja AJ, Gorham JD, et al. Diagnosis and management of autoimmune hepatitis. Hepatology 2010;51(6):2193–213.

35. Czaja AJ. Performance parameters of the diagnostic scoring systems for autoimmune hepatitis. Hepatology 2008;48(5):1540–8.

36. Wong GW, Heneghan MA. Association of extrahepatic manifestations with autoimmune hepatitis. Dig Dis 2015;33(Suppl 2):25–35.

37. van Gerven NM, Verwer BJ, Witte BI, et al. Epidemiology and clinical characteristics of autoimmune hepatitis in the Netherlands. Scand J Gastroenterol 2014; 49(10):1245–54.

38. Muratori P, Lenzi M, Cassani F, et al. Diagnostic approach to autoimmune hepatitis. Expert Rev Clin Immunol 2017;13(8):769–79.

39. Czaja AJ. Autoimmune liver disease and rheumatic manifestations. Curr Opin Rheumatol 2007;19(1):74–80.

40. Borman MA, Urbanski S, Swain MG. Anti-TNF-induced autoimmune hepatitis. J Hepatol 2014;61(1):169–70.

41. French JB, Bonacini M, Ghabril M, et al. Hepatotoxicity associated with the use of anti-TNF-alpha agents. Drug Saf 2016;39(3):199–208.
42. Rodrigues S, Lopes S, Magro F, et al. Autoimmune hepatitis and anti-tumor necrosis factor alpha therapy: a single center report of 8 cases. World J Gastroenterol 2015;21(24):7584–8.
43. Sebode M, Hartl J, Vergani D, et al, International Autoimmune Hepatitis Group (IAIHG). Autoimmune hepatitis: from current knowledge and clinical practice to future research agenda. Liver Int 2017. [Epub ahead of print].
44. Liberal R, Mieli-Vergani G, Vergani D. Clinical significance of autoantibodies in autoimmune hepatitis. J Autoimmun 2013;46:17–24.
45. Cancado EL, Abrantes-Lemos CP, Terrabuio DR. The importance of autoantibody detection in autoimmune hepatitis. Front Immunol 2015;6:222.
46. Muratori L, Deleonardi G, Lalanne C, et al. Autoantibodies in autoimmune hepatitis. Dig Dis 2015;33(Suppl 2):65–9.
47. Selmi C, Ceribelli A, Generali E, et al. Serum antinuclear and extractable nuclear antigen antibody prevalence and associated morbidity and mortality in the general population over 15 years. Autoimmun Rev 2016;15(2):162–6.
48. Mullin S, Rabah R, Malas S, et al. Autoimmune hepatitis type 2 associated with positive antimitochondrial antibodies: an overlap syndrome? Clin Pediatr (Phila) 2016;55(5):479–82.
49. Liaskos C, Rigopoulou E, Zachou K, et al. Prevalence and clinical significance of anticardiolipin antibodies in patients with type 1 autoimmune hepatitis. J Autoimmun 2005;24(3):251–60.
50. Linares P, Vivas S, Olcoz JL. Autoimmune hepatitis associated with the antiphospholipid syndrome and ulcerative colitis. Eur J Intern Med 2005;16(5):376.
51. Czaja AJ. Autoantibodies as prognostic markers in autoimmune liver disease. Dig Dis Sci 2010;55(8):2144–61.
52. Czaja AJ, Ming C, Shirai M, et al. Frequency and significance of antibodies to histones in autoimmune hepatitis. J Hepatol 1995;23(1):32–8.
53. Czaja AJ, Morshed SA, Parveen S, et al. Antibodies to single-stranded and double-stranded DNA in antinuclear antibody-positive type 1-autoimmune hepatitis. Hepatology 1997;26(3):567–72.
54. Czaja AJ. Evolving paradigm of treatment for autoimmune hepatitis. Expert Rev Clin Immunol 2017;13(8):781–98.
55. Haridy J, Nicoll A, Sood S. Methotrexate therapy for autoimmune hepatitis. Clin Gastroenterol Hepatol 2017 [pii:S1542-3565(17)30821-2].
56. Efe C, Hagstrom H, Ytting H, et al. Efficacy and safety of mycophenolate mofetil and tacrolimus as second-line therapy for patients with autoimmune hepatitis. Clin Gastroenterol Hepatol 2017 [pii:S1542-3565(17)30685-7].
57. Weiler-Normann C, Schramm C, Quaas A, et al. Infliximab as a rescue treatment in difficult-to-treat autoimmune hepatitis. J Hepatol 2013;58(3):529–34.
58. Burak KW, Swain MG, Santodomingo-Garzon T, et al. Rituximab for the treatment of patients with autoimmune hepatitis who are refractory or intolerant to standard therapy. Can J Gastroenterol 2013;27(5):273–80.
59. Than NN, Jeffery HC, Oo YH. Autoimmune hepatitis: progress from global immunosuppression to personalised regulatory T cell therapy. Can J Gastroenterol Hepatol 2016;2016:7181685.
60. Schramm C, Bubenheim M, Adam R, et al. Primary liver transplantation for autoimmune hepatitis: a comparative analysis of the European Liver Transplant Registry. Liver Transpl 2010;16(4):461–9.

61. Cho CW, Kwon CHD, Kim JM, et al. Comparative analysis of the clinical outcomes of liver transplantation for probable and definite auto-immune hepatitis by international diagnostic scoring criteria. Transplant Proc 2017;49(5):1126–8.

62. Neuberger J. An update on liver transplantation: a critical review. J Autoimmun 2016;66:51–9.

63. Kerkar N, Yanni G. 'De novo' and 'recurrent' autoimmune hepatitis after liver transplantation: a comprehensive review. J Autoimmun 2016;66:17–24.

64. Shuai Z, Wang J, Badamagunta M, et al. The fingerprint of antimitochondrial antibodies and the etiology of primary biliary cholangitis. Hepatology 2017;65(5):1670–82.

65. Webb GJ, Siminovitch KA, Hirschfield GM. The immunogenetics of primary biliary cirrhosis: a comprehensive review. J Autoimmun 2015;64:42–52.

66. Lleo A, Jepsen P, Morenghi E, et al. Evolving trends in female to male incidence and male mortality of primary biliary cholangitis. Sci Rep 2016;6:25906.

67. Beuers U, Gershwin ME, Gish RG, et al. Changing nomenclature for PBC: from 'cirrhosis' to 'cholangitis'. Clin Gastroenterol Hepatol 2015;13(11):1867–9.

68. Floreani A, Tanaka A, Bowlus C, et al. Geoepidemiology and changing mortality in primary biliary cholangitis. J Gastroenterol 2017;52(6):655–62.

69. Invernizzi P, Floreani A, Carbone M, et al. Primary biliary cholangitis: advances in management and treatment of the disease. Dig Liver Dis 2017;49(8):841–6.

70. Floreani A, Franceschet I, Cazzagon N, et al. Extrahepatic autoimmune conditions associated with primary biliary cirrhosis. Clin Rev Allergy Immunol 2015;48(2–3):192–7.

71. Mills P, MacSween RN, Watkinson G. Arthritis and primary biliary cirrhosis. Br Med J 1977;2(6096):1224.

72. Parikh-Patel A, Gold E, Mackay IR, et al. The geoepidemiology of primary biliary cirrhosis: contrasts and comparisons with the spectrum of autoimmune diseases. Clin Immunol 1999;91(2):206–18.

73. Kung YY, Tsai CY, Tsai YY, et al. Enthesopathy in a case of primary biliary cirrhosis with positive HLA-B27. Clin Exp Rheumatol 1997;15(6):708–9.

74. Philips C, Paramaguru R, Indiran DA, et al. Dermatitis herpetiformis as the initial presentation of primary biliary cholangitis in a male with gluten sensitivity. Cureus 2017;9(5):e1247.

75. Terziroli Beretta-Piccoli B, Guillod C, Marsteller I, et al. Primary biliary cholangitis associated with skin disorders: a case report and review of the literature. Arch Immunol Ther Exp (Warsz) 2017;65(4):299–309.

76. Tsianos EV, Hoofnagle JH, Fox PC, et al. Sjogren's syndrome in patients with primary biliary cirrhosis. Hepatology 1990;11(5):730–4.

77. Uddenfeldt P, Danielsson A, Forssell A, et al. Features of Sjogren's syndrome in patients with primary biliary cirrhosis. J Intern Med 1991;230(5):443–8.

78. Liberal R, Grant CR, Sakkas L, et al. Diagnostic and clinical significance of anti-centromere antibodies in primary biliary cirrhosis. Clin Res Hepatol Gastroenterol 2013;37(6):572–85.

79. Gershwin ME, Mackay IR, Sturgess A, et al. Identification and specificity of a cDNA encoding the 70 kd mitochondrial antigen recognized in primary biliary cirrhosis. J Immunol 1987;138(10):3525–31.

80. Bowlus CL, Gershwin ME. The diagnosis of primary biliary cirrhosis. Autoimmun Rev 2014;13(4–5):441–4.

81. Leung PS, Wang J, Naiyanetr P, et al. Environment and primary biliary cirrhosis: electrophilic drugs and the induction of AMA. J Autoimmun 2013;41:79–86.

82. Chantran Y, Ballot E, Johanet C. Autoantibodies in primary biliary cirrhosis: anti-mitochondrial autoantibodies. Clin Res Hepatol Gastroenterol 2013;37(4):431–3.
83. Liu H, Norman GL, Shums Z, et al. PBC screen: an IgG/IgA dual isotype ELISA detecting multiple mitochondrial and nuclear autoantibodies specific for primary biliary cirrhosis. J Autoimmun 2010;35(4):436–42.
84. Rigopoulou EI, Davies ET, Bogdanos DP, et al. Antimitochondrial antibodies of immunoglobulin G3 subclass are associated with a more severe disease course in primary biliary cirrhosis. Liver Int 2007;27(9):1226–31.
85. Worman HJ, Courvalin JC. Antinuclear antibodies specific for primary biliary cirrhosis. Autoimmun Rev 2003;2(4):211–7.
86. Powell FC, Winkelmann RK, Venencie-Lemarchand F, et al. The anticentromere antibody: disease specificity and clinical significance. Mayo Clin Proc 1984; 59(10):700–6.
87. Chan HL, Lee YS, Hong HS, et al. Anticentromere antibodies (ACA): clinical distribution and disease specificity. Clin Exp Dermatol 1994;19(4):298–302.
88. Tovoli F, Granito A, Giampaolo L, et al. Nailfold capillaroscopy in primary biliary cirrhosis: a useful tool for the early diagnosis of scleroderma. J Gastrointestin Liver Dis 2014;23(1):39–43.
89. Guillen-Del Castillo A, Callejas-Moraga EL, Garcia G, et al. High sensitivity and negative predictive value of the DETECT algorithm for an early diagnosis of pulmonary arterial hypertension in systemic sclerosis: application in a single center. Arthritis Res Ther 2017;19(1):135.
90. Agmon-Levin N, Shapira Y, Selmi C, et al. A comprehensive evaluation of serum autoantibodies in primary biliary cirrhosis. J Autoimmun 2010;34(1):55–8.
91. von Landenberg P, Baumgartner M, Schoelmerich J, et al. Clinical relevance of antiphospholipid antibodies in primary biliary cirrhosis. Ann N Y Acad Sci 2005; 1051:20–8.
92. Floreani A, Mangini C. Primary biliary cholangitis: old and novel therapy. Eur J Intern Med 2017 [pii:S0953-6205(17)30264-9].
93. Bonis PA, Kaplan MM. Low-dose methotrexate in primary biliary cirrhosis. Gastroenterology 1999;117(6):1510–3.
94. Selmi C, Generali E, Cantarini L. Tumor necrosis factor-alpha at the crossroad between rheumatoid arthritis and autoimmune cholangitis. Isr Med Assoc J 2015;17(2):112–3.
95. Del Ross T, Ruffatti A, Floreani A, et al. The efficacy of adalimumab in psoriatic arthritis concomitant to overlapping primary biliary cholangitis and primary sclerosing cholangitis: a case report. BMC Musculoskelet Disord 2016;17(1):485.
96. Wang YH, Yang W, Yang JB, et al. Systems biologic analysis of T regulatory cells genetic pathways in murine primary biliary cirrhosis. J Autoimmun 2015;59: 26–37.
97. Mousa HS, Carbone M, Malinverno F, et al. Novel therapeutics for primary biliary cholangitis: toward a disease-stage-based approach. Autoimmun Rev 2016; 15(9):870–6.
98. Yang XC, Fujino M, Cai SJ, et al. Genetic polymorphisms of cytotoxic T-lymphocyte antigen 4 in primary biliary cholangitis: a meta-analysis. J Immunol Res 2017;2017:5295164.
99. Dhirapong A, Yang GX, Nadler S, et al. Therapeutic effect of cytotoxic T lymphocyte antigen 4/immunoglobulin on a murine model of primary biliary cirrhosis. Hepatology 2013;57(2):708–15.
100. Sarkar S, Bowlus CL. Primary sclerosing cholangitis: multiple phenotypes, multiple approaches. Clin Liver Dis 2016;20(1):67–77.

101. Gidwaney NG, Pawa S, Das KM. Pathogenesis and clinical spectrum of primary sclerosing cholangitis. World J Gastroenterol 2017;23(14):2459–69.
102. Bowlus CL. Cutting edge issues in primary sclerosing cholangitis. Clin Rev Allergy Immunol 2011;41(2):139–50.
103. Yimam KK, Bowlus CL. Diagnosis and classification of primary sclerosing cholangitis. Autoimmun Rev 2014;13(4–5):445–50.
104. Palmela C, Peerani F, Castaneda D, et al. Inflammatory bowel disease and primary sclerosing cholangitis: a review of the phenotype and associated specific features. Gut Liver 2017. [Epub ahead of print].
105. Vavricka SR, Schoepfer A, Scharl M, et al. Extraintestinal manifestations of inflammatory bowel disease. Inflamm Bowel Dis 2015;21(8):1982–92.
106. Xu X, Su L, Gao Y, et al. The prevalence of nonalcoholic fatty liver disease and related metabolic comorbidities was associated with age at onset of moderate to severe plaque psoriasis: a cross-sectional study. PLoS One 2017;12(1): e0169952.
107. Viguier M, Allez M, Zagdanski AM, et al. High frequency of cholestasis in generalized pustular psoriasis: evidence for neutrophilic involvement of the biliary tract. Hepatology 2004;40(2):452–8.
108. Seibold F, Slametschka D, Gregor M, et al. Neutrophil autoantibodies: a genetic marker in primary sclerosing cholangitis and ulcerative colitis. Gastroenterology 1994;107(2):532–6.
109. Metcalf JV, Mitchison HC, Palmer JM, et al. Natural history of early primary biliary cirrhosis. Lancet 1996;348(9039):1399–402.
110. Lazaridis KN, LaRusso NF. Primary sclerosing cholangitis. N Engl J Med 2016; 375(25):2501–2.
111. Saffioti F, Gurusamy KS, Hawkins N, et al. Pharmacological interventions for primary sclerosing cholangitis: an attempted network meta-analysis. Cochrane Database Syst Rev 2017;(3):CD011343.
112. Fickert P, Hirschfield GM, Denk G, et al. norUrsodeoxycholic acid improves cholestasis in primary sclerosing cholangitis. J Hepatol 2017;67(3):549–58.
113. Franceschet I, Cazzagon N, Del Ross T, et al. Primary sclerosing cholangitis associated with inflammatory bowel disease: an observational study in a southern Europe population focusing on new therapeutic options. Eur J Gastroenterol Hepatol 2016;28(5):508–13.
114. Olmedo Martin RV, Amo Trillo V, Gonzalez Grande R, et al. Efficacy and safety of vedolizumab as a treatment option for moderate to severe refractory ulcerative colitis in two patients after liver transplant due to primary sclerosing cholangitis. Rev Esp Enferm Dig 2017;109(9):659–62.
115. Czaja AJ, Carpenter HA. Autoimmune hepatitis overlap syndromes and liver pathology. Gastroenterol Clin North Am 2017;46(2):345–64.
116. Guanabens N, Pares A. Management of osteoporosis in liver disease. Clin Res Hepatol Gastroenterol 2011;35(6–7):438–45.
117. Luxon BA. Bone disorders in chronic liver diseases. Curr Gastroenterol Rep 2011;13(1):40–8.
118. Giannini S, Nobile M, Ciuffreda M, et al. Long-term persistence of low bone density in orthotopic liver transplantation. Osteoporos Int 2000;11(5):417–24.
119. Zhao J, Li W, Cao J, et al. Association between primary biliary cholangitis and fracture: a meta-analysis. Clin Res Hepatol Gastroenterol 2017 [pii:S2210-7401(17) 30139-0].
120. Santos LA, Romeiro FG. Diagnosis and management of cirrhosis-related osteoporosis. Biomed Res Int 2016;2016:1423462.

121. Leslie WD, Bernstein CN, Leboff MS, American Gastroenterological Association Clinical Practice Committee. AGA technical review on osteoporosis in hepatic disorders. Gastroenterology 2003;125(3):941–66.
122. Lopez-Larramona G, Lucendo AJ, Gonzalez-Castillo S, et al. Hepatic osteodystrophy: an important matter for consideration in chronic liver disease. World J Hepatol 2011;3(12):300–7.
123. Pares A, Guanabens N. Treatment of bone disorders in liver disease. J Hepatol 2006;45(3):445–53.
124. Pereira SP, O'Donohue J, Moniz C, et al. Transdermal hormone replacement therapy improves vertebral bone density in primary biliary cirrhosis: results of a 1-year controlled trial. Aliment Pharmacol Ther 2004;19(5):563–70.
125. Crippin JS, Jorgensen RA, Dickson ER, et al. Hepatic osteodystrophy in primary biliary cirrhosis: effects of medical treatment. Am J Gastroenterol 1994;89(1): 47–50.
126. Yurci A, Kalkan AO, Ozbakir O, et al. Efficacy of different therapeutic regimens on hepatic osteodystrophy in chronic viral liver disease. Eur J Gastroenterol Hepatol 2011;23(12):1206–12.
127. Guanabens N, Cerda D, Monegal A, et al. Low bone mass and severity of cholestasis affect fracture risk in patients with primary biliary cirrhosis. Gastroenterology 2010;138(7):2348–56.
128. Guanabens N, Monegal A, Cerda D, et al. Randomized trial comparing monthly ibandronate and weekly alendronate for osteoporosis in patients with primary biliary cirrhosis. Hepatology 2013;58(6):2070–8.
129. Allen CS, Yeung JH, Vandermeer B, et al. Bisphosphonates for steroid-induced osteoporosis. Cochrane Database Syst Rev 2016;(10):CD001347.
130. Kan SL, Yuan ZF, Li Y, et al. Alendronate prevents glucocorticoid-induced osteoporosis in patients with rheumatic diseases: a meta-analysis. Medicine (Baltimore) 2016;95(25):e3990.
131. Rudic JS, Poropat G, Krstic MN, et al. Hormone replacement for osteoporosis in women with primary biliary cirrhosis. Cochrane Database Syst Rev 2011;(12):CD009146.
132. Dubreuil M, Ruiz-Gaspa S, Guanabens N, et al. Ursodeoxycholic acid increases differentiation and mineralization and neutralizes the damaging effects of bilirubin on osteoblastic cells. Liver Int 2013;33(7):1029–38.

Gastrointestinal and Hepatic Disease in Rheumatoid Arthritis

Ethan Craig, MD, MHS, Laura C. Cappelli, MD, MHS*

KEYWORDS

- Rheumatoid arthritis • Gastrointestinal disease • Hepatic disease
- Antirheumatic medications (DMARDs)

KEY POINTS

- Gastrointestinal and hepatic disease are rare extra-articular manifestations of rheumatoid arthritis.
- Treatment of rheumatoid arthritis can lead to digestive and hepatic dysfunction, either as a direct effect of medications, or from the infections to which patients with RA are susceptible.
- Although rare in the modern era, complications of long-standing, poorly controlled RA (including rheumatoid vasculitis, Felty syndrome, and amyloidosis) may be associated with significant GI morbidity.

INTRODUCTION

The importance of the gastrointestinal (GI) tract in development of autoimmunity has been increasingly appreciated in human diseases.[1,2] Many autoimmune diseases primarily affect the GI tract or the liver, including inflammatory bowel disease (IBD), celiac disease, and various autoimmune liver diseases. Rheumatoid arthritis (RA) is a systemic autoimmune disease that can affect multiple organ systems. Understanding the range and prevalence of GI manifestations associated with RA itself, with related autoimmune disorders, and with RA treatments is essential for rheumatologists and other clinicians caring for patients with RA. All organs of the GI tract can be affected either directly from RA, through related autoimmune diseases, or as consequences of treatment (**Fig. 1**). This article discusses the presentation, epidemiology, and diagnosis of GI disease in patients with RA.

Disclosures: The authors have no relevant financial disclosures.

Research reported in this publication was supported by the National Institute of Arthritis and Musculoskeletal and Skin Diseases of the National Institutes of Health under Award Number T32AR048522. The content is solely the responsibility of the authors and does not necessarily represent the official views of the National Institutes of Health.

Johns Hopkins University School of Medicine, Division of Rheumatology, 5501 Hopkins Bayview Circle, Baltimore, MD 21224, USA

* Corresponding author. 5501 Hopkins Bayview Circle, Suite 1.B.1, Baltimore, MD 21224.

E-mail address: lcappel1@jhmi.edu

Rheum Dis Clin N Am 44 (2018) 89–111
https://doi.org/10.1016/j.rdc.2017.09.005
0889-857X/18/© 2017 Elsevier Inc. All rights reserved.

rheumatic.theclinics.com

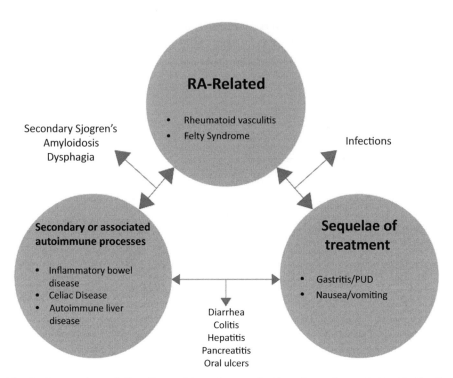

Fig. 1. An overview of digestive and hepatic complications from rheumatoid arthritis, its treatment, and related disorders. PUD, peptic ulcer disease.

EPIDEMIOLOGY OF RHEUMATOID ARTHRITIS

RA is a common rheumatologic disorder that affects up to 1.29 million adults in the United States.[3] Estimates of RA prevalence range between 0.5% and 1% of adults.[3] Lifetime risk among Americans has been reported as 1.7% for men and 3.6% for women.[4] The prevalence of RA seems to be decreasing since the early 1960s. In a 2008 study of RA in Olmstead County, Minnesota, prevalence had decreased over time for most age groups. An increased prevalence was noted only in older age groups, suggesting an increase in chronicity, and decrease in incidence.[3]

Several factors have been associated with an increased risk for RA, including female sex; smoking; and certain infectious agents, such as GI pathogens, as discussed later. Genetic risk has also been identified, with higher risk for RA among those with the shared epitope, a sequence of five amino acids in the hypervariable segment common to several HLA-DRB chains.[5] However, there remains considerable discordance even between identical twins in development of RA, speaking to a possible role of environmental risk factors.[6] Numerous other mutations have been identified that predispose to RA, although none as strongly as the shared epitope, and none that are necessary or sufficient for development of disease.[7,8]

THE GASTROINTESTINAL TRACT IN RHEUMATOID ARTHRITIS PATHOGENESIS

A growing literature suggests that the GI tract may play a major role in the pathogenesis of RA. This hypothesis was initially derived from an epidemiologic association between RA and periodontitis, a link that led early investigators to suspect a causal role of periodontitis in the development of RA.[9]

There are other clear cases of induction of arthritis in humans by GI pathogens. Reactive arthritis is triggered by certain pathogens, such as *Campylobacter*, *Chlamydia*, and *Salmonella*.[10] Following ileojejunal bypass, intestinal bacterial overgrowth has been tied to a high rate of inflammatory arthritis, occurring in up to 50% of patients after this procedure.[11] Whipple disease is a prototypical case of inflammatory arthritis occurring in the setting of intestinal colonization by a single bacterial species in a susceptible host.[12]

Modern molecular investigative techniques have demonstrated a complex interplay between microbes, particularly of the gut, and the human immune system. *Bacteroides fragilis* and certain *Clostridia* species are able to directly upregulate T-regulatory cell activity, inducing an anti-inflammatory effect through production of interleukin (IL)-10.[13,14] Segmented filamentous bacteria have been demonstrated to induce TH-17 cell activity; these cells have been implicated in the pathogenesis of RA and secrete proinflammatory cytokines, including IL-17, tumor necrosis factor (TNF)-α, IL-21, IL-22, and granulocyte-macrophage colony–stimulating factor.[15–19]

It is hypothesized that dysbiosis, or relative change in the homeostatic balance of commensal bacteria, results in altered balance of anti-inflammatory and proinflammatory interactions, and leads to dysregulation of a local immune response. As a result of this dysregulation, local T cells may migrate to distant lymphatic tissue, enabling them to exert effects distant to the site of activation in the intestine.

A growing literature supports this dysbiosis hypothesis in human and animal models. Germ-free or gnotobiotic mouse models (those raised in a germ-free environment with specific organisms introduced selectively) have been used in conjunction with mouse models of RA. Both *Lactobacillus bifidus* and segmented filamentous bacteria are able to produce arthritis in germ-free animals, associated with upregulation of TH-17 and downregulation of T-regulatory cells.[20,21]

Human evidence reflects similar findings. Fecal samples from patients with RA, compared with those with fibromyalgia, have significantly less *Bifidobacteria* and bacteria from the *Bacteroides-Porphyromonas-Prevotella*, *B fragilis*, and *Eubacterium rectale–Clostridium coccoides* groups.[22] Another investigation showed higher levels of *Lactobacillus* in those with early RA versus control subjects.[23] Two studies have shown increased levels of *Prevotella copri* in patients with early RA compared with control subjects, which corresponded with a decrease in *B fragilis* populations.[24,25] Both of these studies suggested a pathogenic role of *P copri*, with induction of disease and a TH-17 response following introduction of *P copri* into a mouse model. A recent study comparing patients with RA with healthy control subjects showed lower abundance of *Hemophilus* species, which correlated with higher levels of autoantibodies in serum.[26] Intriguingly, those with RA treated with disease-modifying antirheumatic drugs (DMARDs) had partial restoration of a "healthy" microbiome.[26]

Finally, recent evidence points to the oral commensal bacteria *Aggregatibacter actinomycetemcomitans* as a potential driver of anti–citrullinated peptide antibody formation.[27] Through leukotoxin A, a pore-forming toxin, *Aggregatibacter* seems to induce dysregulation of citrullination in neutrophils, resulting in hypercitrullination of proteins. Exposure to leukotoxin Aa strains also correlated with anti–citrullinated peptide antibody levels in patients with RA. Further supporting this hypothesis, the effect of shared epitope alleles on anti–citrullinated peptide antibody positivity in this study was seen only in those patients with RA exposed to the leukotoxin A strain of *Aggregatibacter*.[27]

These findings, taken together, suggest a complex role of the oral and intestinal microbiome in RA pathogenesis. The effect of the microbiome is likely modulated by the host environment and genome, the balance with other commensal bacteria, and other environmental factors. This remains an active and rapidly evolving field of research.

Rheumatoid Arthritis–Related Gastrointestinal Manifestations: Epidemiology, Presentation, and Treatment

Patients with RA may develop digestive and hepatic complications of their disease. They can also develop related autoimmune diseases affecting the GI tract. A summary of these conditions by organ system is presented in **Table 1** and selected conditions are detailed next.

RHEUMATOID VASCULITIS
Epidemiology

The incidence of rheumatoid vasculitis (RV) has declined considerably since the time of its initial description. The first estimated incidence from the 1970s in Bristol, United Kingdom, was approximately 6 per million patients.[28] Between 1998 and 2000, incidence in the same UK cohort was reported as 3 per million, and 3.9 per million between 2001 and 2010.[29,30] Several hypotheses have been advanced to explain this drop in incidence, including improvements in RA therapy, decreased used of long-term high-dose steroids, declines in smoking, and changes in oral microbiota.[29–31]

GI involvement from RV remains a rare complication. In 1981, GI events caused by RV, including acute abdomen or colitis, were reported in up to 10% of patients with RV.[28] In contrast, in the same cohort between 2001 and 2010, no GI events were seen among 18 patients; and only two events were seen among 47 patients between 1988 and 2000.[30]

Clinical Manifestations

The clinical presentation of RV is heterogeneous, ranging from mild cutaneous or nailbed disease to life-threatening organ involvement. The typical patient has long-standing seropositive, erosive, and nodular RA.[32] RV is rare among those with seronegative

Table 1
Overview of RA-related and concomitant autoimmune disease–related GI manifestations, by organ involvement

Organ	Involvement
Mouth	Secondary Sjögren syndrome (sicca) Oral ulcerations in associated inflammatory bowel disease
Esophagus	Dysphagia (from amyloidosis, skeletal deformities, and other causes)
Stomach	GI bleeding or dysmotility from amyloidosis
Small intestine	Rheumatoid vasculitis Celiac disease Amyloidosis Associated inflammatory bowel disease
Large intestine (including rectum)	Rheumatoid vasculitis Associated inflammatory bowel disease Amyloidosis
Pancreas	Autoimmune pancreatitis
Liver/gallbladder	Hepatomegaly (in Felty syndrome, rheumatoid vasculitis) Hepatitis, cirrhosis, portal hypertension (in amyloidosis, autoimmune hepatitis, primary biliary cholangitis, or primary sclerosing cholangitis)

RA.[33] Uncommonly, cases with less than 5 years of RA disease duration have been described, as have occasional cases of RV as an initial manifestation of RA.[34]

Constitutional signs including weight loss and hepatosplenomegaly are common, and fevers may occur in a smaller subset of patients. The most commonly affected organs are the skin and peripheral nervous system. Skin manifestations occur in 78% to 88% of patients, and may include purpuric lesions, cutaneous leukocytoclastic vasculitis, nonhealing ulcerations similar to those seen in polyarteritis nodosa, or gangrene.[28,30] Neurologic involvement, including peripheral neuropathy or mononeuritis multiplex, occurs in up to 50% of patients.[28,30] Other commonly affected organs include the heart (pericarditis), lung (alveolitis, interstitial lung disease), kidney (necrotizing glomerulonephritis), and eye (scleritis, corneal melt).

Literature describing characteristics of GI involvement from RV is primarily limited to case reports and case series. GI involvement has been described in association with other systemic manifestations and as an isolated presentation. The presentation is similar to that of other vasculitides known to affect the GI tract, particularly polyarteritis nodosa, which must be considered in the differential diagnosis.

Among a case series of patients with GI involvement from varied systemic vasculitides, common characteristics arise. Abdominal pain is nearly universal.[35] Nausea, vomiting, or diarrhea occur in about one-third of patients.[35] Hematochezia/melena occur in 16% of cases. Ulcerations of the stomach or small bowel are found in up to 27% of patients, and esophageal or colorectal ulcers in about 10%. More severe presentations, such as surgical abdomen, ischemia/infarct, or bowel perforation, were reported in about 15%.[35]

Involvement of several portions of the GI tract has been described in RV. Luminal involvement has been reported, with ulcerations of the small and large intestine.[36,37] Medium vessel involvement may lead to infarction, bowel perforation, and acute abdomen.[38–46] In the large intestine, pancolitis resembling ulcerative colitis, and appendicitis have been described.[47,48] One case presented with recurrent ileal strictures, which may mimic Crohn disease.[49] Within the pancreas, early reports described pancreatic necrosis secondary to medium vessel vasculitis.[37] Intrahepatic hemorrhage, hepatic capsule rupture, and abdominal aneurysmal rupture with syncope have all been described.[50–52]

Treatment

Because of the rarity of RV and lack of validated classification criteria, there is a paucity of evidence-based treatment recommendations. As such, treatment decisions are largely empirical and based on observational evidence.

Perhaps the most widely cited regimen, particularly for severe manifestations of RV, is that outlined by Scott and coworkers[28] in 1981, a combination of intravenous cyclophosphamide and glucocorticoids.

Other approaches have been used, including the use of biologics. In a 2012 report of 17 patients treated with rituximab for RV, 71% achieved complete remission by 6 months, and 82% had complete sustained remission by 12 months.[53] Other biologics, including abatacept and tocilizumab, have been used in selected cases, although data supporting their efficacy are limited.[54,55]

The use of TNF inhibitors has been controversial. These agents clearly play a role in therapy for RA, and have been used successfully in cases of refractory vasculitis.[56] However, observational data suggest that these agents may paradoxically trigger vasculitis.[54,55] Confounding by indication is a significant concern in these data, because those with more severe disease are at higher risk for vasculitis and have higher likelihood of receiving TNF inhibitors. However, in light of these several reports, a degree of caution should be exercised in consideration of these agents for patients with a history of RV.

GASTROINTESTINAL DYSMOTILITY

Several authors have reported high rates of subjective dysphagia in patients with RA, with early studies demonstrating manometric changes including low peristaltic pressures, reduced lower esophageal sphincter pressures, and abnormal peristalsis.[57–59] However, these studies were small, and controls for medications and comorbidities, such as amyloidosis and Sjögren syndrome (SS), which are independently associated with esophageal dysfunction, were limited. A subsequent study of 2131 patients with RA or osteoarthritis showed no difference in subjective dysphagia or gastroesophageal reflux disease between these groups after controlling for use of nonsteroidal anti-inflammatory drugs and prednisone.[60]

Oropharyngeal dysphagia is common in patients with temporomandibular joint involvement, as are impaired masticatory function and masticatory pain and fatigue.[61] Dysphagia secondary to cranial nerve compression in atlantoaxial subluxation may occur, and several reports have described dysphagia in the setting of cervical deformities in RA.[62–66] Amyloidosis may cause dysmotility, and has been associated with goiter leading to extrinsic esophageal compression.[67–69]

Although there is some suggestion that autonomic neuropathy may occur in patients with RA, GI involvement has not been described, as seen in other rheumatic diseases.[70,71] Gastroparesis and bowel dysmotility, although well-described in scleroderma, SS, and systemic lupus erythematosus, have not been associated with RA.

AMYLOIDOSIS

Amyoid A (AA) amyloidosis is a rare complication of chronic inflammatory diseases, including RA. It is caused by deposition of the acute-phase reactant serum amyloid A protein.

Epidemiology

Historically, the most common underlying cause of AA amyloidosis was chronic infections, such as tuberculosis (TB) and osteomyelitis. However, the contribution of chronic infections has declined, and RA now stands as one of the most common causes of this disease.[72]

Estimates of the prevalence of AA amyloidosis in RA vary widely depending on population, year, and method used for detection. Because of a prolonged preclinical phase, estimates of clinical amyloidosis tend to be lower than those from autopsy studies or biopsies. Prevalence of clinical disease is estimated as 0.6% to 1.1% of patients with RA[73,74]; estimates of subclinical disease from random fat pad biopsy have been reported in up to 29% of patients with RA.[75–77] The prevalence of AA amyloidosis in patients with RA in the biologic era is not well-described.

Clinical Manifestations

AA amyloidosis presents with GI manifestations in 10% to 70% of patients.[78] GI symptoms of amyloidosis include weight loss, diarrhea, abdominal pain, esophageal reflux, dysmotility, or bleeding resulting from vessel friability. GI bleeding may be severe, and fatal hemorrhage has been described.[79] Rare cases of protein-losing enteropathy and malabsorption have been reported.[80,81] Hepatic involvement leads to hepatosplenomegaly; obstructive symptoms, such as jaundice and steatorrhea; and portal hypertension and its myriad complications.

Treatment

Treatment of AA amyloidosis involves treatment of the underlying inflammatory disorder. Both TNF inhibitors and the IL-6 receptor inhibitor, tocilizumab, have a body of literature supporting their efficacy in lowering serum AA protein levels, and in some cases, inducing remission of disease.[82–90]

HEPATIC DISEASE IN FELTY SYNDROME

Felty syndrome is a rare complication of RA characterized by the triad of arthritis, splenomegaly, and neutropenia. This syndrome generally occurs in the presence of severe, poorly controlled RA with nodulosis and extra-articular features.

Liver abnormalities are common in Felty syndrome. About two-thirds of patients develop hepatomegaly, and more than half have at least one abnormal liver function test.[91,92] Several findings have been described on biopsy, including nodular regenerative hyperplasia, sinusoidal lymphocytosis, and portal hypertension related to splenomegaly.[92,93] About 35% of patients with Felty syndrome with an abnormal liver enzyme have been found to have nodular regenerative hyperplasia on autopsy.[94] Distortion of the portal architecture caused by nodular regenerative hyperplasia, along with splenomegaly, result in portal hypertension with its attendant complications, especially varices and ascites.[95]

SECONDARY SJÖGRENS SYNDROME

SS and its GI manifestations are addressed in detail elsewhere in this issue (See Yevgeniy Popov and Karen Salomon-Escoto's article, "Gastrointestinal and Hepatic Disease in Sjogren's," in this issue). SS occurs in a primary form (pSS), unassociated with other autoimmune diseases, and a secondary form (sSS), which occurs in conjunction with other autoimmune disease. This section specifically addresses sSS associated with RA.

Epidemiology

RA is the most common autoimmune disease associated with sSS, with reports showing that between 4% and 31% of patients with RA develop sSS, depending on classification criteria used and population included.[96–101]

Clinical Manifestations

The clinical presentations of pSS and sSS are similar. Sicca symptoms remain the predominant manifestation. When compared with patients with pSS, patients with sSS seem to have a slightly lower rate of xerostomia (98% vs 85% in sSS) and parotid enlargement (56% vs 9% in sSS).[101] In addition, patients with sSS are less likely to have anti-SSA or SSB antibodies, and have lower titers of these antibodies, compared with those with pSS.[101] Extraglandular manifestations including vasculitis, adenopathy, renal involvement, neuropathy, and arthritis seem similar between those with sSS and pSS.[101]

GI manifestations are commonly reported in SS. **Table 2** summarizes associated abnormalities and frequency of these findings.

GASTROINTESTINAL MALIGNANCY IN RHEUMATOID ARTHRITIS

The topic of risk for malignancy in RA, both related to the disease itself and to its treatment, has been widely studied. Based on a large meta-analysis, patients with RA do

Table 2
GI manifestations of Sjögren syndrome

	References	Notes
Mouth		
Xerostomia	101–103	Included in classification criteria
Dysgeusia	102,103	
Dental caries	102,103	
Esophagus		
Dysphagia	104–109	May relate to oropharyngeal function because of xerostomia, or esophageal dysmotility
Gastroesophageal reflux disease	104–109	
Esophageal dysmotility	104–109	
Stomach		
Chronic atrophic gastritis	110–113	Up to 81% of patients on EGD
Achlorhydria/ hypopepsinoginemia	114	
Intestine		
Protein-losing enteropathy	115–119	Rare
Celiac disease	114,120,121	Among those with CD, 3.3% may have SS; among those with SS, up to 14.7% may have CD on biopsy, although lower in cohort studies
Cryoglobulinemic vasculitis		Rare
Pancreas		
Pancreatitis	122–125	Often subclinical. Presence of chronic pancreatitis (especially sclerosing) and salivary gland symptoms should raise suspicion for IgG4-related disease
Pancreatic exocrine insufficiency	126,127	Often subclinical
Liver		
Hepatomegaly	128	
Abnormal liver enzymes	128–130	Usually mild, low grade. May follow multiple patterns of elevation
Primary biliary cirrhosis	128–135	Of those with PBC, 18%–38% have SS; of those with SS, 2%–7% have positive antimitochondrial antibody, and 92% of these patients have histologic findings of PBC
Autoimmune hepatitis	136,137	In one study, of those with SS with elevated LFT's, 47% had AIH on biopsy

Abbreviations: AIH, autoimmune hepatitis; CD, celiac disease; EGD, Esophagogastroduodenoscopy; LFT, liver function tests; PBC, primary biliary cholangitis.

seem to be at modestly increased risk for all malignancies compared with the general population, with a standardized incidence ratio (SIR) of 1.09 (1.06–1.13).[138] However, when divided by specific cancer, this increased risk was explained mostly by higher incidences of lymphoma (SIR, 2.26 [1.82–2.81]), melanoma (SIR, 1.23 [1.01–1.49]), and lung cancer (SIR, 1.64 [1.51–1.79]) compared with the general population. In contrast, the incidence of colorectal cancer seemed to be lower in patients with RA (SIR, 0.78 [0.71–0.86]). The mechanism behind the decreased risk of colorectal cancer has been hypothesized to be related to higher use of nonsteroidal anti-inflammatory drugs in patients with RA, which may have a protective effect for colorectal cancer.[138]

Risk for other GI cancers is less clear. In a large registry-based study of Japanese patients with RA, no significant difference in risk for gastric, esophageal, or pancreatic cancer was observed between patients with RA and the general population.[139] Surprisingly, in this cohort, a considerably lower incidence of liver cancer was observed among those with RA, with SIR of 0.33 (0.15–0.51). However, it should be noted that overall risk of malignancy seemed lower in this group relative to those seen in other studies, with overall SIR of 0.89 (0.82–0.97) for those with RA compared with overall population, raising a question of generalizeability.[139]

CONCOMITANT AUTOIMMUNE DISEASES

Given the increased risk of certain autoimmune diseases in patients known to have RA,[140,141] it is important to consider autoimmune conditions as a cause of digestive, liver, or gallbladder dysfunction. This relationship is bidirectional, and those with certain GI autoimmune diseases are also at increased risk of developing RA. The concurrence of GI autoimmune disease with RA is reviewed briefly next.

Autoimmune Liver Diseases

Autoimmune hepatitis is a rare disease causing chronic inflammation of the liver that can ultimately lead to hepatic dysfunction and cirrhosis. RA has been seen in 2% to 4% of patients with autoimmune hepatitis.[142] In another study, anti–cyclic citrullinated peptide antibodies and rheumatoid factor were seen in 8% to 10% of patients with autoimmune liver diseases (autoimmune hepatitis, primary biliary cholangitis, primary sclerosing cholangitis), whereas 5% of those patients actually had a clinical diagnosis of RA.[143] There may be some shared genetic risk between RA and autoimmune hepatitis, because STAT4 polymorphisms have been associated with both conditions.[144]

Like autoimmune hepatitis, primary biliary cholangitis and primary sclerosing cholangitis also share risk loci with RA and thus may have some relationship in terms of pathogenesis.[145] Patients with primary sclerosing cholangitis often have concomitant IBD (more commonly ulcerative colitis than Crohn disease), but can also have other autoimmune diseases. RA was seen in only 1% of a cohort of 287 patients with primary sclerosing cholangitis, but represented 7.9% of non-IBD autoimmune disease in that cohort.[146]

Inflammatory Bowel Disease

IBD, an autoimmune disease that can affect nearly every part of the digestive tract, includes Crohn disease and ulcerative colitis subtypes. In most studies evaluating risk for RA, the two subtypes of IBD are grouped together. In studies of patients with IBD and matched control subjects, the patients with IBD had 1.9 to 2 times higher odds of developing RA as compared with the control subjects.[147,148] IBD is also associated with arthropathy, so careful evaluation of clinical phenotype along with laboratory testing for rheumatoid factor and anti–cyclic citrullinated peptide antibodies is helpful in distinguishing the two entities.

Celiac Disease

Celiac disease is an autoimmune disorder of the intestines precipitated by gluten exposure that can cause diarrhea and nutritional deficiencies. Celiac disease and

RA share certain epidemiologic and genetic associations and can occur in the same patient.[149] As with IBD, arthralgias and inflammatory arthritis can also be seen in patients with celiac disease.

DIGESTIVE AND HEPATIC CONSEQUENCES OF TREATMENT OF RHEUMATOID ARTHRITIS

Although RA and its related diseases may be associated with GI manifestations, it should again be noted that most of the conditions listed to this point are rare findings in RA. Complications from the medications used in treatment of RA, in contrast, are not uncommon. The diagnosis and management of these attendant complications constitutes a major part of the daily practice of rheumatology. The GI effects from medications used in RA are addressed in detail elsewhere in this issue (See Patrick Wood and Liron Caplan's article, "Drug-induced Gastrointestinal and Hepatic Disease Associated with Biologics and Non-Biologic Disease Modifying Anti-Rheumatic Drugs [DMARDS]," in this issue). **Table 3** reviews the known adverse drug reactions associated with common medications used in the management of RA.

INFECTIONS

Antirheumatic therapies, particularly steroids and biologic agents, are associated with an increased risk for opportunistic infections. Here, we briefly review several infections known to prominently affect the GI tract. A full review of infections associated with DMARD therapy is outside the scope of this article, as is treatment of these diseases.

Tuberculosis

TB, caused by *Mycobacterium tuberculosis*, most commonly affects the lung. Extrapulmonary disease is more common with immunosuppression. Among those that develop TB while being treated with biologics, 30% to 57% present with extrapulmonary manifestations, compared with a reported 20% among immunocompetent patients.[150–152] Patients with RA treated with biologic therapies are at significantly increased risk for TB, with about 3.7 to 4 times increased risk for active TB.[153,154]

Tuberculous enteritis may affect any part of the GI tract, and may occur as a primary site of infection, or in the setting of disseminated, or miliary disease. It most commonly affects the peritoneum, ileum, colon, anorectum, and jejunum.[155] The symptoms of tuberculous enteritis are nonspecific, making diagnosis challenging even in endemic regions. Patients present with colicky abdominal pain related to obstruction (90%–100%), weight loss (66%), fever (35%–50%), and changes in bowel habits. Other symptoms may include malabsorption, anorexia, nausea, vomiting, or GI bleeding.[156]

The lesions seen on imaging and colonoscopy may vary. Ulcerative lesions are most common, with multiple segments of ulcerations with or without nodules.[155] Hypertrophic lesions of the intestines including stricture and fibrosis may mimic Crohn disease. A combination of these findings may also occur, with thickening, ulceration, and inflammation of the intestinal wall and ileocecal valve, which may mimic carcinoma.[155]

Nontuberculous Mycobacteria

Nontuberculous mycobacteria (NTM) are a broad group of mycobacterial organisms including *Mycobacterium avium*, *Mycobacterium marinum*, and rapidly growing *Mycobacteria*, among other species. As with TB, infection with NTM most commonly involves the lung, but may involve extrapulmonary sites. These infections are rare even among immunocompromised patients. In a study of 8418 patients treated with

TNF inhibitors, an NTM infection rate of 74 cases per 100,000 person years was observed. Of these cases, 69% were pulmonary, whereas 25% were extrapulmonary.[157] Among patients in clinical trials for multiple biologics, this rate was considerably lower, with only 1 case of NTM observed among 32,504 patients.[153] This lower rate may relate to the comparably shorter follow-up times in clinical trials.

Symptoms of NTM infection vary by the site involved and specific organism. GI involvement may result in diarrhea, abdominal pain, hepatosplenomegaly, and elevation of liver enzymes.

Endemic Mycoses

Histoplasma capsulatum is a dimorphic fungus endemic to the Midwestern and South Central United States.[158] Initial infection is often asymptomatic or associated with a mild flulike illness. Immunocompromised patients may be prone to more severe, disseminated infections, either caused by primary infection, or reactivation of previous infection. Immunosuppressive agents, including TNF inhibitors (especially infliximab), steroids, and conventional DMARDs, seem to be associated with an increased risk for histoplasmosis.[159–162]

Constitutional signs including fevers, weight loss, lymphadenopathy, and hepatosplenomegaly are common.[161] Patients most typically present with pulmonary involvement, often as a pneumonia that fails to respond to typical antibiotic therapy. GI involvement may occur in up to 70% to 90% of those with progressive disseminated disease, although it may remain asymptomatic and go undiagnosed.[163] Histoplasmosis may involve any part of the GI tract. Hepatosplenomegaly and abdominal lymphadenopathy are common. Esophageal involvement may occur because of direct infection with ulcer formation, or from external compression from fibrosing mediastinitis or mediastinal adenitis.[163] Involvement of the stomach and intestine may present with ulcers, GI bleeding, or as inflammatory masses that may mimic carcinoma.[163]

Coccidioiodomycosis has also been reported in association with TNF inhibitor use (especially infliximab).[160,164] Coccidioidomycosis is endemic to the southwestern United States, although cases have been reported outside of this typical area.[165] GI manifestations are rare, although there have been cases reported of liver and pancreas involvement in disseminated coccidioidomycosis.[166]

Patients on TNF inhibitors may also be at risk for blastomycosis. *Blastomyces dermatitidis* is endemic to the Ohio and Mississippi river valleys and the Great Lakes region, although cases have been reported outside this region.[167] The most commonly involved organs are the lung, skin, genitourinary tract, and osteoarticular structures.[167] GI manifestations are rare, but reported. Several cases of oral lesions have been described.[168–173] Other case reports have also described involvement of the esophagus[174,175] and pancreas.[176]

Herpes Simplex Virus

The risk of viral infections seems to be modestly increased in patients using biologic therapies, with about 1.9 times higher odds for viral infection in those treated with biologics compared with other RA treatments (95% confidence interval, 1.02–3.58).[153] In a large meta-analysis of 70 clinical trials for biologic agents, 11 cases of herpes simplex virus were described, and three were noted in a French registry study over 3 years.[153,177] Herpes simplex virus is most commonly associated with recurrent painful oral or anal lesions. It has been described to involve much of the GI tract, including pharyngeal ulcerations, esophagitis, proctitis, and scattered reports of gastritis,

Table 3
GI side effects of medications used in the treatment of RA

Medication	GI Effects
NSAIDs	Ulcerations GI bleeding Colitis Hepatotoxicity
Corticosteroids	Thrush Ulcerations Visceral perforation Hepatic steatosis, NASH Hepatitis B reactivation
csDMARDs	
Methotrexate	Stomatitis Nausea Abdominal pain Diarrhea Hepatotoxicity
Leflunomide	Nausea Abdominal pain Diarrhea Hepatotoxicity
Hydroxychloroquine	Abdominal pain Nausea
Sulfasalazine	Abdominal pain Nausea/vomiting Diarrhea Hepatotoxicity
Azathioprine	Anorexia Nausea/vomiting Hepatotoxicity Hypersensitivity reaction
JAK inhibitor	
Tofacitinib	Abdominal pain Nausea/vomiting Gastritis Diarrhea Opportunistic infections GI perforations LFT abnormalities Hepatic steatosis
Biologics	
TNF inhibitors (adalimumab, etanercept, infliximab, golimumab, certolizumab)	Nausea Abdominal pain Opportunistic infections Hepatotoxicity (especially infliximab) Hepatitis B reactivation
Abatacept	Dyspepsia

(continued on next page)

Table 3 (*continued*)	
Medication	**GI Effects**
Rituximab	Abdominal pain Nausea/vomiting Diarrhea Hepatitis B reactivation Bowel obstruction Bowel perforation Opportunistic infections LFT abnormalities
Tocilizumab	Oral ulceration Abdominal pain Gastritis Bowel perforation Opportunistic infections Hepatotoxicity

Abbreviations: csDMARD, conventional synthetic DMARD; LFT, liver function tests; NASH, nonalcoholic steatohepatitis; NSAIDs, nonsteroidal anti-inflammatory drugs.

jejunitis, and colitis.[178] Both herpes simplex virus 1 and 2 are rare causes of potentially fulminant viral hepatitis.[178]

Cytomegalovirus

Although a common concern in other immunocompromised populations, such as organ transplant recipients and patients with acquired immune deficiency syndrome, cytomegalovirus (CMV) infection is an extremely rare complication in patients treated for RA. In a large meta-analysis of 70 clinical trials for biologic agents, only one case of CMV infection was identified among 32,504 patients; and in a French registry of 57,711 patients, only four cases were noted over 3 years.[153] Several case reports of CMV reactivation with GI manifestations are found in the literature, including in patients treated with methotrexate (MTX) alone.[179–182]

CMV has been described to cause myriad manifestations within the GI tract, including colitis, ulcerations, gastritis, esophagitis, ileitis, appendicitis, and hepatitis.[180–192] Patients may present with fever, abdominal pain, diarrhea, nausea/vomiting, or melena/hematochezia.

MANAGEMENT PRINCIPLES OF RHEUMATOID ARTHRITIS IN THOSE WITH GASTROINTESTINAL DISEASE

Successful treatment of syndromes involving the GI tract in RA depends on identification of the underlying cause. It is therefore important to maintain high index of suspicion for more common causes of GI symptoms that are unrelated to RA. For example, acute diarrhea is most likely infectious and often self-limited, regardless of whether the patient has RA. Similarly, gastroesophageal reflux disease is a common problem in the general population, and management in patients with RA should proceed as in the general population, with empiric therapy and lifestyle modifications as a first line before progression to evaluation for more esoteric causes.

There are some unique issues to consider in treating patients with RA for their GI disease. In those with concomitant autoimmune diseases, choosing treatment that has efficacy both in RA and in the other autoimmune disease is a logical goal. For example, azathioprine can be used in IBD and autoimmune hepatitis and may help improve RA. Similarly, TNF-inhibitors, methotrexate and sulfasalazine, may be used to treat IBD and are effective for RA.

Conversely, treatment of RA itself can be tailored when patients have GI comorbidities. In a patient with gastritis or peptic ulcer disease, injectable methotrexate may be preferable to the oral formulation. In patients with prior diverticulitis, providers should be cautious when using tocilizumab and tofacitinib because of risk of bowel perforation. Any major liver function abnormality is a relative contraindication for such medications as methotrexate and leflunomide.

SUMMARY

The GI tract and liver are uncommon sites for extra-articular manifestations of RA, but patients with RA may experience digestive and hepatic dysfunction for a variety of reasons. Evaluating potential medication side effects or infectious causes of GI dysfunction is important for patients with RA on DMARDs, particularly corticosteroids, methotrexate, and TNF-inhibitors. Considering sequelae of long-standing or untreated RA, such as amyloidosis and RV, is appropriate in the right clinical setting. Patients with RA are also at increased risk for other GI and hepatic autoimmune diseases. These unique features can help clinicians consider a full differential diagnosis when evaluating new digestive and hepatic disease in the setting of RA.

REFERENCES

1. Ciccia F, Ferrante A, Guggino G, et al. The role of the gastrointestinal tract in the pathogenesis of rheumatic diseases. Best Pract Res Clin Rheumatol 2016;30(5): 889–900.
2. Chen K, Liu J, Cao X. Regulation of type I interferon signaling in immunity and inflammation: a comprehensive review. J Autoimmun 2017;83:1–11.
3. Helmick CG, Felson DT, Lawrence RC, et al. Estimates of the prevalence of arthritis and other rheumatic conditions in the United States part I. Arthritis Rheum 2008;58(1):15–25.
4. Crowson CS, Matteson EL, Myasoedova E, et al. The lifetime risk of adult-onset rheumatoid arthritis and other inflammatory autoimmune rheumatic diseases. Arthritis Rheum 2011;63(3):633–9.
5. Kurkó J, Besenyei T, Laki J, et al. Genetics of rheumatoid arthritis: a comprehensive review. Clin Rev Allergy Immunol 2013;45(2):170–9.
6. Silman AJ, MacGregor AJ, Thomson W, et al. Twin concordance rates for rheumatoid arthritis: results from a nationwide study. Br J Rheumatol 1993;32:903–7.
7. Stahl EA, Raychaudhuri S, Remmers EF, et al. Genome-wide association study meta-analysis identifies seven new rheumatoid arthritis risk loci. Nat Genet 2010;42(6):508–14.
8. Svendsen AJ, Holm NV, Kyvik K, et al. Relative importance of genetic effects in rheumatoid arthritis: historical cohort study of Danish nationwide twin population. BMJ 2002;324(7332):264–6.
9. Hunter W. Oral sepsis as a cause of disease. Br Med J 1900;2(2065):215–6.
10. Schmitt SK. Reactive arthritis. Infect Dis Clin North Am 2017;31(2):265–77.
11. Ross CB, Scott HW, Pincus T. Jejunoileal bypass arthritis. Baillieres Clin Rheumatol 1989;3(2):339–55.
12. Moos V, Schneider T. Changing paradigms in Whipple's disease and infection with Tropheryma whipplei. Eur J Clin Microbiol Infect Dis 2011;30:1151–8.

13. Telesford KM, Yan W, Ochoa-Reparaz J, et al. A commensal symbiotic factor derived from *Bacteroides fragilis* promotes human CD39+ Foxp3+ T cells and T reg function. Gut Microbes 2015;6(4):234–42.
14. Atarashi K, Tanoue T, Shima T, et al. Induction of colonic regulatory T cells by indigenous *Clostridium* species. Science 2011;331:337–42.
15. Ivanov II, Atarashi K, Manel N, et al. Induction of intestinal Th17 cells by segmented filamentous bacteria. Cell 2009;139:485–98.
16. Jovanovic DV, Di Battista JA, Martel-Pelletier J, et al. IL-17 stimulates the production and expression of proinflammatory cytokines, IL-beta and TNF-alpha, by human macrophages. J Immunol 1998;160(7):3513–21.
17. Moran EM, Mullan R, McCormick J, et al. Human rheumatoid arthritis tissue production of IL-17A drives matrix and cartilage degradation: synergy with tumour necrosis factor-α, oncostatin M and response to biologic therapies. Arthritis Res Ther 2009;11(4):R113.
18. Kim KW, Kim HR, Park JY, et al. Interleukin-22 promotes osteoclastogenesis in rheumatoid arthritis through induction of RANKL in human synovial fibroblasts. Arthritis Rheum 2012;64(4):1015–23.
19. Lubberts E, van den Bersselaar L, Oppers-Walgreen B, et al. IL-17 promotes bone erosion in murine collagen-induced arthritis through loss of the receptor activator of NF- B ligand/osteoprotegerin balance. J Immunol 2003;170(5): 2655–62.
20. Abdollahi-Roodsaz S, Joosten LAB, Koenders MI, et al. Stimulation of TLR2 and TLR4 differentially skews the balance of T cells in a mouse model of arthritis. J Clin Invest 2008;118(1):205–16.
21. Wu HJ, Ivanov II, Darce J, et al. Gut-residing segmented filamentous bacteria drive autoimmune arthritis via T helper 17 cells. Immunity 2010;32:815–27.
22. Vaahtovuo J, Munukka E, Luukkainen R, et al. Fecal microbiota in early rheumatoid arthritis. J Rheumatol 2008;35(8):1500–5.
23. Liu X, Zou Q, Zeng B, et al. Analysis of fecal *Lactobacillus* community structure in patients with early rheumatoid arthritis. Curr Microbiol 2013;67:170–6.
24. Scher JU, Sczesnak A, Longman RS, et al. Expansion of intestinal *Prevotella copri* correlates with enhanced susceptibility to arthritis. Elife 2013;2:e01202.
25. Maeda Y, Kurakawa T, Umemoto E, et al. Dysbiosis contributes to arthritis development via activation of autoreactive T cells in the intestine. Arthritis Rheum 2016;68(11):2646–61.
26. Zhang X, Zhang D, Jia H, et al. The oral and gut microbiomes are perturbed in rheumatoid arthritis and partly normalized after treatment. Nat Med 2015;21(8): 895–905.
27. Konig MF, Abusleme L, Reinholdt J, et al. *Aggregatibacter actinomycetemcomitans*-induced hypercitrullination links periodontal infection to autoimmunity in rheumatoid arthritis. Sci Transl Med 2016;8(369):369ra176.
28. Scott D, Bacon P, Tribe C. Systemic rheumatoid vasculitis: a clinical and laboratory study of 50 cases. Medicine (Baltimore) 1981;60(4):288–97.
29. Watts RA, Mooney J, Lane SE, et al. Rheumatoid vasculitis: becoming extinct? Rheumatology (Oxford) 2004;43(7):920–3.
30. Ntatsaki E, Mooney J, Scott DGI, et al. Systemic rheumatoid vasculitis in the era of modern immunosuppressive therapy. Rheumatology (Oxford) 2014;53(1): 145–52.
31. Makol A, Crowson CS, Wetter DA, et al. Vasculitis associated with rheumatoid arthritis: a case-control study. Rheumatology (Oxford) 2014;53(5):890–9.

32. Voskuyl AE, Zwinderman AH, Westedt ML, et al. Factors associated with the development of vasculitis in rheumatoid arthritis: results of a case-control study. Ann Rheum Dis 1996;55(3):190–2.

33. Mongan ES, Cass RM, Jacox RF, et al. A study of the relation of seronegative and seropositive rheumatoid arthritis to each other and to necrotizing vasculitis. Am J Med 1969;47(1):23–35.

34. Gray RG, Poppo MJ. Necrotizing vasculitis as the initial manifestation of rheumatoid arthritis. J Rheumatol 1983;10(2):326–8.

35. Pagnoux C, Mahr A, Cohen P, et al. Presentation and outcome of gastrointestinal involvement in systemic necrotizing vasculitides: analysis of 62 patients with polyarteritis nodosa, microscopic polyangiitis, Wegener granulomatosis, Churg-Strauss syndrome, or rheumatoid arthritis-associated. Medicine (Baltimore) 2005;84(2):115–28.

36. Takeuchi K, Kuroda Y. Rheumatoid vasculitis with multiple intestinal ulcerations: report of a case. Ryumachi 2000;40(3):639–43.

37. Bywaters EGL. Peripheral vascular obstruction in rheumatoid arthritis and its relationship to other vascular lesions. Ann Rheum Dis 1957;16(1):84–103.

38. Babian M, Nasef S, Soloway G. Gastrointestinal infarction as a manifestation of rheumatoid vasculitis. Am J Gastroenterol 1998;93(1):119–20.

39. Lee SY, Lee SW, Chung WT. Jejunal vasculitis in patient with rheumatoid arthritis: case report and literature review. Mod Rheumatol 2012;22(6):924–7.

40. Golding D, Goodwill M. Ileal perforation and acute peripheral neuropathy in rheumatoid arthritis. Postgrad Med J 1965;41:27–30.

41. Adler R, Norcross B, Lockie L. Arteritis and infarction of the intestine in rheumatoid arthritis. JAMA 1962;180(11):922–6.

42. Bienenstock H, Minick C, Rogoff B. Mesenteric arteritis and intestinal infarction in rheumatoid disease. Arch Intern Med 1967;119(4):359–64.

43. Parker R, Thomas P. Intestinal perforation and widespread arteritis in rheumatoid arthritis during treatment with cortisone. Br Med J 1959;1(5121):540–2.

44. Wilsher M, Smeeton WM, Koelmeyer TD, et al. Complete heart block and bowel infarction secondary to rheumatoid disease. Ann Rheum Dis 1985;44(6):425–8.

45. Lindsay MK, Tavadia HB, Whyte AS, et al. Acute abdomen in rheumatoid arthritis due to necrotizing arteritis. Br Med J 1973;2(5866):592–3.

46. Tsai J. Perforation of the small bowel with rheumatoid arthritis. South Med J 1980;73(7):939–40.

47. Burt R, Berenson M, Samuelson C, et al. Rheumatoid vasculitis of the colon presenting as pancolitis. Dig Dis Sci 1983;28(2):183–8.

48. van Laar JM, Smit VT, de Beus WM, et al. Rheumatoid vasculitis presenting as appendicitis. Clin Exp Rheumatol 1998;16(6):736–8.

49. Tago M, Naito Y, Aihara H, et al. Recurrent stenosis of the ileum caused by rheumatoid vasculitis. Intern Med 2016;55(7):819–23.

50. Hocking W, Lasser K, Ungerer R, et al. Spontaneous hepatic rupture in rheumatoid arthritis. Arch Intern Med 1981;141:792–4.

51. Mizuno K, Ikeda K, Saida Y, et al. Hepatic hemorrhage in malignant rheumatoid arthritis. Am J Gastroenterol 1996;91(12):2624–5.

52. Achkar A, Stanson A, Johnson C, et al. Rheumatoid arthritis manifesting as intraabdominal hemorrhage. Mayo Clin Proc 1995;70(6):565–9.

53. Puéchal X, Gottenberg JE, Berthelot JM, et al. Rituximab therapy for systemic vasculitis associated with rheumatoid arthritis: results from the Autoimmunity and Rituximab Registry. Arthritis Care Res (Hoboken) 2012;64(3):331–9.

54. Saint Marcoux B, De Bandt M. Vasculitides induced by TNFα antagonists: a study in 39 patients in France. Joint Bone Spine 2006;73(6):710–3.
55. Jarrett S, Cunnane G, Conaghan P, et al. Anti-tumor necrosis factor- α therapy-induced vasculitis: case series. J Rheumatol 2003;30(10):2287–91.
56. Puechal X, Miceli-Richard C, Mejjad O, et al. Anti-tumour necrosis factor treatment in patients with refractory systemic vasculitis associated with rheumatoid arthritis. Ann Rheum Dis 2008;67(6):880–4.
57. Sun DC, Roth SH, Mitchell CS, et al. Upper gastrointestinal disease in rheumatoid arthritis. Am J Dig Dis 1974;19(5):405–10.
58. Peretz A, Muller G, Praet J-P, et al. Oesophageal involvement in rheumatoid arthritis patients: a study with oesophageal radionuclide transit using 81Krm. Nucl Med Commun 1991;12(10):901–6.
59. Bassotti G, Gaburri M, Biscarini L, et al. Oesophageal motor activity in rheumatoid arthritis: a clinical and manometric study. Digestion 1988;39(3):144–50.
60. Wolfe F, Hawley DJ. The comparative risk and predictors of adverse gastrointestinal events in rheumatoid arthritis and osteoarthritis: a prospective 13 year study of 2131 patients. J Rheumatol 2000;27(7):1668–73.
61. Gilheaney Ó, Zgaga L, Harpur I, et al. The prevalence of oropharyngeal dysphagia in adults presenting with temporomandibular disorders associated with rheumatoid arthritis: a systematic review and meta-analysis. Dysphagia 2017. [Epub ahead of print].
62. Ebata S, Hatsushika K, Ohba T, et al. Swallowing function after occipitocervical arthrodesis for cervical deformity in patients with rheumatoid arthritis. NeuroRehabilitation 2015;37(2):299–304.
63. Kinney WC, Scheetz RJ, Strome M. Rheumatoid pannus of the cervical spine: a case report of an unusual cause of dysphagia. Ear Nose Throat J 1999;78(4):284, 289–91.
64. Kinney WC, Scheetz RJ, Strome M. Rheumatoid pannus of the cervical spine: an unusual cause of dysphagia. Otolaryngol Head Neck Surg 1996;115(2):P208–9.
65. Ekberg O, Redlund-Johnell I, Sjöblom KG. Pharyngeal function in patients with rheumatoid arthritis of the cervical spine and temporomandibular joint. Acta Radiol 1987;28(1):35–9.
66. Gow PJ, Gibson T. Dysphagia due to vertical subluxation of the axis in rheumatoid arthritis. Rheumatol Rehabil 1977;16(3):155–7.
67. Uzum G, Kaya FO, Uzum AK, et al. Amyloid goiter associated with amyloidosis secondary to rheumatoid arthritis. Case Rep Med 2013;2013:1–3.
68. Estrada C, Lewandowski C, Schubert T, et al. Esophageal involvement in secondary amyloidosis mimicking achalasia. J Clin Gastroenterol 1990;12(4):447–50.
69. Dubbins P. Secondary amyloidosis involving the stomach in rheumatoid arthritis. J Clin Ultrasound 1992;20(5):364.
70. Edmonds ME, Jones TC, Saunders WA, et al. Autonomic neuropathy in rheumatoid arthritis. Br Med J 1979;2:173–5.
71. Vaisrub S. Autonomic neuropathy complicating rheumatoid arthritis. JAMA 1980;243(2):152.
72. Real de Asua D, Costa R, Galvan J, et al. Systemic AA amyloidosis: epidemiology, diagnosis, and management. Clin Epidemiol 2014;6:369–77.
73. Carmona L, Gonzalez-Alvaro I, Balsa A, et al. Rheumatoid arthritis in Spain: occurrence of extra-articular manifestations and estimates of disease severity. Ann Rheum Dis 2003;62:897–900.

74. Çalgüneri M, Üreten K, Akif Öztürk M, et al. Extra-articular manifestations of rheumatoid arthritis: results of a university hospital of 526 patients in Turkey. Clin Exp Rheumatol 2006;24(3):305–8.

75. Wiland P, Wojtala R, Goodacre J, et al. The prevalence of subclinical amyloidosis in Polish patients with rheumatoid arthritis. Clin Rheumatol 2004;23(3): 193–8.

76. El Mansoury T, Hazenberg B, El Badawy S, et al. Screening for amyloid in subcutaneous fat tissue of Egyptian patients with rheumatoid arthritis: clinical and laboratory characteristics. Ann Rheum Dis 2002;61:42–7.

77. Gomes-Casanovas E, Sanmarti R, Sole M, et al. The clinical significance of amyloid fat deposits in rheumatoid arthritis. Arthritis Rheum 2001;44(1):66–72.

78. Joss N, McLaughlin K, Simpson K, et al. Presentation, survival and prognostic markers in AA amyloidosis. QJM 2000;93(8):535–42.

79. Rowe K, Pankow J, Nehme F, et al. Gastrointestinal amyloidosis: review of the literature. Cureus 2017;9(5):1–6.

80. Shin J-K, Jung Y-H, Bae M-N, et al. Successful treatment of protein-losing enteropathy due to AA amyloidosis with octreotide in a patient with rheumatoid arthritis. Mod Rheumatol 2013;23(2):406–11.

81. Babb RR, Alarcon-Segovia D, Diessner GR, et al. Malabsorption in rheumatoid arthritis: an unusual complication caused by amyloidosis. Arthritis Rheum 1967; 10(1):63–70.

82. Perry ME, Stirling A, Hunter JA. Effect of etanercept on serum amyloid A protein (SAA) levels in patients with AA amyloidosis complicating inflammatory arthritis. Clin Rheumatol 2008;27(7):923–5.

83. Keersmaekers T, Claes K, Kuypers D, et al. Long-term efficacy of infliximab treatment for AA-amyloidosis secondary to chronic inflammatory arthritis. Ann Rheum Dis 2009;68(5):759–61.

84. Nakamura T, Higashi SI, Tomoda K, et al. Etanercept can induce resolution of renal deterioration in patients with amyloid A amyloidosis secondary to rheumatoid arthritis. Clin Rheumatol 2010;29(12):1395–401.

85. Fernández-Nebro A, Tomero E, Ortiz-Santamaría V, et al. Treatment of rheumatic inflammatory disease in 25 patients with secondary amyloidosis using tumor necrosis factor alpha antagonists. Am J Med 2005;118(5):552–6.

86. Gottenberg JE, Merle-Vincent F, Bentaberry F, et al. Anti-tumor necrosis factor a therapy in fifteen patients with AA amyloidosis secondary to inflammatory arthritides: a followup report of tolerability and efficacy. Arthritis Rheum 2003;48(7): 2019–24.

87. Miyagawa I, Nakayamada S, Saito K, et al. Study on the safety and efficacy of tocilizumab, an anti-IL-6 receptor antibody, in patients with rheumatoid arthritis complicated with AA amyloidosis. Mod Rheumatol 2014;24(3):405–9.

88. Courties A, Grateau G, Philippe P, et al. AA amyloidosis treated with tocilizumab: case series and updated literature review. Amyloid 2015;22(2):84–92.

89. Yamada S, Tsuchimoto A, Kaizu Y, et al. Tocilizumab-induced remission of nephrotic syndrome accompanied by secondary amyloidosis and glomerulonephritis in a patient with rheumatoid arthritis. CEN Case Rep 2014;3(2):237–43.

90. Inoue D, Arima H, Kawanami C, et al. Excellent therapeutic effect of tocilizumab on intestinal amyloid a deposition secondary to active rheumatoid arthritis. Clin Rheumatol 2010;29(10):1195–7.

91. Sema K, Takei M, Uenogawa K, et al. Felty's syndrome with chronic hepatitis and compatible autoimmune hepatitis: a case presentation. Intern Med 2005;44(4): 335–41.

92. Thorne C, Urowitz M, Wanless I, et al. Liver disease in Felty's syndrome. Am J Med 1982;73:35–40.
93. Cohen M, Manier J, Bredfeldt J. Sinusoidal lymphocytosis of the liver in Felty's syndrome with a review of the liver involvement in Felty's syndrome. J Clin Gastroenterol 1989;11(1):92–4.
94. Wanless IR. Micronodular transformation (nodular regenerative hyperplasia) of the liver: a report of 64 cases among 2,500 autopsies and a new classification of benign hepatocellular nodules. Hepatology 1990;11(5):787–97.
95. Cohen M, Ginsburg W, Allen G. Nodular regenerative hyperplasia of the liver and bleeding esophageal varices in Felty's syndrome. A case report and literature review. J Rheumatol 1982;9:716–8.
96. Hajiabbasi A, Masooleh IS, Alizadeh Y, et al. Secondary Sjogren's syndrome in 83 patients with rheumatoid arthritis. Acta Med Iran 2016;54(7):448–53.
97. Lins E Silva M, Carvalho CN, Carvalho AA, et al. Effect of xerostomia on the functional capacity of subjects with rheumatoid arthritis. J Rheumatol 2016;43(10): 1795–800.
98. Santosh K, Dhir V, Singh S, et al. Prevalence of secondary Sjogren's syndrome in Indian patients with rheumatoid arthritis: a single-center study. Int J Rheum Dis 2017;20(7):870–4.
99. Gilboe I-M, Kvien T, Uhlig T, et al. Sicca symptoms and secondary Sjogren's syndrome in systemic lupus erythematosus: comparison with rheumatoid arthritis and correlation with disease variables. Ann Rheum Dis 2001;60:1103–9.
100. Uhlig T, Kvien TK, Jensen JL, et al. Sicca symptoms, saliva and tear production, and disease variables in 636 patients with rheumatoid arthritis. Ann Rheum Dis 1999;58(7):415–22.
101. Hernandez-Molina G, Avila-Casado C, Cardenas-Velazquez F, et al. Similarities and differences between primary and secondary Sjogren's syndrome. J Rheumatol 2010;37(4):800–8.
102. Soto-Rojas AE, Villa AR, Sifuentes-Osornio J, et al. Oral manifestations in patients with Sjögren's syndrome. J Rheumatol 1998;25(5):906–10.
103. Doig JA, Whaley K, Dick WC, et al. Otolaryngological aspects of Sjogren's syndrome. Br Med J 1971;4:460–3.
104. Türk T, Pirildar T, Tunç E, et al. Manometric assessment of esophageal motility in patients with primary Sjögren's syndrome. Rheumatol Int 2005;25(4):246–9.
105. Volter F, Fain O, Mathieu E, et al. Esophageal function and Sjogren's syndrome. Dig Dis Sci 2004;49(2):248–53.
106. Anselmino M, Zaninotto G, Costantini M, et al. Esophageal motor function in primary Sjogren's syndrome: correlation with dysphagia and xerostomia. Dig Dis Sci 1997;42(1):113–8.
107. Kjellén G, Fransson SG, Lindström F, et al. Esophageal function, radiography, and dysphagia in Sjögren's syndrome. Dig Dis Sci 1986;31(3):225–9.
108. Mandl T, Ekberg O, Wollmer P, et al. Dysphagia and dysmotility of the pharynx and oesophagus in patients with primary Sjogren's syndrome. Scand J Rheumatol 2007;36(5):394–401.
109. Grande L, Lacima G, Ros E, et al. Esophageal motor function in primary Sjögren's syndrome. Am J Gastroenterol 1993;88(3):378–81.
110. Maury C, Tornroth T, Teppo A. Atrophic gastritis in Sjogren's syndrome. Morphologic, biochemical, and immunologic findings. Arthritis Rheum 1985;28(4): 388–94.
111. Pokorny G, Karacsony G, Lonovics J, et al. Types of atrophic gastritis in patients with primary Sjogren's syndrome. Ann Rheum Dis 1991;50(2):97–100.

112. Collin P, Karvonen AL, Korpela M, et al. Gastritis classified in accordance with the Sydney system in patients with primary Sjögren's syndrome. Scand J Gastroenterol 1997;32(2):108–11.
113. Ostuni PA, Germana B, Di Mario F, et al. Gastric involvement in primary Sjögren's syndrome. Clin Exp Rheumatol 1993;11(1):21–5.
114. Szodoray P, Barta Z, Lakos G, et al. Coeliac disease in Sjögren's syndrome: a study of 111 Hungarian patients. Rheumatol Int 2004;24(5):278–82.
115. Mok MY. Protein losing enteropathy and primary Sjögren's syndrome. Clin Exp Rheumatol 1997;15(6):705.
116. Nagashima T, Hoshino M, Shimoji S, et al. Protein-losing gastroenteropathy associated with primary Sjögren's syndrome: a characteristic oriental variant. Rheumatol Int 2009;29(7):817–20.
117. Uraoka Y, Tanigawa T, Watanabe K, et al. Complete remission of protein-losing gastroenteropathy associated with Sjögren's syndrome by B cell-targeted therapy with rituximab. Am J Gastroenterol 2012;107(8):1266–8.
118. Yamashita H, Muto G, Hachiya R, et al. A case of Sjögren's syndrome complicated by protein-losing gastroenteropathy with unprecedented pulmonary interstitial lesions. Mod Rheumatol 2014;24(5):877–9.
119. Liao C-Y, Chien S-T, Wang C-C, et al. Sjögren's syndrome associated with protein losing gastroenteropathy manifested by intestinal lymphangiectasia successfully treated with prednisolone and hydroxychloroquine. Lupus 2015; 24(14):1552–6.
120. Iltanen S, Collin P, Korpela M, et al. Celiac disease and markers of celiac disease latency in patients with primary Sjögren's syndrome. Am J Gastroenterol 1999;94(4):1042–6.
121. Collin P, Reunala T, Pukkala E, et al. Coeliac disease–associated disorders and survival. Gut 1994;35(9):1215–8.
122. Hayakawa T, Naruse S, Kitagawa M, et al. Clinical aspects of autoimmune pancreatitis in Sjogren's syndrome. JOP 2001;2(3):88–92.
123. Rueda JC, Duarte-Rey C, Casas N. Successful treatment of relapsing autoimmune pancreatitis in primary Sjogren's syndrome with rituximab: report of a case and review of the literature. Rheumatol Int 2009;29(12):1481–5.
124. Lindstrom E, Lindstrom F, von Schenck H, et al. Pancreatic ductal morphology and function in primary Sjogren's syndrome. Int J Pancreatol 1991;8(2):141–9.
125. Nishimori I, Morita M, Kino J, et al. Pancreatic involvement in patients with Sjogren's syndrome and primary biliary cirrhosis. Int J Pancreatol 1995;17(1):47–54.
126. Coll J, Navarro S, Tomas R, et al. Exocrine pancreatic function in Sjögren's syndrome. Arch Intern Med 1989;149(4):848.
127. Afzelius PIA, Fallentin EMVAM, Larsen S, et al. Pancreatic function and morphology in Sjögren's syndrome. Scand J Gastroenterol 2010;45(6):752–8.
128. Csepregi A, Szodoray P, Zeher M. Do autoantibodies predict autoimmune liver disease in primary Sjogren's syndrome? Data of 180 patients upon a 5 year follow-up. Scand J Immunol 2002;56:623–9.
129. Kaplan MJ, Ike RW. The liver is a common non-exocrine target in primary Sjögren's syndrome: a retrospective review. BMC Gastroenterol 2002;2:21.
130. Montano-Loza AJ, Crispin-Acuna JC, Remes-Troche JM, et al. Abnormal hepatic biochemistries and clinical liver disease in patients with primary Sjogren's syndrome. Ann Hepatol 2007;6(3):150–5.
131. Wang L, Zhang F-C, Chen H, et al. Connective tissue diseases in primary biliary cirrhosis: a population-based cohort study. World J Gastroenterol 2013;19(31): 5131–7.

132. Uddenfeldt P, Danielsson Å, Forsell Å, et al. Features of Sjögren's syndrome in patients with primary biliary cirrhosis. J Intern Med 1991;230:443–8.

133. Skopouli F, Barbatis C, Moutsopoulos H. Liver involvement in primary Sjögren's syndrome. Br J Rheumatol 1994;33:745–8.

134. Tsianos E, Hoofnagle J, Fox P, et al. Sjogren's syndrome in patients with primary biliary cirrhosis. Hepatology 1990;11:730–4.

135. Sun Y, Zhang W, Li B, et al. The coexistence of Sjögren's syndrome and primary biliary cirrhosis: a comprehensive review. Clin Rev Allergy Immunol 2015; 48(2–3):301–15.

136. Matsumoto T, Morizane T, Aoki Y, et al. Autoimmune hepatitis in primary Sjogren's syndrome: pathological study of the livers and labial salivary glands in 17 patients with primary Sjogren's syndrome. Pathol Int 2005;55(2):70–6.

137. Karp JK, Akpek EK, Anders RA. Autoimmune hepatitis in patients with primary Sjögren's syndrome: a series of two-hundred and two patients. Int J Clin Exp Pathol 2010;3(6):582–6.

138. Simon TA, Thompson A, Gandhi KK, et al. Incidence of malignancy in adult patients with rheumatoid arthritis: a meta-analysis. Arthritis Res Ther 2015;17:212.

139. Hashimoto A, Chiba N, Tsuno H, et al. Incidence of malignancy and the risk of lymphoma in Japanese patients with rheumatoid arthritis compared to the general population. J Rheumatol 2015;42(4):564–71.

140. Somers EC, Thomas SL, Smeeth L, et al. Are individuals with an autoimmune disease at higher risk of a second autoimmune disorder? Am J Epidemiol 2009;169:749–55.

141. Somers EC, Thomas SL, Smeeth L, et al. Autoimmune diseases co-occurring within individuals and within families: a systematic review. Epidemiology 2006; 17(2):202–17.

142. Wong GW, Heneghan MA. Association of extrahepatic manifestations with autoimmune hepatitis. Dig Dis 2015;33(suppl 2):25–35.

143. Utiyama SRR, Zenatti KB, Nóbrega HAJ, et al. Rheumatic disease autoantibodies in autoimmune liver diseases. Immunol Invest 2016;45(6):566–73.

144. Migita K, Nakamura M, Abiru S, et al. Association of STAT4 polymorphisms with susceptibility to type-1 autoimmune hepatitis in the Japanese population. Sookoian SC. PLoS One 2013;8(8):e71382.

145. Carbone M, Neuberger JM. Autoimmune liver disease, autoimmunity and liver transplantation. J Hepatol 2014;60(1):210–23.

146. Jegadeesan R, Navaneethan U, Bharadwaj S, et al. Impact of concurrent non-IBD immunological diseases on the outcome of primary sclerosing cholangitis. Inflamm Bowel Dis 2016;22(4):948–54.

147. Weng X, Liu L, Barcellos LF, et al. Clustering of inflammatory bowel disease with immune mediated diseases among members of a northern California-managed care organization. Am J Gastroenterol 2007;102(7):1429–35.

148. Cohen R, Robinson D, Paramore C, et al. Autoimmune disease concomitance among inflammatory bowel disease patients in the United States, 2001-2002. Inflamm Bowel Dis 2008;14(6):738–43.

149. Lerner A, Matthias T. Rheumatoid arthritis-celiac disease relationship: joints get that gut feeling. Autoimmun Rev 2015;14(11):1038–47.

150. Keane J, Gershon S, Wise R, et al. Tuberculosis associated with infliximab, a tumor necrosis factor alpha-neutralizing agent. N Engl J Med 2001;345(15): 1098–104.

151. Farer LS, Lowell AM, Meador MP. Extrapulmonary tuberculosis in the United States. Am J Epidemiol 1979;109(2):205–17.

152. Yoshinaga Y, Kanamori T, Ota Y, et al. Clinical characteristics of *Mycobacterium tuberculosis* infection among rheumatoid arthritis patients. Mod Rheumatol 2004;14(2):143–8.
153. Kourbeti IS, Ziakas PD, Mylonakis E. Biologic therapies in rheumatoid arthritis and the risk of opportunistic infections: a meta-analysis. Clin Infect Dis 2014; 58(12):1649–57.
154. Ai J-W, Zhang S, Ruan Q-L, et al. The risk of tuberculosis in patients with rheumatoid arthritis treated with tumor necrosis factor- antagonist: a metaanalysis of both randomized controlled trials and registry/cohort studies. J Rheumatol 2015;42(12):2229–37.
155. Marshall JB. Tuberculosis of the gastrointestinal tract and peritoneum. Am J Gastroenterol 1993;88(7):989–99.
156. Horvath KD, Whelan RL. Intestinal tuberculosis: return of an old disease. Am J Gastroenterol 1998;93(5):692–6.
157. Winthrop KL, Chang E, Yamashita S, et al. Nontuberculous mycobacteria infections and anti-tumor necrosis factor-α therapy. Emerg Infect Dis 2009;15(10): 1556–61.
158. Assi MA, Sandid MS, Baddour LM, et al. Systemic histoplasmosis: a 15-year retrospective institutional review of 111 patients. Medicine (Baltimore) 2007; 86:162–9.
159. Winthrop KL, Yamashita S, Beekmann SE, et al. Mycobacterial and other serious infections in patients receiving anti–tumor necrosis factor and other newly approved biologic therapies: case finding through the emerging infections network. Clin Infect Dis 2008;46(11):1738–40.
160. Wallis RS, Broder MS, Wong JY, et al. Granulomatous infectious diseases associated with tumor necrosis factor antagonists. Clin Infect Dis 2004;38(9):1261–5.
161. Hage CA, Bowyer S, Tarvin SE, et al. Recognition, diagnosis, and treatment of histoplasmosis complicating tumor necrosis factor blocker therapy. Clin Infect Dis 2010;50(1):85–92.
162. Lee JH, Slifman NR, Gershon SK, et al. Life-threatening histoplasmosis complicating immunotherapy with tumor necrosis factor alpha antagonists infliximab and etanercept. Arthritis Rheum 2002;46(10):2565–70.
163. Kahi CJ, Wheat LJ, Allen SD, et al. Gastrointestinal histoplasmosis. Am J Gastroenterol 2005;100(1):220–31.
164. Bergstrom L, Yocum DE, Ampel NM, et al. Increased risk of coccidioidomycosis in patients treated with tumor necrosis factor alpha antagonists. Arthritis Rheum 2004;50(6):1959–66.
165. Dweik M, Baethge BA, Duarte AG. Coccidioidomycosis pneumonia in a nonendemic area associated with infliximab. South Med J 2007;100(5):517–8.
166. Rogan MP, Thomas K. Fatal miliary coccidioidomycosis in a patient receiving infliximab therapy: a case report. J Med Case Rep 2007;1:79.
167. Castillo CG, Kauffman CA, Miceli MH. Blastomycosis. Infect Dis Clin North Am 2016;30(1):247–64.
168. Mincer HH, Oglesby RJ. Intraoral North American blastomycosis. Oral Surg Oral Med Oral Pathol 1966;22(1):36–41.
169. Bell WA, Gamble J, Garrington GE. North American blastomycosis with oral lesions. Oral Surg Oral Med Oral Pathol 1969;28(6):914–23.
170. Simon GB, Berson SD, Young CN. Blastomycosis of the tongue: a case report. S Afr Med J 1977;52(2):82–3.
171. Page LR, Drummond JF, Daniels HT, et al. Blastomycosis with oral lesions. Report of two cases. Oral Surg Oral Med Oral Pathol 1979;47(2):157–60.

172. Rose HD, Gingrass DJ. Localized oral blastomycosis mimicking actinomycosis. Oral Surg Oral Med Oral Pathol 1982;54(1):12–4.

173. Damm DD, Fantasia JE. Exophytic mass of buccal mucosa. Blastomycosis. Gen Dent 2002;50(6):561, 564.

174. Khandekar A, Moser D, Fidler WJ. Blastomycosis of the esophagus. Ann Thorac Surg 1980;30(1):76–9.

175. McKenzie R, Khakoo R. Blastomycosis of the esophagus presenting with gastrointestinal bleeding. Gastroenterology 1985;88(5 Pt 1):1271–3.

176. Deutsch J, Burke T, Nelson T. Pancreatic and splenic blastomycosis in an immune-competent woman diagnosed by endoscopic ultrasonography-guided fine-needle aspiration. Endoscopy 2007;39(Suppl 1):E272–3.

177. Salmon-Ceron D, Tubach F, Lortholary O, et al. Drug-specific risk of non-tuberculosis opportunistic infections in patients receiving anti-TNF therapy reported to the 3-year prospective French RATIO registry. Ann Rheum Dis 2011; 70(4):616–23.

178. Lavery EA, Coyle WJ. Herpes simplex virus and the alimentary tract. Curr Gastroenterol Rep 2008;10(4):417–23.

179. Mourgues C, Henquell C, Tatar Z, et al. Monitoring of Epstein-Barr virus (EBV)/cytomegalovirus (CMV)/varicella-zoster virus (VZV) load in patients receiving tocilizumab for rheumatoid arthritis. Joint Bone Spine 2016;83(4):412–5.

180. Vallet H, Houitte R, Azria A, et al. Cytomegalovirus colitis and hypo-IgG after rituximab therapy for rheumatoid arthritis. J Rheumatol 2011;38(5):965–6.

181. Komura T, Ohta H, Nakai R, et al. Cytomegalovirus reactivation induced acute hepatitis and gastric erosions in a patient with rheumatoid arthritis under treatment with an anti-IL-6 receptor antibody, tocilizumab. Intern Med 2016;55(14): 1923–7.

182. Panteris V, Karakosta A, Merikas E, et al. Gastric outlet obstruction due to cytomegalovirus infection in an immunocompromised patient. Case Rep Gastroenterol 2009;3(3):280–5.

183. Goodgame RW. Gastrointestinal cytomegalovirus disease. Ann Intern Med 1993;119:924–35.

184. Disorders O. Cytomegalovirus infection of the human gastrointestinal tract. J Gastroenterol Hepatol 1999;14:973–6.

185. Bernard S, Germi R, Lupo J, et al. Symptomatic cytomegalovirus gastrointestinal infection with positive quantitative real-time PCR findings in apparently immunocompetent patients: a case series. Clin Microbiol Infect 2015;21(12):1121.e1-7.

186. Stam F, Kolkman JJ, Jiwa MM, et al. Cytomegalovirus gastritis in an immunocompetent patient. J Clin Gastroenterol 1996;22(4):322–4.

187. Dinesh BV, Selvaraju K, Kumar S, et al. Cytomegalovirus-induced colonic stricture presenting as acute intestinal obstruction in an immunocompetent adult. BMJ Case Rep 2013;2013 [pii:bcr-2013-200944].

188. Canterino JE, McCormack M, Gurung A, et al. Cytomegalovirus appendicitis in an immunocompetent host. J Clin Virol 2016;78:9–11.

189. Villar LA, Massanari R, Mitros F. Cytomegalovirus infection with acute erosive esophagitis. Am J Med 1984;76:924–8.

190. Venkataramani A, Schlueter A, Spech T, et al. Cytomegalovirus esophagitis in an immunocompetent host. Gastrointest Endosc 1994;40(3):392–3.

191. Klauber E, Briski LE, Khatib R. Cytomegalovirus colitis in the immunocompetent host: an overview. Scand J Infect Dis 1998;30(6):559–64.

192. Kim SY, Solomon DH. Tumor necrosis factor blockade and the risk of viral infection. Nat Rev Rheumatol 2010;6(3):165–74.

Gastrointestinal and Hepatic Disease in the Inflammatory Myopathies

Chiranjeevi Gadiparthi, MD, MPH[a], Amneet Hans, MD[b],
Kyle Potts, MD[b], Mohammad K. Ismail, MD[c],*

KEYWORDS

- Corticosteroids • Creatine kinase • Dermatomyositis • Inclusion body myositis
- Oropharyngeal dysphagia • Polymyositis

KEY POINTS

- Oropharyngeal dysphagia due to the involvement of pharyngeal and proximal esophageal musculature is the most common gastrointestinal symptom in myositis, and severe cases are generally associated with inclusion body myositis.
- Inflammatory myopathy should be considered in the differential diagnosis of unexplained dysphagia because it may occur without other muscular or skin manifestations.
- Because of increased risk of occult malignancies, especially in the first year, age-appropriate cancer screening such as colonoscopy is recommended upon the diagnosis of inflammatory myopathy.
- Recurrent or worsening myopathy or skin symptoms in dermatomyositis patients warrants reevaluation for occult malignancy.
- Elevation of aminotransferases in inflammatory myopathy patients can be of skeletal muscle origin rather than from the liver.

Conflicts of Interest: All authors declare no conflicts of interest for this article, including financial, consultant, institutional, and other relationships that might lead to bias or conflict of interest.
Financial Support: There was no financial or grant support for this study.
Author Contributions: C. Gadiparthi, A. Hans, and M.K. Ismail were responsible for drafting, critical revision, and approval of the final article.
All authors were involved in the final approval of the version of the article submitted and have agreed to be accountable for all aspects of the work.
Potential Competing Interests: None.
^a Division of Gastroenterology and Hepatology, University of Tennessee Health Science Center, 1211 Union Avenue, Suite # 340, Memphis, TN 38104, USA; ^b University of Colorado School of Medicine, 13001 E 17th Pl, Aurora, CO 80045, USA; ^c Division of Gastroenterology and Hepatology, University of Tennessee Health Sciences Center, 1211 Union Avenue, Suite #460, Memphis, TN 38104, USA
* Corresponding author.
E-mail address: mismail@uthsc.edu

INTRODUCTION

The idiopathic inflammatory myopathies are a group of acquired heterogeneous autoimmune disorders characterized by the hallmark feature of muscle weakness. Proximal muscle weakness, when present, is often disabling. Because of insidious nature of the disease and nonspecific symptoms such as malaise and fatigue, diagnosis can frequently be delayed. The diagnosis is particularly challenging when the nonmuscular organ involvement such as gastrointestinal, pulmonary, or cardiac manifestations precedes muscle weakness. The extent and severity of associated systemic organ involvement varies with each type of inflammatory myopathy. Dermatomyositis (DM), due to the characteristic skin rash, may be better recognized than other inflammatory myopathies. Because of such challenges and the heterogeneity of inflammatory myopathies, understanding the pathogenesis and nonmuscular systemic organ involvement is critical for the diagnosis and management of this unique group of patients. The diagnosis of inflammatory myopathies is based on elevated serum muscle enzymes, electromyographic abnormalities, and presence of inflammatory infiltrate in the skeletal muscle resulting in symmetric proximal muscle weakness.[1]

The inflammatory myopathies are classified into 3 major categories: polymyositis (PM), DM, and inclusion body myositis (IBM). However, 2 other subtypes, necrotizing autoimmune myositis and overlap syndrome have been increasingly recognized as distinct entities.[2] This classification is largely based on clinical, immunopathologic, and dermatologic characteristics.[3]

Epidemiology

The prevalence of inflammatory myopathies is not very precisely known and estimated largely based on epidemiologic studies that do not perform systematic sampling of the general population. Nevertheless, the evidence suggests that PM and DM are very rare diseases with estimated incidence of 1 to 10 new cases per million persons per year.[4–8] In the United States, based on the medical claims data from a large managed care database, the adjusted annual incidence rate of inflammatory myopathies is 5.8 to 7.9 per 100,000 person-years and annual prevalence is 14.0 to 17.4 per 100,000, which is higher than elsewhere.[9] Women are affected at a higher rate than men, generally at 2:1 ratio, and as high as 5:1 during childbearing years.[4,8] The adult inflammatory myopathies usually occur in middle age with an average age of onset for DM and PM ranging from 52 to 56 years. In contrast, IBM occurs in later years with mean age of onset of 67 years, and it is more common in men.[8,10] On the other hand, juvenile DM is the most common (85% cases) form of juvenile inflammatory myopathies with a median age of onset of 7.5 years.[11]

The systemic organ involvement associated with inflammatory myopathies includes arthritis, cardiac arrhythmias, pulmonary and gastrointestinal symptoms. A myriad of gastrointestinal disorders involving oropharynx, esophagus, stomach, liver, small intestine, colon, and rectum has been reported in inflammatory myopathy patients (**Table 1**). In addition, there is a substantial increase in risk of occult malignancies, including the gastrointestinal cancers in myopathy patients, especially in those with DM. In this review, the authors focus on the gastrointestinal and hepatic manifestations associated with inflammatory myopathies.

Table 1
Gastrointestinal and hepatic manifestations of inflammatory myopathies based on the area of involvement

	Involvement	Comments
Oropharynx and esophagus	1. Dysphagia 2. Gastrointestinal reflux 3. Atonic esophagus	1. Severe dysphagia in IBM 2. Increased underlying malignancy 3. Higher mortality
Stomach	1. Delayed gastric emptying and gastroparesis 2. Vasculitis of stomach and ulceration[a] 3. Gastric cancer	1. Vasculitis is common in children 2. Gastric cancer is associated with DM
Pancreas	Pancreatic cancer[b]	Pancreatic cancer is the most common gastrointestinal malignancy
Small intestine	1. Pneumatosis cytoides intestinalis 2. Intestinal motility disorders 3. CIP 4. Celiac disease	
Colon and rectum	1. Vasculopathy of colon[b] 2. Crohn's disease [bc] 3. Ulcerative colitis 4. Colon and rectal cancer	Treating IBD symptoms improve myopathy symptoms
Liver	1. Elevated transaminases 2. Fatty liver disease 3. AIH 4. PBC	1. Elevated transaminases are frequently from muscle injury 2. Fatty liver is most common

Abbreviations: AIH, Auto-immune hepatitis; CIP, chronic intestinal pseudo-obstuction; IBD, inflammatory bowel disease; PBC, primary biliary cholangitis.
[a] Juvenile dermatomyositis.
[b] Adult dermatomyositis.
[c] Polymyositis.

OROPHARYNGEAL AND ESOPHAGEAL MANIFESTATIONS

Oropharynx and upper esophagus are the most common areas of gastrointestinal involvement associated with inflammatory myopathies. In myopathy patients, dysphagia is the most common gastrointestinal symptom, with various studies reporting a wide range of prevalence, 10% to 73%.[12–14] Dysphagia typically refers to difficulty in eating because of disruption in the swallowing process. It is a subjective sensation suggesting the presence of an organic abnormality in the passage of liquids or solids from the oral cavity to the stomach. Patients' complaints range from the inability to initiate a swallow to the sensation of solids or liquids being hindered during their passage through the esophagus into the stomach.

Dysphagia can be classified as either oropharyngeal or esophageal. Oropharyngeal dysphagia, also called transfer dysphagia, arises from disorders that affect the function of the oropharynx, larynx, and upper esophageal sphincter. Neurogenic and myogenic disorders as well as oropharyngeal tumors are the most common underlying causes for oropharyngeal dysphagia. Esophageal dysphagia arises within the body of the esophagus, the lower esophageal sphincter, or cardia, and is most commonly due to mechanical causes or a motility disturbance.

Dysphagia is more prevalent in patients with IBM, often is more severe and refractory to treatment.[13] Dysphagia in inflammatory myopathies is predominantly due to the involvement of striated muscle of hypopharynx and upper esophageal sphincter leading to oropharyngeal dysphagia. The underlying pathophysiologic mechanisms are similar to the involvement of skeletal muscle elsewhere—chronic inflammation, edema, muscular atrophy, and very rarely spontaneous esophageal rupture.[15,16] In a longitudinal study conducted in Japan, there was an increased incidence of underlying malignancy in DM patients who had concomitant dysphagia.[17] Although there is no evidence to support routine screening for cancers in dysphagia patients, other cancer-related symptoms should prompt further evaluation. Presence of dysphagia increases the risk of death in patients with inflammatory myopathy. In a retrospective study by Williams and colleagues,[14] 31% of inflammatory myopathy patients with dysphagia died at 12 months. Respiratory failure resulting from aspiration pneumonia was the most common cause of death in dysphagia patients.

Symptoms

Dysphagia can be for both solids and liquids. Patients may experience hoarseness of voice, inability to swallow food bolus, coughing while eating, nasal speech and nasal regurgitation, reflux symptoms, and laryngitis. According to a Mayo Clinic study by Oh and colleagues[13] evaluating 783 patients with inflammatory myopathy, 62 patients had dysphagia, and the most commonly reported symptoms were difficulty with solid and dry foods (96%), feeling of food stuck in the throat (85%), and coughing while eating (75%). Severe and persistent dysphagia in inflammatory myositis patients can have serious consequences including malnutrition and aspiration pneumonia.

Diagnosis

Dysphagia may sometimes be the only manifestation of inflammatory myopathy, and the absence of involvement of facial, bulbar, or proximal muscles can lead to considerable delay in the diagnosis. Although rare, inflammatory myopathies should be considered in differential diagnosis of unexplained dysphagia. Physical examination findings are nonspecific and include nasal voice, weakness of vocal cords, and inability to elevate the palate.

The diagnostic sensitivity of elevated serum creatine kinase (CK) is about 75% in inflammatory myopathy patients with dysphagia (ie, one-fourth of patients may have normal CK levels), and it has high positive predictive value.[14] Myositis-specific antibodies, although insensitive, tend to be specific for particular clinical manifestations and can be useful in establishing the diagnosis.[18] Other laboratory parameters include elevated erythrocyte sedimentation rate and antinuclear antibody (ANA).[14]

Modified barium swallow with videofluoroscopy in conjunction with an oropharyngeal examination by a speech pathologist can provide a more objective measure of swallowing.[19] The videofluoroscopy with barium swallow involves the swallowing of barium suspension of varying consistency, fluid and semi-solid, by the patient. This procedure may reveal a prolonged pharyngeal phase, regurgitation and tracheal aspiration, barium retention in the hypopharynx along with atony of pyriform fossa, and rarely Zenker diverticulum.[20,21] Esophageal motility studies with manometry may show abnormally low esophageal sphincter pressures with normal relaxation and low-amplitude nonperistaltic contractions.[22] The findings of upper endoscopy may be non-specific, showing esophagitis and strictures.[22] A combination of video-fibrolaryngoscopy and videofluoroscopy is probably the best approach for evaluating the dysphagia in myopathy patients. Cricopharyngeal dysfunction may mimic oropharyngeal dysphagia of myositis due to similar anatomic involvement of the cricopharyngeus muscle. However, Cricopharyngeal dysfunction is characterized by rigid contraction of the muscle resulting in blockage of the food during deglutition, whereas in myositis-associated dysphagia, the musculature is too weak to propel the food bolus forward.[23]

The muscular dysphagia associated with inflammatory myopathies should be differentiated from dysphagia in acute stroke and other neuromuscular disorders, such as muscular dystrophy, myasthenia gravis, Parkinson disease, poliomyelitis, and motor neuron diseases. Poliomyelitis usually occurs in children and results in flaccid paresis of the lower extremities more frequently than upper extremities. Muscular dystrophies are a group of genetic disorders that cause progressive irreversible weakness and loss of muscle mass and are associated with dysphagia at later stages. Parkinson disease is a neurodegenerative disease with insidious onset and slow progression, associated with rigidity, tremor, and bradykinesia. Dysphagia usually occurs in later stages in Parkinson patients and can be very disabling. Steroid-induced myopathy resulting from long-term steroid use is another entity that may emulate inflammatory myopathy because of its characteristic proximal muscle weakness. Unlike the muscle inflammation in myositis patients, muscle biopsy in steroid-induced myopathy may show atrophy. Therefore biopsy of involved muscles in dysphagia patients, as with any other inflammatory myopathy, is the gold standard in establishing the diagnosis. In practice, however, it is cumbersome and not performed routinely in dysphagia patients because of the proximity of pharyngeal musculature to vital organs.

Treatment

As with any dysphagia, initial management includes modification of food and fluid consistency, evaluation of the patient by a speech pathologist, and providing advice on the consistency and quantity of food and fluid in the diet, as well as education regarding various positioning techniques (chin tuck) to improve swallowing. There are no randomized control trials that have evaluated the efficacy of glucocorticoids or immunosuppressive agents (disease modifying anti-rheumatic drugs) in inflammatory myopathy patients with dysphagia. However, glucocorticoids remain a mainstay of treatment, despite evidence is largely anecdotal. Immunosuppressive agents, including methotrexate, cyclosporine, azathioprine, and cyclophosphamide can be used in addition to glucocorticoids.[12]

In steroid-resistant PM and DM patients, intravenous immunoglobulin (IVIG) has been used successfully for life-threatening esophageal involvement. In a study by Marie and colleagues,[24] 73 steroid-resistant patients including 25 who had life-threatening esophageal impairment necessitating exclusive enteral feeding, received 2 mg/kg IVIG infusions monthly. Sixty patients (82.2%) had complete resolution of esophageal symptoms, enabling the return of normal oral feeding.

Glucocorticoid and immunosuppressive agents are usually ineffective in treating IBM patients with dysphagia. Such patients may benefit from extended myotomy involving the constrictor muscle above and the esophageal musculature below.[13,25] Other interventions, such as balloon dilatation and botulinum toxin injections have been tried with variable success.[13] If these measures fail, then evaluation for an alternative route for nutritional support must be considered. Enteral nutrition can be achieved through various means including nasogastric or nasoenteric tube, the percutaneous endoscopic (or radiologically placed) gastrostomy (PEG) or jejunostomy tubes.[26] These tubes are placed through the abdominal wall into the stomach (gastrostomy) or the intestine (jejunostomy). Although these are generally safe, one study reported a higher mortality (64%) in patients who required PEG tube.[13] However, the higher mortality in this study probably suggests the severity of the underlying dysphagia rather than complications related to PEG tube.

Stomach and Small Intestine

Although oropharynx and esophagus are the most commonly affected regions in the gastrointestinal tract, stomach and small intestinal involvement is seen infrequently as well. Vasculitis involving the gastrointestinal tract may occur in juvenile DM patients, leading to acute noninflammatory enteropathy. Pathogenic mechanisms causing acute enteropathy in juvenile DM patients are arterial and venous hyperplasia as well as occlusive thrombi in the submucosal and serosal blood vessels of the gastrointestinal tract.[12] Acute ischemia results from small and medium-sized arterial narrowing and occlusion.[27,28] These patients experience severe abdominal pain, constipation, vomiting, including hematemesis; ischemic ulcers and perforation can occur in severe cases.[29–32]

Several case reports of pneumatosis cystoides intestinalis have been reported in patients with DM and PM due to alveolar rupture of affected lung leading to retroperitoneal dissection.[33–38] A rare case of Juvenile DM has been reported with atonic esophagus associated with delayed gastric emptying and intestinal mucosal thickening with a characteristic radiographic appearance of "stacked coins" on upper gastrointestinal series with small bowel follow-through.[39] This patient was successfully treated with prednisone and other immunosuppressive agents, including daily azathioprine and weekly methotrexate, resulting in resolution of symptoms. Delayed gastric emptying suggestive of gastroparesis has been reported in patients with PM and DM in old case reports; however, to the best of the authors' knowledge, no recent cases have been reported.[40]

INTESTINAL PSEUDO-OBSTRUCTION

Chronic intestinal pseudo-obstruction (CIP) is an uncommon disorder characterized by recurrent obstructive symptoms without a mechanical obstruction causing significant morbidity and mortality. Typical clinical presentation of CIP varies widely based on the functional derangement of the affected region in the gastrointestinal tract. Although abdominal pain, nausea, and vomiting are more predominant with upper gastrointestinal involvement, abdominal distension and constipation are suggestive of a more distal involvement. Diarrhea and steatorrhea can occur as a result of small intestinal bacterial overgrowth. Because of recurrent symptoms, CIP patients often undergo unnecessary exploratory laparotomy.

The involvement of small intestine in systemic sclerosis and scleroderma is well recognized. Although very rare, inflammatory myositis has been implicated in patients with CIP.[41] Barium study with small intestinal follow-through may assist in differentiating systemic sclerosis from inflammatory myopathy affecting the small intestine.[42] PM usually involves the duodenum and jejunum, causing dilatation and mucosal crowding, resulting in segmental ileus. The pseudodiverticulae, which are pathognomonic of systemic sclerosis, are usually not seen in PM. The circular valvulae of the small intestine become thin in systemic sclerosis, whereas they may be thickened in PM.

In a cross-sectional study involving 20 adult patients with CIP, 65% had visceral myopathy; however, one patient had inflammatory myositis.[43] Dewit and colleagues[44] reported another case of CIP in a 37-year-old woman, who underwent full-thickness intestinal biopsy that revealed diffuse infiltration of smooth muscle by T-lymphocytes and plasma cells, thus confirming the inflammatory myositis. Although therapy with glucocorticoids was unsuccessful, treatment with cyclosporine resulted in spontaneous bowel movement 3 months after persistent pseudo-obstruction. Although glucocorticoids are usually effective for musculoskeletal manifestations of inflammatory myopathy patients, they may be not adequate in treating visceral myopathy symptoms. In one case report, a DM patient with anti-EJ autoanti-body who developed CIP showed an improvement in symptoms when treated with octreotide. Although this strategy appears to be promising, more evidence is needed to validate the effectiveness of octreotide in these patients.[45]

CELIAC DISEASE

Celiac disease is a chronic inflammatory autoimmune disease of the small intestine precipitated by an abnormal immune response to peptides found in gluten-rich dietary products in susceptible individuals. Although celiac disease is associated with several other autoimmune diseases, its true prevalence in inflammatory myopathy patients is not known. According to a study by Selva-O'Callaghan and colleagues[46] in Spain, among 51 consecutive adult patients diagnosed with inflammatory myopathy who were followed for a 2-year period, 17 (31%) patients had immunoglobulin A (IgA)-class antigliadin antibodies (AGA). However, none of them had positive antitissue transglu-taminase or antiendomysial antibodies, which are more specific for celiac disease. Out of 5 patients who underwent jejunal biopsy, 3 had villous atrophy and crypt hyperpla-sia consistent with celiac disease; however, the myopathy symptoms of these patients did not respond to a gluten-free diet. Based on these observations, the investigators concluded that AGA are more frequently found in myopathy patients than in the gen-eral population, and celiac disease appears to be more prevalent in these patients. Positive status to HLA-DQ2 allele, which is known to be more frequent in patients with inflammatory myopathies, could explain the high prevalence of AGA in this pop-ulation, but the diagnostic value of HLA-DQ2 or -DQ8 haplotypes to detect celiac dis-ease in patients with inflammatory myopathy is limited.

In another study, patients with gluten sensitivity who had myopathy symptoms and elevated CK reported improvement of muscle symptoms with gluten-free diet.[47] However, the results of this study should be applied with caution because only 1 out of 13 patients had IBM on muscle biopsy, suggesting a possible alternative etiology for myopathy (such as vitamin D deficiency or hypothyroidism) in the remain-ing patients. Nevertheless, large population-based studies are required to estimate the true prevalence of celiac disease in inflammatory myopathy patients and to eval-uate the effect of a gluten free diet on myopathy symptoms.

COLON AND RECTUM

DM associated vasculopathy of the colon, associated with noninflammatory acute endarteropathy, is more frequently reported in children. Only 1% to 6% of adult DM patients may have vasculopathy. A case of vasculopathy of the colon was reported in a 63-year-old patient admitted with severe abdominal pain and distention.[48] There were multiple ischemic ulcers in the transverse and descending colon, complicated by perforation. A variety of vascular changes were noted in the microscopic examination including lymphoplasmocytic infiltration around and within the vessel walls, various degrees of venous occlusion, and intimal hyperplasia of the arteries. However, another study reported endoscopic findings of edematous hyperemic bowel wall, multiple ero-sions, and ulcerative lesions with histology demonstrating diffuse mucosal inflamma-tion and multiple vascular ectasias without vasculitis in adults with DM.[49]

INFLAMMATORY BOWEL DISEASE

Crohn's disease and ulcerative colitis are reported in patients with inflammatory myopathy; however, the true prevalence is unknown. Crohn's disease with concurrent

DM or PM has been described in case reports.[50,51] Interestingly, the myopathy symptoms resolved and CK normalized in these patients with successful treatment of Crohn's disease. Thus, in patients with coexistent Crohn's and inflammatory myopathy, it appears that treating the inflammatory bowel disease may be a more prudent approach than using glucocorticoids for treating myopathy symptoms.

A few case reports have suggested an association between ulcerative colitis and DM.[52-54] In addition, Tseng and colleagues,[55] using a nationwide cohort in Taiwan, reported that ulcerative colitis was associated with an increased cumulative incidence of DM, independent of age, sex, and concomitant autoimmune diseases such as rheumatoid arthritis or systemic lupus erythematosus (hazard ratio: 6.19, 95% confidence interval (CI): 1.77–21.29; $P = .004$). In this large national cohort of patients from 1998 to 2011, the cumulative incidence of DM and PM were compared between ulcerative colitis patients (n = 3133) and control (n = 14,726) subjects. Although cumulative incidence of DM increased in the ulcerative colitis group compared with the control group ($P = .026$), PM had similar incidence among the two groups ($P = .596$). The exact underlying mechanism for increased cumulative incidence of DM and ulcerative colitis is unknown; however, in genetically susceptible individuals, a dysregulated mucosal immune response to commensal gut microbiota is thought to play a role.[55] At the molecular level, ulcerative colitis and DM share common susceptibility loci such as interferon regulatory factor 5 and vitamin D receptor.[56-59] The Tseng study has a small sample size; thus, more studies are needed to verify the findings and evaluate if the severity and course of ulcerative colitis are different in DM patients. These studies would be necessary before justifying a modified therapeutic approach. However, because of the relatively rare incidence of both DM and ulcerative colitis, identifying a large cohort of patients with coincidence of these 2 conditions may not be feasible.

GASTROINTESTINAL MALIGNANCIES

An increased risk of malignancy is associated with inflammatory myopathies, particularly with DM and less frequently with PM. Of DM patients, 24% have underlying malignancy, commonly adenocarcinoma, and the risk of cancer is highest during the first year of diagnosis of myositis.[60]

Epidemiology

Increased risk of cancer associated with inflammatory myopathies was first reported several decades ago. In Western countries, ovarian, cervical, lung, and gastrointestinal cancers, as well as lymphoma are commonly associated with inflammatory myopathies, whereas nasopharyngeal cancer is more common in China, Southeast Asia, and Northern Africa. Based on several large population-based cohort studies conducted in Australia, Scandinavian countries, and Scotland, the frequency of cancers in inflammatory myopathy patients is 10% to 30%, with a stronger association with DM.[61-64] Among 618 patients with DM from a pooled national discharge data from Sweden, Finland, and Denmark, 198 patients were diagnosed with cancers.[62] In DM patients, there was an increased relative risk of gastrointestinal and nongastrointestinal cancers with a cumulative standardized incidence ratio (SIR) of 3.0 (95% CI: 2.5–3.6). The gastrointestinal cancers with high SIR were pancreatic cancer (3.8; 95% CI: 1.6–9.0), gastric cancer (3.5; 95% CI: 1.7–7.3), and colorectal cancer (2.5; 95% CI: 1.4–4.4). Although PM was associated with non-Hodgkin lymphoma and bladder cancer, there was no significant risk associated with gastrointestinal malignancies. It is important to note that these epidemiologic studies largely examined Caucasians and may not be generalizable to other ethnicities.

Huang and colleagues,[65] using a national database in Taiwan, showed that among DM patients of Chinese descent, there was an increased risk of nasopharyngeal, lung, and breast cancers but not of gastrointestinal cancers. The combined relative risk of cancers, according to a meta-analysis by Zantos and colleagues,[66] is 4.4 (95% CI: 3.0–6.6) with DM and 2.1 (95% CI: 1.4–3.3) with PM. Although the risk of cancer is higher in adult myopathy patients, there is no increased risk reported in juvenile DM or other myopathies in children. Several studies have identified the risk factors that increase the likelihood of underlying malignancy in inflammatory myopathy patients. These demographic, clinical, and laboratory features are summarized in **Box 1**.[59,62,64,67–69]

Pathogenesis

The underlying molecular mechanisms implicated in the increased cancer risk associated with myopathy (CAM) are not very clear. However, a complex interaction of several factors, including host factors, infectious and toxic triggers, and paraneoplastic syndromes, may play a role in carcinogenesis in these patients.[60] Despite the absence of robust evidence of genetic predisposition, the association between *HLADQA1*0301* and anti-p155/140 antibodies in Caucasian patients suggests some genetic basis for cancer in inflammatory myopathy.[70] Other mechanisms, such as "crossover" immunity, are proposed, whereby the autoantibodies directed against the autoantigens expressed in tumor cells may cross over and act as myositis-specific antibodies, leading to myositis. For example, in a study of patients with colorectal cancer, Zampieri and colleagues[71] demonstrated an increased activity of muscle inflammation and regeneration of myofibrils in the rectus abdominis muscle without clinical evidence of myositis based on the biopsy findings performed at the time of surgery. This supports the hypothesis of crossover immunity due to cancer-induced muscle injury leading to subclinical myositis in patients with colorectal cancer. More recent study demonstrated that DM and CAM exhibit similarities in gene expression and immunohistochemical findings, suggesting that humoral immunity is the main underlying mechanism implicated in both myopathies.[72] This adds to existing evidence for the importance of cancer screening in inflammatory myopathy patients, particularly those with DM.

Box 1
Demographic, clinical, and laboratory risk factors associated with malignancy in inflammatory myopathies

High-risk features

1. Older age

2. Male sex

3. Severe and rapid muscle weakness

4. Severe skin involvement with necrosis and ulceration

5. Dysphagia

6. Elevated ESR and CRP

7. Low complement level

8. Antitranscriptional intermediary factor (TIF1γ/α)

Abbreviations: CRP, C-reactive protein; ESR, erythrocyte sedimentation rate.

Screening and Diagnosis

According to Hill's study, the risk of cancer is highest during the first year (60%–70%) after the diagnosis of DM and decreases thereafter; however, it continues to remain higher than that of the general population.[62] DM is also considered to be a paraneoplastic syndrome because the severity of muscular and skin manifestations tends to follow the course of cancer, improving or resolving after the treatment of cancer and worsening during cancer relapse. Patients with DM-associated rectal cancer noted resolution of cutaneous symptoms following the resection of the rectal cancer.[73,74] However, during the follow-up, DM flare indicated metastatic disease, supporting the hypothesis of paraneoplastic manifestation of DM. Cancer recurrence should always be suspected in inflammatory myopathy patients who experience sudden exacerbation of previously well-controlled CAM or cutaneous symptoms; and such patients should undergo careful evaluation for metastatic disease or relapse of the primary cancer.

Comprehensive history and physical examination are mandatory in patients with newly diagnosed inflammatory myopathy, and clinicians should maintain a high index of suspicion for an underlying malignancy. Age-appropriate cancer screening such as colonoscopy should be performed at the time of diagnosis of myopathy, especially DM. Computerized tomography scan and upper gastrointestinal endoscopy in myopathy patients for the screening of other gastrointestinal cancers, including gastric and pancreatic cancers in the absence of other symptoms (unexplained weight loss or abdominal pain), are controversial. Some studies have identified high-risk features of malignancy, such as older age, presence of dysphagia, severe myopathy that is glucocorticoid refractory, and severe skin rash associated with necrosis.[61,67–69,75]

The utility of myositis-related autoantibody testing in predicting the risk of CAM was studied in a cross-sectional study in the United Kingdom.[76] According to this study, a positive anti-p150/144 antibody was highly specific and moderately sensitive with high negative predictive value for CAM. On the other hand, a negative myositis associated antibody panel (anti-Jo-1, anti-PM-Scl, anti-U1-RNP, anti-U3-RNP, and anti-Ku antibodies) was highly sensitive and had high negative predictive value. Overall, a combination of these 2 approaches will be highly sensitive and have high negative predictive value for CAM. Therefore, patients who fall into the high-risk category based on the autoantibody testing may need more intense and thorough evaluation for cancer screening and surveillance. More recent studies showed that myositis-specific autoantibodies, particularly antitranscriptional intermediary factor (TIF1γ/α) in DM, were associated with underlying malignancy.[77,78]

HEPATIC MANIFESTATIONS

A variety of hepatic manifestations in inflammatory myopathy patients have been described, including elevated liver enzymes and an association with other conditions, such as viral hepatitis, fatty liver disease, primary biliary cholangitis (PBC), and autoimmune hepatitis (AIH). Matsumoto and colleagues[79] reported several liver histopathology findings in a large case series of 160 patients with collagen vascular diseases that included 18 patients with PM and DM. Hepatic manifestations in these 18 patients were fatty liver 12 (66.7%), hepatic congestion 9 (50%), nonspecific reactive hepatitis 2 (11.1%), hepatic arteritis 1 (5.6%), and PBC 1 (5.6%). According to this study, fatty liver disease seems to be the most common manifestation in inflammatory myopathy patients.

PBC is a chronic autoimmune cholestatic liver disease, frequently (90%–95%) associated with the characteristic marker of positive antimitochondrial antibodies (AMA).

Although positive AMA can be a common occurrence in inflammatory myopathy patients, the prevalence of PBC in these patients is rarely reported. In one study, inflammatory myopathy patients with positive AMA had unique characteristics, such as chronic disease course, muscle atrophy, cardiac involvement, and granulomatous inflammation on histopathology, compared with those with negative AMA.[80]

AIH, which is frequently associated with other rheumatic disorders such as rheumatoid arthritis and Sjögren syndrome, is uncommon in inflammatory myopathy patients. A few cases of AIH in PM/DM patients have been reported; however, except for one case report, these cases were associated with other conditions including hepatitis C virus (HCV) infection, myasthenia gravis, sarcoidosis, Sjögren syndrome, and systemic sclerosis.[81–85] Therefore, a strong association between AIH and inflammatory myopathies is unlikely.

Elevated Transaminases

Elevation of aspartate aminotransferase and alanine aminotransferase is usually a marker of hepatocellular injury. However, the elevated transaminases can be of extrahepatic origin, including skeletal muscle, heart, kidney, and pancreas.[86] Elevated transaminases are frequently found in inflammatory myopathy patients. This elevation generally follows the trend of serum CK level, suggesting that the skeletal muscle as most likely source of transaminases, rather than the liver. In a large series of 85 patients with inflammatory myopathy attending a rheumatology clinic at a county hospital, 80% had elevated serum transaminases at the time of presentation.[87] Following the treatment of inflammatory myopathy and normalization of CK levels, 85% of the patients with elevated transaminases demonstrated normalization, suggesting a strong correlation between CK level and transaminases. Several other studies also suggested strong correlation between CK level and transaminases.[88,89] Therefore, evaluation for hepatic dysfunction is not routinely required if elevated aminotransferases improve with normalization of CK and resolution of myopathy symptoms. However, if elevated liver enzymes in these patients do not temporally follow the CK level, and in the presence of other signs of liver disease, further evaluation into other causes of liver involvement is warranted.

Hepatitis B and C

A few cases of chronic HCV infection have been reported in patients with IBM.[90–93] A recent case-control study in Japanese patients showed increased prevalence of HCV in IBM patients compared with those with PM (28% vs 4.5%).[94] More importantly, there was occurrence of myositis symptoms after treatment with interferon-α and ribavirin treatment in IBM patients with HCV, suggesting the possible role of medications in development of myositis symptoms. These results may be unique to the Japanese population, because similar studies have not been conducted among other ethnicities or in other geographic areas, limiting the generalizability of the findings.

Hepatitis B virus infection (HBV) has been reported, albeit rarely, in patients with PM.[95] Rare case reports of DM associated with HBV and hepatocellular carcinoma are also published.[96,97] Myositis symptoms in a patient with HBV infection worsened with exacerbation of hepatitis, suggesting that the activity of HBV is closely related to myositis symptoms.[98]

SUMMARY

The principal manifestation of idiopathic inflammatory myopathies is muscle weakness. However, extramuscular organ involvement is also well documented and frequently seen in clinical practice. In addition to considerable heterogeneity in the onset, presentation, and prognosis of various types of myopathies, the extent and severity of systemic organ involvement also varies substantially in each category. The onset of nonmuscular systemic symptoms may precede muscular or cutaneous manifestations, resulting in considerable delay in the diagnosis. More importantly, myopathy patients frequently present to nonrheumatology practices that may not be well equipped to recognize the vague symptoms associated with these rare disorders. Therefore, a thorough understanding of the disease course and the systemic manifestations is crucial for accurate diagnosis and institution of appropriate therapy to improve the outcomes. Gastrointestinal symptoms, such as difficulty in swallowing, dyspepsia, nausea, early satiety, abdominal pain, and gastrointestinal bleeding, may suggest a serious underlying abnormality. Thus, comprehensive evaluation and prompt referral to a gastroenterologist may be warranted.

Severe cases of dysphagia that are associated with IBM need aggressive therapy and a multidisciplinary care because of the substantial risk of morbidity and mortality. Although rare, myositis should be considered in the differential diagnosis of CIP. In myopathy patients with associated Crohn's disease and ulcerative colitis, treating the inflammatory bowel disease frequently improves the myositis symptoms. Although the association between occult malignancy and DM justifies early screening, patients with PM should also undergo thorough and age-appropriate cancer screening, including colonoscopy, as part of standard of care.

Elevated transaminases in myopathy patients can be from underlying muscle injury especially in the setting of elevated CK level; therefore, evaluation for underlying liver disease should be approached conservatively. Although the evidence is not robust, glucocorticoids remain the mainstay of treatment in myopathy patients for both muscular and nonmuscular systemic symptoms including the gastrointestinal disorders. In addition, other immunosuppressive agents, such as azathioprine, methotrexate, cyclophosphamide, and cyclosporine can be used, depending on the severity and extent of myopathy. IVIG has a role in severe and life-threatening cases of dysphagia that are refractory to therapy.

REFERENCES

1. Dalakas MC, Hohlfeld R. Polymyositis and dermatomyositis. Lancet 2003; 362(9388):971–82.

2. Dalakas MC. Inflammatory muscle diseases. N Engl J Med 2015;372(18): 1734–47.

3. Briani C, Doria A, Sarzi-Puttini P, et al. Update on idiopathic inflammatory myopathies. Autoimmunity 2006;39(3):161–70.

4. Oddis CV, Conte CG, Steen VD, et al. Incidence of polymyositis-dermatomyositis: a 20-year study of hospital diagnosed cases in Allegheny County, PA 1963-1982. J Rheumatol 1990;17(10):1329–34.

5. Benbassat J, Geffel D, Zlotnick A. Epidemiology of polymyositis-dermatomyositis in Israel, 1960-76. Isr J Med Sci 1980;16(3):197–200.

6. Weitoft T. Occurrence of polymyositis in the county of Gavleborg, Sweden. Scand J Rheumatol 1997;26(2):104–6.

7. Koh ET, Seow A, Ong B, et al. Adult onset polymyositis/dermatomyositis: clinical and laboratory features and treatment response in 75 patients. Ann Rheum Dis 1993;52(12):857–61.

8. Dobloug C, Garen T, Bitter H, et al. Prevalence and clinical characteristics of adult polymyositis and dermatomyositis; data from a large and unselected Norwegian cohort. Ann Rheum Dis 2015;74(8):1551-6.
9. Furst DE, Amato AA, Iorga SR, et al. Epidemiology of adult idiopathic inflammatory myopathies in a U.S. managed care plan. Muscle Nerve 2012;45(5):676-83.
10. Tan JA, Roberts-Thomson PJ, Blumbergs P, et al. Incidence and prevalence of idiopathic inflammatory myopathies in South Australia: a 30-year epidemiologic study of histology-proven cases. Int J Rheum Dis 2013;16(3):331-8.
11. Rider LG, Katz JD, Jones OY. Developments in the classification and treatment of the juvenile idiopathic inflammatory myopathies. Rheum Dis Clin North Am 2013; 39(4):877-904.
12. Ebert EC. Review article: the gastrointestinal complications of myositis. Aliment Pharmacol Ther 2010;31(3):359-65.
13. Oh TH, Brumfield KA, Hoskin TL, et al. Dysphagia in inflammatory myopathy: clinical characteristics, treatment strategies, and outcome in 62 patients. Mayo Clin Proc 2007;82(4):441-7.
14. Williams RB, Grehan MJ, Hersch M, et al. Biomechanics, diagnosis, and treatment outcome in inflammatory myopathy presenting as oropharyngeal dysphagia. Gut 2003;52(4):471-8.
15. Kleckner FS. Dermatomyositis and its manifestations in the gastrointestinal tract. Am J Gastroenterol 1970;53(2):141-6.
16. Dougenis D, Papathanasopoulos PG, Paschalis C, et al. Spontaneous esophageal rupture in adult dermatomyositis. Eur J Cardiothorac Surg 1996;10(11): 1021-3.
17. Mugii N, Hasegawa M, Matsushita T, et al. Oropharyngeal dysphagia in dermatomyositis: associations with clinical and laboratory features including autoantibodies. PLoS One 2016;11(5):e0154746.
18. Satoh M, Tanaka S, Ceribelli A, et al. A comprehensive overview on myositis-specific antibodies: new and old biomarkers in idiopathic inflammatory myopathy. Clin Rev Allergy Immunol 2017;52(1):1-19.
19. Barbiera F, Condello S, De Palo A, et al. Role of videofluorography swallow study in management of dysphagia in neurologically compromised patients. Radiol Med 2006;111(6):818-27.
20. Belafsky PC, Mims JW, Postma GN, et al. Dysphagia and aspiration secondary to polymyositis. Ear Nose Throat J 2002;81(5):316.
21. Georgalas C, Baer ST. Pharyngeal pouch and polymyositis: association and implications for aetiology of Zenker's diverticulum. J Laryngol Otol 2000;114(10): 805-7.
22. de Merieux P, Verity MA, Clements PJ, et al. Esophageal abnormalities and dysphagia in polymyositis and dermatomyositis. Arthritis Rheum 1983;26(8): 961-8.
23. Dietz F, Logeman JA, Sahgal V, et al. Cricopharyngeal muscle dysfunction in the differential diagnosis of dysphagia in polymyositis. Arthritis Rheum 1980;23(4): 491-5.
24. Marie I, Menard JF, Hatron PY, et al. Intravenous immunoglobulins for steroid-refractory esophageal involvement related to polymyositis and dermatomyositis: a series of 73 patients. Arthritis Care Res 2010;62(12):1748-55.
25. Houser SM, Calabrese LH, Strome M. Dysphagia in patients with inclusion body myositis. Laryngoscope 1998;108(7):1001-5.
26. The role of percutaneous endoscopic gastrostomy in enteral feeding. Guidelines for clinical application. Gastrointest Endosc 1988;34(3 Suppl):35s-6s.

27. Mamyrova G, Kleiner DE, James-Newton L, et al. Late-onset gastrointestinal pain in juvenile dermatomyositis as a manifestation of ischemic ulceration from chronic endarteropathy. Arthritis Rheum 2007;57(5):881–4.

28. Crowe WE, Bove KE, Levinson JE, et al. Clinical and pathogenetic implications of histopathology in childhood polydermatomyositis. Arthritis Rheum 1982;25(2): 126–39.

29. Downey EC Jr, Woolley MM, Hanson V. Required surgical therapy in the pediatric patient with dermatomyositis. Arch Surg 1988;123(9):1117–20.

30. Takeda T, Fujisaku A, Jodo S, et al. Fatal vascular occlusion in juvenile dermatomyositis. Ann Rheum Dis 1998;57(3):172–3.

31. Wang IJ, Hsu WM, Shun CT, et al. Juvenile dermatomyositis complicated with vasculitis and duodenal perforation. J Formos Med Assoc 2001;100(12):844–6.

32. Ramirez G, Asherson RA, Khamashta MA, et al. Adult-onset polymyositis-dermatomyositis: description of 25 patients with emphasis on treatment. Semin Arthritis Rheum 1990;20(2):114–20.

33. Pasquier E, Wattiaux MJ, Peigney N. First case of pneumatosis cystoides intestinalis in adult dermatomyositis. J Rheumatol 1993;20(3):499–503.

34. Fischer TJ, Cipel L, Stiehm ER. Pneumatosis intestinalis associated with fatal childhood dermatomyositis. Pediatrics 1978;61(1):127–30.

35. Braunstein EM, White SJ. Pneumatosis intestinalis in dermatomyositis. Br J Radiol 1980;53(634):1011–2.

36. Oliveros MA, Herbst JJ, Lester PD, et al. Pneumatosis intestinalis in childhood dermatomyositis. Pediatrics 1973;52(5):711–2.

37. Kuroda T, Ohfuchi Y, Hirose S, et al. Pneumatosis cystoides intestinalis in a patient with polymyositis. Clin Rheumatol 2001;20(1):49–52.

38. Zarbalian Y, von Rosenvinge EC, Twadell W, et al. Recurrent pneumatosis intestinalis in a patient with dermatomyositis. BMJ Case Rep 2013;2013 [pii: bcr2013200308].

39. Laskin BL, Choyke P, Keenan GF, et al. Novel gastrointestinal tract manifestations in juvenile dermatomyositis. J Pediatr 1999;135(3):371–4.

40. Weston S, Thumshirn M, Wiste J, et al. Clinical and upper gastrointestinal motility features in systemic sclerosis and related disorders. Am J Gastroenterol 1998; 93(7):1085–9.

41. Boardman P, Nolan DJ. Case report: small intestinal pseudo-obstruction: an unusual manifestation of polymyositis. Clin Radiol 1998;53(9):706–7.

42. Feldman F, Marshak RH. Dermatomyositis with significant involvement of the gastrointestinal tract. Am J Roentgenol Radium Ther Nucl Med 1963;90:746–52.

43. Mann SD, Debinski HS, Kamm MA. Clinical characteristics of chronic idiopathic intestinal pseudo-obstruction in adults. Gut 1997;41(5):675–81.

44. Dewit S, de Hertogh G, Geboes K, et al. Chronic intestinal pseudo-obstruction caused by an intestinal inflammatory myopathy: case report and review of the literature. Neurogastroenterol Motil 2008;20(4):343–8.

45. Yamada C, Sato S, Sasaki N, et al. A case of dermatomyositis and Anti-EJ autoantibody with chronic intestinal pseudoobstruction successfully treated with octreotide. Case Rep Rheumatol 2016;2016:9510316.

46. Selva-O'Callaghan A, Casellas F, de Torres I, et al. Celiac disease and antibodies associated with celiac disease in patients with inflammatory myopathy. Muscle Nerve 2007;35(1):49–54.

47. Hadjivassiliou M, Chattopadhyay AK, Grunewald RA, et al. Myopathy associated with gluten sensitivity. Muscle Nerve 2007;35(4):443–50.

48. Pulham NJ, Cho M, Chan F. A 63-year-old woman with muscle weakness and abdominal pain. Gastroenterology 2016;150(4):e12–3.
49. Tweezer-Zaks N, Ben-Horin S, Schiby G, et al. Severe gastrointestinal inflammation in adult dermatomyositis: characterization of a novel clinical association. Am J Med Sci 2006;332(6):308–13.
50. Szabo N, Lukacs S, Kulcsar I, et al. Association of idiopathic inflammatory myopathy and Crohn's disease. Clin Rheumatol 2009;28(1):99–101.
51. Shimoyama T, Tamura Y, Sakamoto T, et al. Immune-mediated myositis in Crohn's disease. Muscle Nerve 2009;39(1):101–5.
52. Rayamajhi SJ, Gorla AKR, Basher RK, et al. Unsuspected active ulcerative colitis in a patient with dermatomyositis: a rare association detected on 18F-FDG PET/CT during the search for an occult malignancy. Indian J Nucl Med 2017; 32(2):130–2.
53. Hayashi T, Nakamura T, Kurachi K, et al. Ulcerative colitis accompanied with sarcoidosis and dermatomyositis: report of a case. Dis Colon Rectum 2008; 51(4):474–6.
54. Bodoki L, Nagy-Vincze M, Griger Z, et al. Anti-NXP2-positive dermatomyositis associated with ulcerative colitis and celiac disease. Orv Hetil 2014;155(26): 1033–8 [in Hungarian].
55. Tseng CC, Chang SJ, Liao WT, et al. Increased cumulative incidence of dermatomyositis in ulcerative colitis: a nationwide cohort study. Sci Rep 2016;6:28175.
56. Xue LN, Xu KQ, Zhang W, et al. Associations between vitamin D receptor polymorphisms and susceptibility to ulcerative colitis and Crohn's disease: a meta-analysis. Inflamm Bowel Dis 2013;19(1):54–60.
57. Jostins L, Ripke S, Weersma RK, et al. Host-microbe interactions have shaped the genetic architecture of inflammatory bowel disease. Nature 2012; 491(7422):119–24.
58. Dzhebir G, Kamenarska Z, Hristova M, et al. Association of vitamin D receptor gene BsmI B/b and FokI F/f polymorphisms with adult dermatomyositis and systemic lupus erythematosus. Int J Dermatol 2016;55(8):e465–8.
59. Chen S, Wang Q, Wu Z, et al. Genetic association study of TNFAIP3, IFIH1, IRF5 polymorphisms with polymyositis/dermatomyositis in Chinese Han population. PLoS One 2014;9(10):e110044.
60. Zahr ZA, Baer AN. Malignancy in myositis. Curr Rheumatol Rep 2011;13(3): 208–15.
61. Buchbinder R, Forbes A, Hall S, et al. Incidence of malignant disease in biopsy-proven inflammatory myopathy. A population-based cohort study. Ann Intern Med 2001;134(12):1087–95.
62. Hill CL, Zhang Y, Sigurgeirsson B, et al. Frequency of specific cancer types in dermatomyositis and polymyositis: a population-based study. Lancet 2001; 357(9250):96–100.
63. Airio A, Pukkala E, Isomaki H. Elevated cancer incidence in patients with dermatomyositis: a population based study. J Rheumatol 1995;22(7):1300–3.
64. Stockton D, Doherty VR, Brewster DH. Risk of cancer in patients with dermatomyositis or polymyositis, and follow-up implications: a Scottish population-based cohort study. Br J Cancer 2001;85(1):41–5.
65. Huang YL, Chen YJ, Lin MW, et al. Malignancies associated with dermatomyositis and polymyositis in Taiwan: a nationwide population-based study. Br J Dermatol 2009;161(4):854–60.
66. Zantos D, Zhang Y, Felson D. The overall and temporal association of cancer with polymyositis and dermatomyositis. J Rheumatol 1994;21(10):1855–9.

67. Andras C, Ponyi A, Constantin T, et al. Dermatomyositis and polymyositis associated with malignancy: a 21-year retrospective study. J Rheumatol 2008;35(3): 438–44.
68. Fardet L, Dupuy A, Gain M, et al. Factors associated with underlying malignancy in a retrospective cohort of 121 patients with dermatomyositis. Medicine (Baltimore) 2009;88(2):91–7.
69. Ponyi A, Constantin T, Garami M, et al. Cancer-associated myositis: clinical features and prognostic signs. Ann N Y Acad Sci 2005;1051:64–71.
70. Targoff IN, Mamyrova G, Trieu EP, et al. A novel autoantibody to a 155-kd protein is associated with dermatomyositis. Arthritis Rheum 2006;54(11):3682–9.
71. Zampieri S, Valente M, Adami N, et al. Polymyositis, dermatomyositis and malignancy: a further intriguing link. Autoimmun Rev 2010;9(6):449–53.
72. Noda T, Iijima M, Noda S, et al. Gene expression profile of inflammatory myopathy with malignancy is similar to that of dermatomyositis rather than polymyositis. Intern Med 2016;55(18):2571–80.
73. Ono K, Shimomura M, Toyota K, et al. Successful resection of liver metastasis detected by exacerbation of skin symptom in a patient with dermatomyositis accompanied by rectal cancer: a case report and literature review. Surg Case Rep 2017;3(1):3.
74. Nagano Y, Inoue Y, Shimura T, et al. Exacerbation of dermatomyositis with recurrence of rectal cancer: a case report. Case Rep Oncol 2015;8(3):482–6.
75. Basset-Seguin N, Roujeau JC, Gherardi R, et al. Prognostic factors and predictive signs of malignancy in adult dermatomyositis. A study of 32 cases. Arch Dermatol 1990;126(5):633–7.
76. Chinoy H, Fertig N, Oddis CV, et al. The diagnostic utility of myositis autoantibody testing for predicting the risk of cancer-associated myositis. Ann Rheum Dis 2007;66(10):1345–9.
77. Ceribelli A, Isailovic N, De Santis M, et al. Myositis-specific autoantibodies and their association with malignancy in Italian patients with polymyositis and dermatomyositis. Clin Rheumatol 2017;36(2):469–75.
78. Hida A, Yamashita T, Hosono Y, et al. Anti-TIF1-gamma antibody and cancer-associated myositis: a clinicohistopathologic study. Neurology 2016;87(3): 299–308.
79. Matsumoto T, Kobayashi S, Shimizu H, et al. The liver in collagen diseases: pathologic study of 160 cases with particular reference to hepatic arteritis, primary biliary cirrhosis, autoimmune hepatitis and nodular regenerative hyperplasia of the liver. Liver 2000;20(5):366–73.
80. Maeda MH, Tsuji S, Shimizu J. Inflammatory myopathies associated with anti-mitochondrial antibodies. Brain 2012;135(Pt 6):1767–77.
81. Ko KF, Ho T, Chan KW. Autoimmune chronic active hepatitis and polymyositis in a patient with myasthenia gravis and thymoma. J Neurol Neurosurg Psychiatry 1995;59(5):558–9.
82. Marie I, Levesque H, Courtois H, et al. Polymyositis, cranial neuropathy, autoimmune hepatitis, and hepatitis C. Ann Rheum Dis 2000;59(10):839–40.
83. Lis-Swiety A, Brzezinska-Wcislo L, Pierzchala E, et al. Systemic sclerosis-polymyositis overlap syndrome accompanied by autoimmune hepatitis and sarcoidosis of mediastinal lymphnodes. J Eur Acad Dermatol Venereol 2006; 20(1):107–8.
84. Stefanidis I, Giannopoulou M, Liakopoulos V, et al. A case of membranous nephropathy associated with Sjogren syndrome, polymyositis and autoimmune hepatitis. Clin Nephrol 2008;70(3):245–50.

85. Hounoki H, Shinoda K, Ogawa R, et al. Simultaneously developed polymyositis and autoimmune hepatitis. BMJ Case Rep 2011;2011 [pii:bcr0920114763].
86. Bohlmeyer TJ, Wu AH, Perryman MB. Evaluation of laboratory tests as a guide to diagnosis and therapy of myositis. Rheum Dis Clin North Am 1994;20(4):845–56.
87. Mathur T, Manadan AM, Thiagarajan S, et al. Serum transaminases are frequently elevated at time of diagnosis of idiopathic inflammatory myopathy and normalize with creatine kinase. J Clin Rheumatol 2014;20(3):130–2.
88. Edge K, Chinoy H, Cooper RG. Serum alanine aminotransferase elevations correlate with serum creatine phosphokinase levels in myositis. Rheumatology (Oxford) 2006;45(4):487–8.
89. Volochayev R, Csako G, Wesley R, et al. Laboratory test abnormalities are common in polymyositis and dermatomyositis and differ among clinical and demographic groups. Open Rheumatol J 2012;6:54–63.
90. Alexander JA, Huebner CJ. Hepatitis C and inclusion body myositis. Am J Gastroenterol 1996;91(9):1845–7.
91. Kase S, Shiota G, Fujii Y, et al. Inclusion body myositis associated with hepatitis C virus infection. Liver 2001;21(5):357–60.
92. Tsuruta Y, Yamada T, Yoshimura T, et al. Inclusion body myositis associated with hepatitis C virus infection. Fukuoka Igaku Zasshi 2001;92(11):370–6.
93. Yakushiji Y, Satoh J, Yukitake M, et al. Interferon beta-responsive inclusion body myositis in a hepatitis C virus carrier. Neurology 2004;63(3):587–8.
94. Uruha A, Noguchi S, Hayashi YK, et al. Hepatitis C virus infection in inclusion body myositis: a case-control study. Neurology 2016;86(3):211–7.
95. Mihas AA, Kirby JD, Kent SP. Hepatitis B antigen and polymyositis. JAMA 1978;239(3):221–2.
96. Yang SY, Cha BK, Kim G, et al. Dermatomyositis associated with hepatitis B virus-related hepatocellular carcinoma. Korean J Intern Med 2014;29(2):231–5.
97. Kee SJ, Kim TJ, Lee SJ, et al. Dermatomyositis associated with hepatitis B virus-related hepatocellular carcinoma. Rheumatol Int 2009;29(5):595–9.
98. Nojima T, Hirakata M, Sato S, et al. A case of polymyositis associated with hepatitis B infection. Clin Exp Rheumatol 2000;18(1):86–8.

Gastrointestinal and Hepatic Disease in Fibromyalgia

Richard A. Schatz, MD[a],*, Baharak Moshiree, MD, MS-CI[b]

KEYWORDS

- Irritable bowel syndrome • Central sensitization • Fibromyalgia • Abdominal pain
- Hyperalgesia

KEY POINTS

- Considerable overlap exists between fibromyalgia (FM) and functional gastrointestinal diseases such as irritable bowel syndrome (IBS) in terms of pathophysiology, lack of a biomarkers, and treatment options.
- Central and peripheral sensitization accounts for both visceral and somatic pain experienced by patients with FM and IBS.
- Pharmacologic, psychological, and dietary treatments for FM and IBS are similar and effective. The degree of improvements in patients' quality of life depends on the strength of the patient-physician relationship.
- Hepatic disease in patients with FM is rare, although comorbid conditions such as obesity may increase the risk of nonalcoholic steatohepatitis.

OVERVIEW

Gastrointestinal (GI) symptoms and conditions are common in fibromyalgia (FM), as well as in other rheumatologic diseases, including connective tissue disorders, spondylarthritides, and rheumatoid arthritis. FM has been linked to several GI and hepatology diseases, including but not limited to irritable bowel syndrome (IBS), gastroesophageal reflux disease, functional dyspepsia, and viral hepatitis. The most well-substantiated evidence and literature relates to IBS, a common GI condition characterized by abdominal pain, and altered bowel habits otherwise unexplained by

Disclosure Statement: R. Schatz, no relevant disclosures; B. Moshiree, grant support from Prometheus Lab and Medtronic; advisory boards of Allergan, Ironwood, and Synergy Pharmaceuticals.
[a] Division of Gastroenterology and Hepatology, Medical University of South Carolina, 114 Doughty Street, STB Suite 249, Charleston, SC 29425, USA; [b] Division of Gastroenterology, Carolinas HealthCare System, 1025 Morehead Medical Drive, Suite 300, Charlotte, NC 28204, USA
* Corresponding author.
E-mail address: schatzr@musc.edu

alternative methodologies or diagnoses. Like FM, the underlying pathogenesis for IBS remains unclear, although dysregulation within the brain-gut axis resulting in a hyperalgesic state has been hypothesized.

Aside from its pathogenesis, IBS and FM share many other similarities, including a female predominance, fatigue, insomnia, and well-described psychiatric aspects. These common manifestations and pathogenesis of disease serve as a foundation for overlapping treatment modalities, including pharmacologic and psychological therapies (see later discussion). Indeed, the tremendous heterogeneity in terms of pathogenesis and symptom profile among patients with both disorders prevents the use of a universally applicable treatment algorithm. Instead, treatment using trial-and-error and a multidisciplinary approach is required for optimal management.

GASTROINTESTINAL DISORDERS IN FIBROMYALGIA
Introduction

GI diseases are commonly seen in FM in addition to all other rheumatologic diseases and disorders, including connective tissue disorders such as system lupus erythematosus, scleroderma, Ehler-Danlos syndrome, and rheumatoid arthritis. This article focuses predominantly on the overlap between FM and IBS, a functional disorder that not only overlaps with other GI disorders such as functional dyspepsia but also with non-GI disorders such as temporomandibular joint disorder, interstitial cystitis, and chronic fatigue syndrome. Evidence is lacking about whether patients with FM have higher rates of other common GI disorders (besides IBS). These disorders may include gastroesophageal reflux disease, esophageal hypersensitivity, and functional dyspepsia. Interestingly, studies have suggested an alteration of central brain activation, immune dysfunction, and an enhanced pain perception that is similar for these visceral pain disorders and FM (a somatic pain syndrome) with similar psychosocial risk factors that impair patient's quality of life.[1] This article discusses how IBS and FM have shared multifactorial bases and how, therefore, their treatments are similar.

Irritable bowel syndrome

Overview IBS is a common, widely prevalent GI condition characterized by abdominal pain associated with an alteration in bowel habits otherwise unexplained by anatomic, structural, or metabolic pathologic assessment.[2,3] Frequently, nonspecific GI symptoms of bloating, flatulence, nausea, and fecal urgency are also present. The diagnosis is established by the fulfillment of the recently updated Rome IV guidelines in which patients manifest recurrent abdominal pain on average at least 1 day per week in the last 3 months with symptom onset for at least 6 months prior, associated with 2 or more of the following criteria:[4,5]

1. Relation to defecation
2. Change in form (appearance) of stool
3. Change in stool frequency.

The underlying pathogenesis of patients with IBS remains unclear, although dysregulation within the brain-gut axis is generally regarded as the central, unifying hypothesis.[6] The dysregulation is likely multifactorial and results from a combination of impairment in gut motility, visceral hypersensitivity, altered mucosal and immune function, change in gut microbiota, and central processing of sensory input.[7,8]

Classification of irritable bowel syndrome Given that IBS is a clinical diagnosis that involves multiple subjective components, multiple different disease indices have been developed to afford better quality research and treatment outcomes. These scales, among others, include the Irritable Bowel Syndrome Quality of Life Questionnaire (a condition-specific IBS quality of life measure), the Cognitive Scale for Functional Bowel Disorders, and the Functional Bowel Disorder Severity Index (FBDSI).[9] The latter assesses severity of disease based on a scoring system (mild, moderate, or severe) that depends on the presence and intensity of pain, the diagnosis of a functional abdominal pain syndrome, and the number of health care visits in the previous 6 months.[10]

Different subclasses of IBS depend on the predominant bowel habit: constipation-predominant (IBS-C), diarrhea-predominant (IBS-D), mixed bowel habits (IBS-M), and otherwise unclassified IBS (IBS-U).[11] Likewise, treatments for IBS are often tailored to the specific subtype in which the patient is classified.

Association of irritable bowel syndrome and fibromyalgia

There is a longstanding, well-established association between IBS and FM.[12–15] In fact, FM is the most commonly studied IBS comorbidity.[15] In patients with IBS the prevalence of FM is 32.5% (range: 28%–65%) and in patients with FM the prevalence of IBS is 48% (range: 32%–77%) per a comprehensive review by Whitehead and colleagues[15] from 2002. The strength of association seems to correlate well with the level of severity scored by the aforementioned FBDSI.[9,16]

IBS and FM share multiple similarities and comorbidities. Aside from a female predominance, patients with both diseases have higher rates of sleep problems, chronic fatigue, comorbid anxiety, and/or depression. Both disorders can profoundly impair patients' activities of daily living, diminish overall quality of life, and carry high health care expenditures. Likewise, their onset is often associated with a significantly traumatic or stressful event. Such similarities serve as a foundation for overlapping treatment modalities, including psychotherapy and hypnosis, cognitive-behavioral therapies (CBTs), analgesics, and antidepressants (see later discussion).[12,13,17,18]

IBS and FM are traditionally categorized as central sensitivity disorders in which patients tend to aberrantly perceive pain by hyperalgesia and receptive field expansion.[19,20] IBS was classically regarded as a disease of chronic visceral hypersensitivity, whereas FM was characterized by chronic somatic pain discomfort. Newer studies have attempted to debunk this theory by demonstrating widespread somatic hyperalgesia and hypersensitivity in subjects with IBS, providing greater support for a link between the 2 conditions.[13,21–23]

To better understand their association, the etiologic factors of pain interpretation and neural pain regulation has been studied in FM and IBS. Visceral and somatic afferent fibers that affect pain modulation overlap in certain areas of the central nervous system, including both the brain and spinal cord. The anterior cingulate cortex, which is involved in motivational and affective components of pain and is highly stimulated by viscerosomatic afferent input, has been a focal point and highlighted as a common pathway in the disease processing of both disorders.[17,24] The insula and somatosensory cortices also play important roles in sensory and emotional processing and their subsequent integration.[25] Conditioned pain modulation and central processing, and disinhibition of visceral and somatic input, in addition to the attenuation of diffuse noxious inhibitory control (descending pathways), may contribute to symptoms of greater pain intensity in patients with both disorders.[13,26–29]

Secondary hyperalgesia in patients with IBS and FM has also been pronounced at lumbosacral spinal levels, which perhaps helps explain the increased thermal and visceral hypersensitivity seen in patients with IBS and patients with FM plus IBS compared with healthy controls.[22] Increased spinal neuron excitability at lumbosacral levels, possibly due to anatomic convergence from visceral and somatic nociceptive afferents onto a common pool of spinal neurons, combined with long ascending propriospinal interactions, might help further explain such widespread hyperalgesia.[22,30]

The severity of IBS is determined by a complex interplay of multiple different factors:

1. Intensity of GI symptoms
2. Extraintestinal symptoms and comorbidities
3. Psychosocial factors
4. Degree of disability.

It has been proposed that patients on the mild-moderate disease spectrum tend to exhibit more peripherally generated symptoms with gut-based features (ie, relieved by defecation, worse with eating, and intermittent, crampy abdominal pain), whereas those with severe disease tend to have a more noxious, persistent phenotype with psychosocial and somatic comorbidities.[13,26] For example, increased gut motility or visceral afferent firing worsens GI symptoms, thereby exacerbating psychological distress. This may further increase symptom intensity and push patients into a more severe spectrum of disease.[26,31] This hypothesis holds true for many other central sensitivity disorders, specifically FM,[26] and may explain the higher rates of concomitant FM in patients with more severe IBS.[9,16]

Association of fibromyalgia and hepatic disease

A relationship between FM and both viral hepatitis and nonalcoholic steatohepatitis (NASH) has been postulated, although it remains incompletely understood and somewhat controversial.[32–37] One hypothesis links viral disease with FM via the viral-mediated release of inflammatory cytokines (ie, interleukin-1, interleukin-6, and tumor necrosis factor-alpha), resulting in hyperalgesia and dysregulation of the hypothalamic-pituitary-adrenal (HPA) axis.[38] A recent Irish study (2012) estimated a very high prevalence of FM (57%) in subjects with chronic hepatitis C virus (HCV).[35] Although other investigators have described a prevalence typically ranging from 5% to 20%, many have failed to substantiate any significant association.[39,40] Investigators have similarly suggested a relationship between hepatitis B virus (HBV) infection and the presence of FM in subjects with either chronic, active HBV or inactive HBV carriers.[32,34,37] Although these studies describe greater than 20% prevalence of FM in subjects with HBV infections,[32,37] future well-designed studies with larger numbers of subjects are warranted. Nevertheless, these data suggest that both HCV and HBV, as well as NASH, should at least be considered in the evaluation and workup of secondary FM.

Treatments of comorbid irritable bowel syndrome and fibromyalgia

Addressing patient expectations, education, and goals is essential in the treatment of both FM and IBS. Both patient populations tend to most often benefit from a multidisciplinary and multifaceted treatment approach, tailoring a combination of pharmacologic and nonpharmacologic therapies to each individual.[2,18,41–44] The most relevant and studied nonpharmacologic therapies include exercise, patient education, and CBT. Indeed, the development of positive psychological and/or cognitive characteristics may offset neurobiologic factors that contribute to worsening pain and other comorbid negative symptoms.[45] Nevertheless, the tremendous heterogeneity and symptom profile among patients with these disorders does not allow for a universally applicable algorithm. Instead, treatment modalities using trial and error ultimately dictate the most efficacious balance of treatments.

Pharmacotherapies for irritable bowel syndrome and fibromyalgia The basis of concomitant IBS and FM pharmacotherapies is correcting aberrant neural pathways and neurotransmitter imbalances characteristic of both central pain syndromes. Patients with both disorders tend to have an excess of neurotransmitters implicated in the sensation and perception of pain (ie, substance P, glutamate and other excitatory amino acids, serotonin 5HT-2a/3a), with a relative paucity of those involved in pain inhibition (ie, norepinephrine, serotonin 5HT-1a/b, dopamine). Thus, the most frequently prescribed medications for both conditions are tricyclic antidepressants (TCAs), selective serotonin reuptake inhibitors (SSRIs), serotonin norepinephrine reuptake inhibitors (SNRIs), gabapentin, and pregabalin. These medications have shown to reduce pain, fatigue, and insomnia, and improve physician and patient global assessments.[2,41] Aside from their effect on the central pain threshold, antidepressants may also improve certain GI symptoms via their anticholinergic effects (TCAs), regulation of GI transit, and peripheral antineuropathic actions. Interestingly, although multiple classes of medications are used to treat FM, the only US Food and Drug Administration (FDA)-approved medications for FM are duloxetine, milnacipran, and pregabalin.

Opioids and opioid agonists Current evidence does not support use of opioid-agonists in either IBS or FM, and notably can cause hyperalgesia in FM, worsening symptoms and function.[46] The exception is the mu-opioid receptor agonist tramadol, which can help improve pain in FM, though this improvement in pain is not associated with improved function. Tramadol inhibits norepinephrine and serotonin, which help balance potential dysfunction or deficit in these neurotransmitters. Constipation is a common opioid adverse effect that argues against their use in patients with IBS-C or chronic constipation.[41] There are insufficient data to support the prescription of opioids and other simple analgesics for treatment of either condition, although, unfortunately, these are still used frequently for treatment of pain in IBS and FM, a practice that the authors think is not justified.

Tricyclic antidepressants TCAs serve to increase the concentration of both serotonin and norepinephrine by inhibiting reuptake in spinal neurons, thereby inhibiting descending pain pathways. They have shown benefit in both FM and IBS. Doses used for IBS and FM (ie, amitriptyline 25–75 mg bed time) are typically much lower than doses used to treat depression when the target is regulating the brain-gut axis. A large metaanalysis from 2009 concluded that TCAs induce a positive clinical response and reduce abdominal pain scores in patients with IBS,[47] whereas another metaanalysis demonstrated superiority of TCAs over placebo in the treatment of IBS with a number needed to treat (NNT) of 4.[2] TCAs are most effective in treating patients with IBS-D and IBS-M because the anticholinergic side-effects (ie, constipation) often limit their use in IBS-C.[48,49] TCAs have traditionally provided the strongest evidence for medication efficacy in FM, particularly the combination of amitriptyline with cyclobenzaprine.[43,44] A large meta-analysis from 2016 demonstrated the best results for managing pain compared with other pharmacologic approaches.[43]

Selective serotonin reuptake inhibitors and serotonin norepinephrine reuptake inhibitors SSRIs and SNRIs, including fluoxetine, duloxetine (30–60 mg daily), and milnacipran (titrated to 50–100 mg twice a day), continue to be widely prescribed for patients with both FM and IBS. Some studies have suggested modest benefit in pain, function, and potentially in constipation for patients with IBS-C.[39–41] The American College of Gastroenterology IBS taskforce published a systematic review and meta-analysis (2009) from 5 randomized controlled trials and demonstrated the superiority of SSRIs compared with placebo in the treatment of IBS with an NNT of 3.5 (2). Indeed, SSRIs and SNRIs may be best suited to treat those patients with FM and IBS with comorbid anxiety and depression. Larger, well-designed studies are warranted to better understand their clinical utility and tolerability.[50–52]

Pregabalin Pregabalin is a gamma-aminobutyric acid (GABA) analogue that binds to the alpha(2)delta calcium channel, thereby increasing extracellular GABA concentrations. Initially approved for the treatment of neuropathic pain, it was among first pharmacologic agents approved by the FDA for the treatment of FM. Doses of 300 to 600 mg can reduce pain intensity, sleep disturbances, and fatigue in FM patients,[53–56] and also lead to increased visceral pain threshold in patients with IBS without significant adverse effects.[57] At higher doses (1800–3600 mg divided 3 times daily), gabapentin may also have similar benefits in select patients (eg, IBS-D), although evidence is limited.[58,59] Evidence for the use of pregabalin in IBS and FM was further supported by another recent pilot study (Saito and colleagues, 2016)[60] in which 85 IBS subjects were randomized to 225 mg of pregabalin versus placebo twice daily for 12 weeks. The subjects included all subtypes, including 20% with concomitant FM. The investigators found improvement in the symptoms of bloating and diarrhea. Ongoing phase II studies are pending (available at: ClinicalTrials.gov Identifier: NCT00977197).

Probiotics Probiotics are live microorganisms that, when administered in sufficient amounts, may confer positive health benefits and serve to repopulate, reconstitute, and maintain the appropriate gut microbial milieu. The most common available formulations include the genera *Lactobacillus*, *Bifidobacterium*, *Escherichia*, *Enterococcus*, *Bacillus*, and *Streptococcus*.[61] Studies have previously shown probiotics to be effective in a variety of GI conditions, including IBS,[62–64] and these may be considered as part of a multifaceted approach to FM.[61] Indeed, imbalanced gut microbiota may alter epithelial permeability to activate nociceptive vagal sensory pathways and affect the HPA axis, implicated in the pathogenesis of both IBS and FM. The use of probiotics is thought to not only strengthen gut barrier function but also decrease inflammatory response of the bowel, stimulate release of alpha interferons, and mitigate visceral hypersensitivity.[64–66] Although some patients respond favorably with limited side effects, the magnitude of the benefit remains uncertain.[67,68] Furthermore, insufficient research exists to optimally guide which specific probiotic product to prescribe for which patient.

Nonpharmacologic therapies
Cognitive behavioral therapy and hypnotherapy As part of the multidisciplinary approach to these disorders, CBT and hypnotherapy may improve pain-related behavior, self-efficacy, coping strategies, and overall physical function in select patients.[69–72] This approach is particularly effective for short-term pain reduction.[73] The premise of CBT is that dysfunctional thinking and maladaptive responses generate pathologic negative emotions, thereby adversely affecting subsequent behaviors, emotions, and even the visceral response.[69] Thus, the goal of therapy is to assist patients in better understanding these impaired mental patterns and improve on them via educational and behavioral interventions. For IBS, long-term data have shown both CBT[74] and hypnotherapy[75] to be effective. A recent study (2016) demonstrated similar global improvement in GI symptoms with gut-directed hypnotherapy compared with the low fermentable oligo-di-mono-saccharides and polyols (FODMAP) diet. In addition, hypnotherapy was superior to diet for psychological indices (ie, anxiety and depression scores).[76]

Exercise By affording individual positive coping mechanisms and symptom management, CBT may be best used synergistically with concomitant exercise therapy. Improved physical fitness and function via aerobic and strength training serve to reduce pain, improve health-related quality of life, better IBS symptom severity scores, and may decrease fatigue and depression in both IBS and FM.[77–79] Exercise has also been shown to improve colonic motility and intestinal transit time for intestinal gas, which may further benefit patients with IBS.[80] One recent study (2015) also presented data suggesting exercise interventions might serve as an antiinflammatory treatment in FM patients and decrease proinflammatory cytokines[81]; one can assume the same holds true for IBS.

In addition to traditional exercises (eg, cycling, walking, swimming, and jogging), alternative exercise options have also been investigated and likely confer benefit (eg, tai chi, chi gong, yoga, Nordic walking, vibration, and lifestyle physical activity). Heated pool treatment or balneotherapy was reported to be effective in improving pain and function[42,82,83] as were physiotherapy, relaxation, and deep tissue massage. Still, maintenance of an exercise program in both disorders is contingent on the patient being able to deal with stress, pain, barriers to exercise, and underlying disability.[69] A gradual intensity progression is recommended for deconditioned individuals toward a goal of moderate intensity.[77]

Dietary interventions Approximately a decade ago, gluten-free diets were recommended for treatment of IBS-D in cases of suspected gluten sensitivity.[84] However, the current cornerstone of dietary treatments for IBS is the low FODMAP diet, which limits fructose, fructans, galactooligosaccharides, lactose, and polyols. This approach has been found to be very effective in alleviating many of the symptoms of IBS, including bloating and abdominal pain.[85–87] For patients with FM requiring weight loss, the low FODMAP diet has also been shown to improve somatic pain symptoms, even when compared with traditional weight loss methods, without loss of macronutrients or micronutrients.[87]

Miscellaneous Alternative mind-body and holistic therapies, including psychoeducation, biofeedback, mindfulness-based therapies, hypnosis, acupuncture, and other relaxation strategies, have also been explored in patients with IBS and FM.[76,88,89] Evidence supporting their use in IBS patients has been limited due to inadequate research and lack of insurance coverage for such therapies.[90] Indeed, it is important to determine the benefit early during the course of therapy to maximize cost-effectiveness.[91] Aside from the previously described CBT and hypnotherapy, mindfulness-based therapies, biofeedback, and brief psychodynamic therapy all have, at least relatively, the most robust evidence for benefit in patients with IBS and FM.[88,90,92] At this point, however, the evidence for use of acupuncture in IBS is weak.[93,94] Some evidence exists for the use of peppermint oil and melatonin in both conditions.[95,96] However, apart from these 2 exceptions, the evidence in support of herbal medicines remains extremely weak.

SUMMARY

GI conditions are common in FM, with IBS representing by far the most common ailment. Various subtypes have been described, with several factors combining to determine the severity of IBS. The management of IBS uses a combination of non-pharmacologic approaches and an extensive list of pharmacologic therapies has been shown to provide modest benefit to patients.

REFERENCES

1. Malt EA, Berle JE, Olafsson S, et al. Fibromyalgia is associated with panic disorder and functional dyspepsia with mood disorders. A study of women with random sample population controls. J Psychosom Res 2000;49(5):285–9.
2. Brandt LJ, Chey WD, Foxx-Orenstein AE, et al. An evidence-based position statement on the management of irritable bowel syndrome. Am J Gastroenterol 2009; 104(Suppl 1):S1–35.
3. Chang JY, Talley NJ. An update on irritable bowel syndrome: from diagnosis to emerging therapies. Curr Opin Gastroenterol 2011;27(1):72–8.
4. Tack J, Drossman DA. What's new in Rome IV? Neurogastroenterol Motil 2017; 29(9).
5. Whitehead WE, Palsson OS, Simrén M. Irritable bowel syndrome: what do the new Rome IV diagnostic guidelines mean for patient management? Expert Rev Gastroenterol Hepatol 2017;11(4):281–3.
6. Mayer EA, Tillisch K. The brain-gut axis in abdominal pain syndromes. Annu Rev Med 2011;62:381–96.
7. Mayer EA, Labus JS, Tillisch K, et al. Towards a systems view of IBS. Nat Rev Gastroenterol Hepatol 2015;12(10):592–605.
8. Spiller R, Aziz Q, Creed F, et al. Guidelines on the irritable bowel syndrome: mechanisms and practical management. Gut 2007;56(12):1770–98.
9. Sperber AD, Carmel S, Atzmon Y, et al. Use of the Functional Bowel Disorder Severity Index (FBDSI) in a study of patients with the irritable bowel syndrome and fibromyalgia. Am J Gastroenterol 2000;95(4):995–8.
10. Drossman DA, Li Z, Toner BB, et al. Functional bowel disorders. A multicenter comparison of health status and development of illness severity index. Dig Dis Sci 1995;40(5):986–95.
11. Longstreth GF, Thompson WG, Chey WD, et al. Functional bowel disorders. Gastroenterology 2006;130(5):1480–91.
12. Veale D, Kavanagh G, Fielding JF, et al. Primary fibromyalgia and the irritable bowel syndrome: different expressions of a common pathogenetic process. Br J Rheumatol 1991;30(3):220–2.
13. Tremolaterra F, Gallotta S, Morra Y, et al. The severity of irritable bowel syndrome or the presence of fibromyalgia influencing the perception of visceral and somatic stimuli. BMC Gastroenterol 2014;14(1):9002.
14. Wallace DJ, Hallegua DS. Fibromyalgia: the gastrointestinal link. Curr Pain Headache Rep 2004;8(5):364–8.
15. Whitehead WE, Palsson O, Jones KR. Systematic review of the comorbidity of irritable bowel syndrome with other disorders: what are the causes and implications? Gastroenterology 2002;122(4):1140–56.
16. Lubrano E, Iovino P, Tremolaterra F, et al. Fibromyalgia in patients with irritable bowel syndrome. An association with the severity of the intestinal disorder. Int J Colorectal Dis 2001;16(4):211–5.
17. Chang L, Berman S, Mayer EA, et al. Brain responses to visceral and somatic stimuli in patients with irritable bowel syndrome with and without fibromyalgia. Am J Gastroenterol 2003;98(6):1354–61.
18. Chang F-Y. Irritable bowel syndrome: the evolution of multi-dimensional looking and multidisciplinary treatments. World J Gastroenterol 2014;20(10):2499–514.
19. Slim M, Calandre EP, Rico-Villademoros F. An insight into the gastrointestinal component of fibromyalgia: clinical manifestations and potential underlying mechanisms. Rheumatol Int 2015;35(3):433–44.

20. Yunus MB. Fibromyalgia and overlapping disorders: the unifying concept of central sensitivity syndromes. Semin Arthritis Rheum 2007;36(6):339–56.
21. Kim SE, Chang L. Overlap between functional GI disorders and other functional syndromes: what are the underlying mechanisms? Neurogastroenterol Motil 2012;24(10):895–913.
22. Moshiree B, Price DD, Robinson ME, et al. Thermal and visceral hypersensitivity in irritable bowel syndrome patients with and without fibromyalgia. Clin J Pain 2007;23(4):323–30.
23. Riedl A, Schmidtmann M, Stengel A, et al. Somatic comorbidities of irritable bowel syndrome: a systematic analysis. J Psychosom Res 2008;64(6):573–82.
24. Jensen KB, Srinivasan P, Spaeth R, et al. Overlapping structural and functional brain changes in patients with long-term exposure to fibromyalgia pain. Arthritis Rheum 2013;65(12):3293–303.
25. Tracey I, Mantyh PW. The cerebral signature for pain perception and its modulation. Neuron 2007;55(3):377–91.
26. Drossman DA, Chang L, Bellamy N, et al. Severity in irritable bowel syndrome: a Rome Foundation Working Team report. Am J Gastroenterol 2011;106(10): 1749–59 [quiz: 1760].
27. Piche M, Bouin M, Arsenault M, et al. Decreased pain inhibition in irritable bowel syndrome depends on altered descending modulation and higher-order brain processes. Neuroscience 2011;195:166–75.
28. Julien N, Goffaux P, Arsenault P, et al. Widespread pain in fibromyalgia is related to a deficit of endogenous pain inhibition. Pain 2005;114(1–2):295–302.
29. de Souza JB, Potvin S, Goffaux P, et al. The deficit of pain inhibition in fibromyalgia is more pronounced in patients with comorbid depressive symptoms. Clin J Pain 2009;25(2):123–7.
30. Chang L, Mayer EA, Johnson T, et al. Differences in somatic perception in female patients with irritable bowel syndrome with and without fibromyalgia. Pain 2000; 84(2–3):297–307.
31. Creed F. The relationship between psychosocial parameters and outcome in irritable bowel syndrome. Am J Med 1999;107(5A):74S–80S.
32. Ozsahin M, Gonen I, Ermis F, et al. The prevalence of fibromyalgia among patients with hepatitis B virus infection. Int J Clin Exp Med 2013;6(9):804–8.
33. Yazmalar L, Deveci Ö, Batmaz İ, et al. Fibromyalgia incidence among patients with hepatitis B infection. Int J Rheum Dis 2016;19(7):637–43.
34. Kozanoglu E, Canataroglu A, Abayli B, et al. Fibromyalgia syndrome in patients with hepatitis C infection. Rheumatol Int 2003;23(5):248–51.
35. Mohammad A, Carey JJ, Storan E, et al. Prevalence of fibromyalgia among patients with chronic hepatitis C infection: relationship to viral characteristics and quality of life. J Clin Gastroenterol 2012;46(5):407–12.
36. Rogal SS, Bielefeldt K, Wasan AD, et al. Fibromyalgia symptoms and cirrhosis. Dig Dis Sci 2015;60(5):1482–9.
37. Adak B, Tekeoğlu I, Ediz L, et al. Fibromyalgia frequency in hepatitis B carriers. J Clin Rheumatol 2005;11(3):157–9.
38. Thompson ME, Barkhuizen A. Fibromyalgia, hepatitis C infection, and the cytokine connection. Curr Pain Headache Rep 2003;7(5):342–7.
39. Narváez J, Nolla JM, Valverde-García J. Lack of association of fibromyalgia with hepatitis C virus infection. J Rheumatol 2005;32(6):1118.
40. Palazzi C, D'Amico E, D'Angelo S, et al. Hepatitis C virus infection in Italian patients with fibromyalgia. Clin Rheumatol 2008;27(1):101–3.

41. Hauser W, Thieme K, Turk DC. Guidelines on the management of fibromyalgia syndrome - a systematic review. Eur J Pain 2010;14(1):5–10.
42. Carville SF, Arendt-Nielsen L, Bliddal H, et al. EULAR evidence-based recommendations for the management of fibromyalgia syndrome. Ann Rheum Dis 2008;67(4):536–41.
43. Papadopoulou D, Fassoulaki A, Tsoulas C, et al. A meta-analysis to determine the effect of pharmacological and non-pharmacological treatments on fibromyalgia symptoms comprising OMERACT-10 response criteria. Clin Rheumatol 2016; 35(3):573–86.
44. Goldenberg DL, Burckhardt C, Crofford L. Management of fibromyalgia syndrome. JAMA 2004;292(19):2388–95.
45. Hassett AL, Gevirtz RN. Nonpharmacologic treatment for fibromyalgia: patient education, cognitive-behavioral therapy, relaxation techniques, and complementary and alternative medicine. Rheum Dis Clin North Am 2009;35(2):393–407.
46. Gaskell H, Moore RA, Derry S, et al. Oxycodone for neuropathic pain and fibromyalgia in adults. Cochrane Database Syst Rev 2014;(6):CD010692.
47. Rahimi R, Nikfar S, Rezaie A, et al. Efficacy of tricyclic antidepressants in irritable bowel syndrome: a meta-analysis. World J Gastroenterol 2009;15(13):1548–53.
48. Grover M, Drossman DA. Centrally acting therapies for irritable bowel syndrome. Gastroenterol Clin North Am 2011;40(1):183–206.
49. Chey WD, Maneerattaporn M, Saad R. Pharmacologic and complementary and alternative medicine therapies for irritable bowel syndrome. Gut Liver 2011; 5(3):253–66.
50. Arnold LM, Hess EV, Hudson JI, et al. A randomized, placebo-controlled, double-blind, flexible-dose study of fluoxetine in the treatment of women with fibromyalgia. Am J Med 2002;112(3):191–7.
51. Arnold LM, Rosen A, Pritchett YL, et al. A randomized, double-blind, placebo-controlled trial of duloxetine in the treatment of women with fibromyalgia with or without major depressive disorder. Pain 2005;119(1–3):5–15.
52. Vitton O, Gendreau M, Gendreau J, et al. A double-blind placebo-controlled trial of milnacipran in the treatment of fibromyalgia. Hum Psychopharmacol 2004; 19(Suppl 1):S27–35.
53. Ohta H, Oka H, Usui C, et al. A randomized, double-blind, multicenter, placebo-controlled phase III trial to evaluate the efficacy and safety of pregabalin in Japanese patients with fibromyalgia. Arthritis Res Ther 2012;14(5):R217.
54. Crofford LJ, Rowbotham MC, Mease PJ, et al. Pregabalin for the treatment of fibromyalgia syndrome: results of a randomized, double-blind, placebo-controlled trial. Arthritis Rheum 2005;52(4):1264–73.
55. Arnold LM, Russell IJ, Diri EW, et al. A 14-week, randomized, double-blinded, placebo-controlled monotherapy trial of pregabalin in patients with fibromyalgia. J Pain 2008;9(9):792–805.
56. Derry S, Cording M, Wiffen PJ, et al. Pregabalin for pain in fibromyalgia in adults. Cochrane Database Syst Rev 2016;(9):CD011790.
57. Vaishnavi SN, Nemeroff CB, Plott SJ, et al. Milnacipran: a comparative analysis of human monoamine uptake and transporter binding affinity. Biol Psychiatry 2004; 55(3):320–2.
58. Lee KJ, Kim JH, Cho SW. Gabapentin reduces rectal mechanosensitivity and increases rectal compliance in patients with diarrhoea-predominant irritable bowel syndrome. Aliment Pharmacol Ther 2005;22(10):981–8.
59. Moore RA, Wiffen PJ, Derry S, et al. Gabapentin for chronic neuropathic pain and fibromyalgia in adults. Cochrane Database Syst Rev 2014;(4):CD007938.

60. Saito YA, Almazar AE, Tilkes K, et al. A Placebo-Controlled Trial of Pregabalin for Irritable Bowel Syndrome. Am J Gastroenterol 2016;111:S236.

61. Francis DK, Utrobicic A, Choy EHS, et al. Probiotics for fibromyalgia. Cochrane Database of Systematic Reviews 2013;(3):CD010451.

62. Schrezenmeir J, de Vrese M. Probiotics, prebiotics, and synbiotics—approaching a definition. Am J Clin Nutr 2001;73(2):361s–4s.

63. Lee BJ, Bak YT. Irritable bowel syndrome, gut microbiota and probiotics. J Neurogastroenterol Motil 2011;17(3):252–66.

64. Floch MH, Walker WA, Sanders ME, et al. Recommendations for Probiotic use–2015 update: proceedings and consensus opinion. J Clin Gastroenterol 2015; 49(Suppl 1):S69–73.

65. Quigley EM. Bacteria: a new player in gastrointestinal motility disorders–infections, bacterial overgrowth, and probiotics. Gastroenterol Clin North Am 2007; 36(3):735–48, xi.

66. Spiller R. Review article: probiotics and prebiotics in irritable bowel syndrome. Aliment Pharmacol Ther 2008;28(4):385–96.

67. McFarland LV, Dublin S. Meta-analysis of probiotics for the treatment of irritable bowel syndrome. World J Gastroenterol 2008;14(17):2650–61.

68. Moayyedi P, Ford AC, Talley NJ, et al. The efficacy of probiotics in the treatment of irritable bowel syndrome: a systematic review. Gut 2010;59(3):325–32.

69. Bennett R, Nelson D. Cognitive behavioral therapy for fibromyalgia. Nat Clin Pract Rheumatol 2006;2(8):416–24.

70. Alda M, Luciano JV, Andrés E, et al. Effectiveness of cognitive behaviour therapy for the treatment of catastrophisation in patients with fibromyalgia: a randomised controlled trial. Arthritis Res Ther 2011;13(5):R173.

71. Bernardy K, Füber N, Köllner V, et al. Efficacy of cognitive-behavioral therapies in fibromyalgia syndrome - a systematic review and metaanalysis of randomized controlled trials. J Rheumatol 2010;37(10):1991–2005.

72. van Koulil S, Effting M, Kraaimaat FW, et al. Cognitive–behavioural therapies and exercise programmes for patients with fibromyalgia: state of the art and future directions. Ann Rheum Dis 2007;66(5):571–81.

73. Glombiewski JA, Sawyer AT, Gutermann J, et al. Psychological treatments for fibromyalgia: a meta-analysis. Pain 2010;151(2):280–95.

74. Peters E, Crombie T, Agbedjro D, et al. The long-term effectiveness of cognitive behavior therapy for psychosis within a routine psychological therapies service. Front Psychol 2015;6:1658.

75. Laird KT, Tanner-Smith EE, Russell AC, et al. Short-term and long-term efficacy of psychological therapies for irritable bowel syndrome: a systematic review and meta-analysis. Clin Gastroenterol Hepatol 2016;14(7):937–47.e4.

76. Peters SL, Yao CK, Philpott H, et al. Randomised clinical trial: the efficacy of gut-directed hypnotherapy is similar to that of the low FODMAP diet for the treatment of irritable bowel syndrome. Aliment Pharmacol Ther 2016;44(5):447–59.

77. Busch AJ, Webber SC, Brachaniec M, et al. Exercise therapy for fibromyalgia. Curr Pain Headache Rep 2011;15(5):358–67.

78. Busch AJ, Schachter CL, Overend TJ, et al. Exercise for fibromyalgia: a systematic review. J Rheumatol 2008;35(6):1130–44.

79. Daley AJ, Grimmett C, Roberts L, et al. The effects of exercise upon symptoms and quality of life in patients diagnosed with irritable bowel syndrome: a randomised controlled trial. Int J Sports Med 2008;29(9):778–82.

80. Johannesson E, Simrén M, Strid H, et al. Physical activity improves symptoms in irritable bowel syndrome: a randomized controlled trial. Am J Gastroenterol 2011; 106(5):915–22.

81. Sanada K, Díez MA, Valero MS, et al. Effects of non-pharmacological interventions on inflammatory biomarker expression in patients with fibromyalgia: a systematic review. Arthritis Res Ther 2015;17:272.

82. Zijlstra TR, van de Laar MA, Bernelot Moens HJ, et al. Spa treatment for primary fibromyalgia syndrome: a combination of thalassotherapy, exercise and patient education improves symptoms and quality of life. Rheumatology (Oxford) 2005; 44(4):539–46.

83. Adams N, Sim J. Rehabilitation approaches in fibromyalgia. Disabil Rehabil 2005; 27(12):711–23.

84. Vazquez-Roque MI, Camilleri M, Smyrk T, et al. A controlled trial of gluten-free diet in patients with irritable bowel syndrome-diarrhea: effects on bowel frequency and intestinal function. Gastroenterology 2013;144(5):903–11.e3.

85. Rao SS, Yu S, Fedewa A. Systematic review: dietary fibre and FODMAP-restricted diet in the management of constipation and irritable bowel syndrome. Aliment Pharmacol Ther 2015;41(12):1256–70.

86. Shepherd SJ, Halmos E, Glance S. The role of FODMAPs in irritable bowel syndrome. Curr Opin Clin Nutr Metab Care 2014;17(6):605–9.

87. Eswaran SL, Chey WD, Han-Markey T, et al. A randomized controlled trial comparing the low FODMAP diet vs. modified NICE guidelines in US adults with IBS-D. Am J Gastroenterol 2016;111(12):1824–32.

88. Glombiewski JA, Bernardy K, Häuser W. Efficacy of EMG- and EEG-biofeedback in fibromyalgia syndrome: a meta-analysis and a systematic review of randomized controlled trials. Evid Based Complement Alternat Med 2013;2013:962741.

89. Theadom A, Cropley M, Smith HE, et al. Mind and body therapy for fibromyalgia. Cochrane Database Syst Rev 2015;(4):CD001980.

90. Asare F, Storsrud S, Simren M. Meditation over medication for irritable bowel syndrome? On exercise and alternative treatments for irritable bowel syndrome. Curr Gastroenterol Rep 2012;14(4):283–9.

91. Lackner JM, Gudleski GD, Keefer L, et al. Rapid response to cognitive behavior therapy for irritable bowel syndrome. Clin Gastroenterol Hepatol 2010;8(5): 426–32.

92. Cash E, Salmon P, Weissbecker I, et al. Mindfulness meditation alleviates fibromyalgia symptoms in women: results of a randomized clinical trial. Ann Behav Med 2015;49(3):319–30.

93. Manheimer E, Wieland LS, Cheng K, et al. Acupuncture for irritable bowel syndrome: systematic review and meta-analysis. Am J Gastroenterol 2012;107(6): 835–47 [quiz: 848].

94. Deare JC, Zheng Z, Xue CC, et al. Acupuncture for treating fibromyalgia. Cochrane Database Syst Rev 2013;(5):CD007070.

95. Liu JP, Yang M, Liu YX, et al. Herbal medicines for treatment of irritable bowel syndrome. Cochrane Database Syst Rev 2006;(1):CD004116.

96. Cash BD, Epstein MS, Shah SM. A novel delivery system of peppermint oil is an effective therapy for irritable bowel syndrome symptoms. Dig Dis Sci 2016;61(2): 560–71.

Gastrointestinal and Hepatic Disease in Sjogren Syndrome

Yevgeniy Popov, DO, MPH[a],*, Karen Salomon-Escoto, MD[b]

KEYWORDS

- Sjogren syndrome • Sicca • Xerostomia • Dysphagia • Oral involvement • Hepatitis
- Pancreatitis

KEY POINTS

- Sjogren syndrome predominantly affects the salivary glands.
- Diagnosis is challenging due to inconsistent serologies and histopathology.
- Extraglandular manifestations are common and cause morbidity.
- Esophageal, gastric, hepatic, and pancreatic involvement have been described.
- Treatment primarily targets salivary and lacrimal glands.

INTRODUCTION

Sjogren syndrome (SS) is a lymphocyte-mediated, infiltrative autoimmune disorder characterized by destruction of exocrine glands. The glandular damage leads to secretory dysfunction manifesting as dryness of mucosal membranes.[1] This article summarizes the epidemiology, pathogenesis, and pathology of SS. The role of cytokines and autoantibodies in decreasing secretory functions of lacrimal and salivary glands is described. The article then reviews the symptoms and clinical features of SS, according to the involvement of individual gastrointestinal organs. Diagnostic considerations are addressed, including the challenging nature of the differential diagnosis, due to the high prevalence of dry eyes, dry mouth, fatigue, and musculoskeletal pain in other conditions. Furthermore, positive antinuclear antibodies (ANAs) and the histopathology features of sialadenitis may mimic SS. The role of minor salivary gland biopsy as gold standard for diagnosis is reviewed, with emphasis on the requirement of

[a] Department of Medicine, University of Massachusetts Medical School, 119 Belmont Street, Worcester, MA 01605, USA; [b] Rheumatology Division, University of Massachusetts Medical School, 119 Belmont Street, Worcester, MA 01605, USA
* Corresponding author.
E-mail address: yevgeniy.popov@umassmemorial.org

Rheum Dis Clin N Am 44 (2018) 143–151
https://doi.org/10.1016/j.rdc.2017.09.010
rheumatic.theclinics.com

an experienced pathologist's interpretation to avoid confusion caused by nonspecific findings. Finally, the article surveys various treatments, which chiefly consist of drugs that increase salivary secretion and decrease ocular inflammation.[2]

EPIDEMIOLOGY

SS is estimated to affect up to 4 million people in the United States, with a prevalence of 3.3%.[3] It is the second most common autoimmune rheumatic disorder after rheumatoid arthritis, exceeding the prevalence for systemic lupus erythematosus, yet remains underdiagnosed.[4,5] SS has a female predominance with various studies citing a female:male distribution in the range between 9:1 and 24:1.[1,6] All ages of individuals may be affected, but it is more common between the fourth and sixth decades of life. The disease affects all ethnicities, but is typically seen more frequently in Caucasians.

PATHOGENESIS AND PATHOPHYSIOLOGY
Pathogenesis

The pathogenesis of primary SS is not completely understood, but is a complex interplay involving both T-cell and B-cell dysfunction. Monocellular infiltration of glandular structures underlies the basic pathogenesis in primary SS. Th1 cells are implicated as the key constituent of biopsy infiltrates. This is further supported by studies demonstrating an increased quantity of Th1 cytokines from salivary glands and saliva of patients with SS.[7,8] Other studies suggest that helper T cells contribute to the inflammatory process, with multiple studies suggesting that expression of helper T-cell cytokines, such as interleukin (IL)-17 and IL-18 are associated with more advanced disease.[9] B-cell hyperactivity is also implicated in the pathogenesis of primary SS and is thought to be related to the development of extraglandular manifestations.[10] B-cell pathogenesis is primary mediated by B-lymphocyte Activating Factor (BAFF), which promotes survival and maturation. Studies evaluating transgenic mice with BAFF overexpression demonstrated a markedly decreased salivary production and advanced sialadenitis.[11] The role of BAFF in pathogenesis is further supported by studies demonstrating increased BAFF serum levels in patients with primary SS.[12]

Histopathology

Salivary gland biopsy is a cornerstone in the diagnosis of primary SS. The most common anatomic site of salivary gland biopsy is from the lip and, in some instances, parotid gland.[13] Positive findings are based on the presence of focal lymphocytic sialadenitis (FLS), which is characterized by perivascular or periductal mononuclear cell aggregates adjacent to normal-appearing acini. A focus is defined as an aggregate of at least 50 lymphocytes; a positive focus score (FS) is defined by the presence of more than 1 inflammatory aggregation of 50 or more mononuclear cells per 4 mm^2 of glandular tissue. Studies of FSs show there is a correlation between higher FS and more rapid decline in stimulated salivary flow rate.[14]

ANATOMIC DISTRIBUTION OF THE INVOLVEMENT

Organ	Involvement	Evidence	Citation
Mouth/Salivary glands	Xerostomia	Cohort	Vivino,[6] 2017
Esophagus	Dysphagia	Cohort	Palma et al,[28] 1994
Stomach	Gastritis Gastrointestinal motility	Cohort	Maury et al,[29] 1985
Pancreas	Pancreatitis, pancreatic insufficiency	Case control	Afzelius et al,[34] 2010
Liver	Increased risk of hepatitis C complications	Cohort	Zeron et al,[48] 2013
Gall bladder	Primary biliary cirrhosis	Cohort	Selmi et al,[49] 2012
Small Intestine	Duodenal ulcers, Celiac disease	Cohort	Biagini et al,[31] 1991
Colon, etc.	N/A	N/A	N/A

Abbreviation: N/A; Not applicable.

GASTROINTESTINAL SYMPTOMS IN SJOGREN SYNDROME

Xerostomia and xerophthalmia are the classic sicca symptoms associated with SS, occurring in 80% of patients; however, 25% to 30% of patients are known to experience extraglandular involvement as well.[15] In particular, several gastrointestinal manifestations have been reported in patients with SS with varying degrees of dysphagia being common.[16] Other features include various forms of gastric involvement, including gastritis and antiparietal cell antibodies,[17] which collectively has been found in up to 23% of patients. Gastritis typically presents as central upper abdominal pain, as well as nausea, vomiting, bloating, and early satiety. In rare cases, pancreatic involvement has been reported in the forms of pancreatitis and pancreatic insufficiency. This presents with symptoms similar to gastritis, but includes frequent diarrhea and foul-smelling, greasy stools (steatorrhea). Liver manifestations include primary biliary cirrhosis and acceleration of hepatitis C virus. Up to 49% of patients with primary SS have had some form of abnormal liver tests.

SJOGREN SYNDROME AND THE ORAL CAVITY

The prototypical manifestations of SS are best characterized as sicca symptoms, which can manifest as xerophthalmia and xerostomia. Xerostomia gives rise to several consequences for oral health, including acceleration of dental caries, periodontal involvement, angular cheilitis, lip dryness, and nonspecific ulcerations and aphthae. Oral manifestations of xerostomia occur in more than half of patients with primary SS. Extent of xerostomia and oral manifestations are proportional to the duration of disease, as longer time intervals lead to decreased saliva and depletion of protective factors.[18] Studies evaluating salivary content in patients with SS have noted that the enzymatic and buffering properties of saliva diminish over time.[19] Such changes predispose patients to opportunistic infections, such as *Candida albicans*, which may range from asymptomatic infections to tongue fissures, generalized candidiasis, and angular cheilitis.[18] It is estimated that 87% of patients with SS will experience some form of oral candidiasis.[20] Furthermore, the changes in salivary content promote overgrowth of organisms implicated in cariogenesis and acid-resistant plaques including *Lactobacillus* spp and *Streptococcus mutans*.[18] Patients with SS also have a propensity to develop lymphomas, particularly in tissues in which the disease is most active, such as the salivary glands.[21] Studies estimate that patients with SS are 44 times more likely to develop a B-type lymphoma than the general population.[22]

The extent of salivary gland involvement can be further elucidated with diagnostic imaging, including salivary scintigraphy imaging using Technetium 99-sodium pertechnetate, which can differentiate the salivary gland involved and also predict response to therapy.[23] Involvement of the parotid gland may be evaluated by magnetic resonance (MR) sialography.[24] Ultrasound is an emerging imaging modality for the evaluation of SS involvement, with some studies suggesting that ultrasound results correspond to labial minor gland biopsy scores and salivary flow rates.[25]

SJOGREN SYNDROME AND GASTROINTESTINAL MOTILITY

Several clinical observations have been made regarding patients with SS and delayed gastric emptying, prompting the theory that patients with SS may have a unique pathogenesis that affects gastric motility. One proposed hypothesis suggests that immunoglobulin (Ig)G Sjogren autoantibodies may impair the function of muscarinic receptors. Preliminary studies have demonstrated that SS IgG leads to reduced salivary Sjogren gland function and that SS IgG leads to inhibition of muscarinic receptors in the bladder.[26] Some studies have evaluated autonomic nervous system dysfunction in patients with primary SS using edrophonium challenge testing and citric acid stimulation, demonstrating that patients with SS may be experiencing blockade in acetylcholine-mediated activity.[27] Either of these abnormalities could explain dysfunction of the enteric/intrinsic nervous system in SS.

SJOGREN SYNDROME AND DYSPHAGIA

Studies evaluating dysphagia in patients with SS estimate that up to 80% of these patients experience some spectrum of dysphagia. The mechanism of dysphagia is not clear and may reflect a combination of xerostomia versus a motor dysmotility component.[28]

SJOGREN SYNDROME AND GASTRITIS

Gastric involvement presents in various forms among patients with SS, with up to 23% of patients experiencing some form of dyspepsia.[17] Manifestations may include reduced acid production, antiparietal antibodies, and gastritis.

Atrophic gastritis in patients with SS has been reported to have an incidence of up to 65%. Atrophic gastritis appears to be age-related finding in patients with SS, as frequency increases with age.[29] There is some correlation between the degree of atrophic gastritis and lymphocytic infiltration of gastric mucosa; the cellular infiltrations in gastric mucosa display histologic similarly to what is found in salivary glands. In patients with SS, hypopepsinogenemia in atrophic gastritis correlates positively with high SS-B antibody titers, erythrocyte sedimentation rate, and IgA levels. It has been found in up to 69% of patients with SS with gastric involvement.[30]

SJOGREN SYNDROME AND THE SMALL BOWEL

Patients with a co-occurrence of SS and primary biliary cirrhosis (PBC) appear to have a propensity for duodenal ulcers. One study cited an ulcer rate of 85% in SS/PBC overlap compared with 26% with duodenal ulcers in isolated PBC.[31]

Studies investigating the epidemiology of celiac disease have noted more frequent concomitant occurrence with SS than the general population.[32] Szodoray and colleagues[33] discovered celiac in 4.5% of patients with primary SS disease: a prevalence 10-fold higher than the non-SS population. Celiac disease occurring in patients with SS more commonly occurs as the latent form and is more likely to appear in younger patients with SS. Interestingly, some patients with SS may experience gluten sensitivity without celiac disease.[33] Generalized abdominal discomfort was the most commonly observed symptom in the SS and celiac overlap population, adding to the difficulty in diagnosis.[32]

SJOGREN SYNDROME AND THE PANCREAS

The pancreas shares histologic and functional features of the salivary glands, leading studies to evaluate the association of pancreatitis in SS.[34] Current estimates set the prevalence of autoimmune causes of pancreatitis at approximately 5%.[35] There have been no formal studies linking autoimmune pancreatitis to SS; however, investigators have estimated that patients with SS appear to have a 25% to 33% prevalence of chronic pancreatitis–like morphologic changes, which would be markedly elevated compared with control populations.[36]

SJOGREN SYNDROME AND HEPATITIS C

Patients with SS are estimated to have a prevalence of hepatitis C virus (HCV) co-infection of 13%.[37] Patients appear to be predominantly from the Mediterranean area and are more likely to be older men.[1] Several studies have suggested that patients with primary SS have an alternate immunologic response to HCV, leading to the acceleration of liver damage.[15] Compared with those without HCV infection, patients with SS with HCV infection were found to have a higher rate of cryoglobulin markers and alterations in the pattern of autoantibodies (more frequent rheumatoid factor, lower frequency of anti-La and anti-Ro antibodies). These immunologic alterations may reflect changes in neoplastic surveillance that could also explain the increased prevalence of lymphoma in HCV-positive patients with SS.

AUTOIMMUNE HEPATITIS

Patients with SS with autoimmune liver involvement appear to be exceedingly rare compared with hepatitis C or PBC (see Carlo Selmi and colleagues' article, "Rheumatic Manifestations in Autoimmune Liver Disease," in this issue). The immunologic pattern in patients with SS with autoimmune liver disease is predominated by a higher rate of autoantibodies compared with viral involvement, which is driven more by hypocomplementemia and increased cryoglobulin marker expression. Reports regarding autoimmune hepatitis associated with primary SS have predominantly centered on cases arising from Japan, Korea, and China.[3] Autoimmune hepatitis is more likely to affect younger female individuals.

DIAGNOSTIC EVALUATION

The physical examination can help detect lacrimal or salivary gland hypertrophy. Presence of dental caries and decreased salivary pooling under the tongue are signs of underactive salivary glands. Oral candidiasis may be present, too, and appears as white-to-yellow creamy plaques or coating on the tongue or inner cheeks.

The most recent criteria for classification of SS (ie, enrollment of a homogeneous populations into studies or trials) is based on the 2016 consensus statement issued by the American College of Rheumatology and European League against Rheumatism. Although not intended as diagnostic criteria, the criteria do highlight some of the key features of SS, including that 2 of the 5 criteria are based on oral manifestations of disease. The criteria are based on a weighted score of 5 items including positive anti-SSA/Ro antibody (3 points), FLS on labial salivary gland biopsy (3 points), abnormal ocular staining in at least 1 eye (1 point), Schirmer test with result of less than or equal to 5 mm per 5 minutes (1 point), and unstimulated salivary flow rate of less than or equal to 0.1 mL per minute (1 point). A total score of 4 or greater in the setting of clinical signs and symptoms meets criteria for the classification of primary SS.[38]

Item	Score
Labial salivary gland with focal lymphocytic sialadenitis and focus score of greater than or equal to 1 foci/4 mm^2	3
Anti-SSA/SSB positive	3
Ocular staining score of at least 5 (or van Bijsterveld score of at least 4) in at least 1 eye	1
Schirmer test ≤5 mm/5 min in at least 1 eye	1
Unstimulated whole saliva flow rate ≤0.1 mL/min	1

Adapted from Shiboski CH, Shiboski SC, Seror R, et al. 2016 American College of Rheumatology/European League Against Rheumatism classification criteria for primary Sjogren's syndrome: a consensus and data-driven methodology involving three international patient cohorts. Ann Rheum Dis 2017;76(1):9–16.

DIGESTIVE AND HEPATIC ASPECTS RELATED TO TREATMENT OF SJOGREN SYNDROME

Hydroxychloroquine and methotrexate are considered first-line and second-line therapy in the management of inflammatory musculoskeletal pain due to SS.[39] Prolonged methotrexate use, and to a lesser degree hydroxychloroquine use, carries a risk of hepatotoxicity. Transaminitis is estimated to occur in more than 20% of methotrexate-exposed patients and appears to correlate with the duration of treatment.[40] The most current American College of Rheumatology guidelines recommend monitoring bloodwork at a frequency based on the duration of prior methotrexate exposure, ranging anywhere between 2 and 12 weeks.[41]

MANAGEMENT OF THE DIGESTIVE/HEPATIC MANIFESTATIONS

In terms of addressing digestive manifestations of SS, the most recent guidelines for the treatment of SS only specifically examine dry mouth.[39] Based on a modest amount of data, the investigators recommend fluoride use. Based on purely expert opinion, the investigators recommend patients with SS with dry mouth "increase saliva through gustatory, masticatory stimulation, and pharmaceutical agents; for example, sugar-free lozenges and/or chewing gum, xylitol, mannitol, and the prescription medications pilocarpine and cevimeline." Several placebo-controlled trials have evaluated the efficacy of oral pilocarpine in the treatment of oral sicca symptoms with variable degrees of improvement ranging between 42% and 61%.[42] The main adverse effects of pilocarpine treatment included increased frequency of sweating and urinary frequency.[43] Placebo-controlled trials also have evaluated the use of cevimeline in treatment of dry mouth with frequency of improvement ranging between 37% and 45%.[42] There is also suggestion that cevimeline may reduce lymphocytic infiltration and hasten sialography stage.[44] In addition, conservative management of oral sicca symptoms should include avoidance of drying agents, such anticholinergic medications, and reducing the intake of caffeine, alcohol, and nicotine.[45] As previously mentioned, patients with SS are prone to candidiasis due to the lack of salivary protective factors. Oral preparations containing nystatin are typical first-line agents.[46]

Therapies for patients with SS experiencing liver and biliary involvement are limited. The use of ursodeoxycholic acid has been approved for primary biliary cholangitis.[47]

SUMMARY

SS is a common rheumatic disease. Although it has predominantly ocular and oral manifestations, multiple extraglandular symptoms may occur, particularly in the liver and gastrointestinal tract. The diagnosis is challenging, as symptoms, examination, laboratory, and histopathology findings of SS may be present in other systemic diseases. Treatment of SS per se does not target gastrointestinal manifestations specifically, yet monitoring for potential hepatic and gastrointestinal involvement is important, to prevent serious complications.

REFERENCES

1. Ramos-Casals M, Brito-Zeron P, Siso-Almirall A, et al. Primary Sjogren syndrome. BMJ 2012;344:e3821.
2. Fox RI, Stern M, Michelson P. Update in Sjogren syndrome. Curr Opin Rheumatol 2000;12(5):391–8.
3. Ramos-Casals M, Brito-Zeron P, Siso-Almirall A, et al. Primary Sjogren syndrome. Praxis (Bern 1994) 2012;101(24):1565–71 [in German].
4. Helmick CG, Felson DT, Lawrence RC, et al. Estimates of the prevalence of arthritis and other rheumatic conditions in the United States. Part I. Arthritis Rheum 2008;58(1):15–25.
5. Skopouli FN, Dafni U, Ioannidis JP, et al. Clinical evolution, and morbidity and mortality of primary Sjogren's syndrome. Semin Arthritis Rheum 2000;29(5): 296–304.
6. Vivino FB. Sjogren's syndrome: clinical aspects. Clin Immunol 2017 [pii:S1521-6616(16)30678-7].
7. Boumba D, Skopouli FN, Moutsopoulos HM. Cytokine mRNA expression in the labial salivary gland tissues from patients with primary Sjogren's syndrome. Br J Rheumatol 1995;34(4):326–33.
8. Fox RI, Kang HI, Ando D, et al. Cytokine mRNA expression in salivary gland biopsies of Sjogren's syndrome. J Immunol 1994;152(11):5532–9.
9. Sakai A, Sugawara Y, Kuroishi T, et al. Identification of IL-18 and Th17 cells in salivary glands of patients with Sjogren's syndrome, and amplification of IL-17-mediated secretion of inflammatory cytokines from salivary gland cells by IL-18. J Immunol 2008;181(4):2898–906.
10. Gottenberg JE, Lavie F, Abbed K, et al. CD4 CD25high regulatory T cells are not impaired in patients with primary Sjogren's syndrome. J Autoimmun 2005;24(3): 235–42.
11. Groom J, Kalled SL, Cutler AH, et al. Association of BAFF/BLyS overexpression and altered B cell differentiation with Sjogren's syndrome. J Clin Invest 2002; 109(1):59–68.
12. Mariette X. Pathophysiology of Sjogren's syndrome. Ann Med Interne (Paris) 2003;154(3):157–68 [in French].

13. Levenstein MM, Fisher BK, Fisher LL, et al. Simultaneous occurrence of subacute cutaneous lupus erythematosus and Sweet syndrome. A marker of Sjogren syndrome? Int J Dermatol 1991;30(9):640–3.

14. Fisher BA, Jonsson R, Daniels T, et al. Standardisation of labial salivary gland histopathology in clinical trials in primary Sjogren's syndrome. Ann Rheum Dis 2017; 76(7):1161–8.

15. Brito-Zeron P, Gheitasi H, Retamozo S, et al. How hepatitis C virus modifies the immunological profile of Sjogren syndrome: analysis of 783 patients. Arthritis Res Ther 2015;17:250.

16. Sheikh SH, Shaw-Stiffel TA. The gastrointestinal manifestations of Sjogren's syndrome. Am J Gastroenterol 1995;90(1):9–14.

17. Ebert EC. Gastrointestinal and hepatic manifestations of Sjogren syndrome. J Clin Gastroenterol 2012;46(1):25–30.

18. Blochowiak K, Olewicz-Gawlik A, Polanska A, et al. Oral mucosal manifestations in primary and secondary Sjogren syndrome and dry mouth syndrome. Postepy Dermatol Alergol 2016;33(1):23–7.

19. Mathews SA, Kurien BT, Scofield RH. Oral manifestations of Sjogren's syndrome. J Dent Res 2008;87(4):308–18.

20. Yan Z, Young AL, Hua H, et al. Multiple oral *Candida* infections in patients with Sjogren's syndrome–prevalence and clinical and drug susceptibility profiles. J Rheumatol 2011;38(11):2428–31.

21. Nocturne G, Mariette X. Sjogren syndrome-associated lymphomas: an update on pathogenesis and management. Br J Haematol 2015;168(3):317–27.

22. Cornec D, Costa S, Devauchelle-Pensec V, et al. Do high numbers of salivary gland-infiltrating B cells predict better or worse outcomes after rituximab in patients with primary Sjogren's syndrome? Ann Rheum Dis 2016;75(6):e33.

23. Vivino FB, Hermann GA. Role of nuclear scintigraphy in the characterization and management of the salivary component of Sjogren's syndrome. Rheum Dis Clin North Am 2008;34(4):973–86, ix.

24. Vivino FB, Gala I, Hermann GA. Change in final diagnosis on second evaluation of labial minor salivary gland biopsies. J Rheumatol 2002;29(5):938–44.

25. Baldini C, Luciano N, Tarantini G, et al. Salivary gland ultrasonography: a highly specific tool for the early diagnosis of primary Sjogren's syndrome. Arthritis Res Ther 2015;17:146.

26. Waterman SA. Multiple subtypes of voltage-gated calcium channel mediate transmitter release from parasympathetic neurons in the mouse bladder. J Neurosci 1996;16(13):4155–61.

27. Imrich R, Alevizos I, Bebris L, et al. Predominant glandular cholinergic dysautonomia in patients with primary Sjogren's syndrome. Arthritis Rheumatol 2015; 67(5):1345–52.

28. Palma R, Freire A, Freitas J, et al. Esophageal motility disorders in patients with Sjogren's syndrome. Dig Dis Sci 1994;39(4):758–61.

29. Maury CP, Tornroth T, Teppo AM. Atrophic gastritis in Sjogren's syndrome. Morphologic, biochemical, and immunologic findings. Arthritis Rheum 1985; 28(4):388–94.

30. Montefusco PP, Geiss AC, Bronzo RL, et al. Sclerosing cholangitis, chronic pancreatitis, and Sjogren's syndrome: a syndrome complex. Am J Surg 1984; 147(6):822–6.

31. Biagini MR, Milani S, Fedi P, et al. Duodenal ulcer and Sjogren's syndrome in patients with primary biliary cirrhosis: a casual association? Am J Gastroenterol 1991;86(9):1190–3.

32. Szodoray P, Barta Z, Lakos G, et al. Coeliac disease in Sjogren's syndrome–a study of 111 Hungarian patients. Rheumatol Int 2004;24(5):278–82.
33. Liden M, Kristjansson G, Valtysdottir S, et al. Gluten sensitivity in patients with primary Sjogren's syndrome. Scand J Gastroenterol 2007;42(8):962–7.
34. Afzelius P, Fallentin EM, Larsen S, et al. Pancreatic function and morphology in Sjogren's syndrome. Scand J Gastroenterol 2010;45(6):752–8.
35. Greenberger NJ. Autoimmune pancreatitis: time for a collective effort. Gastrointest Endosc 2007;66(6):1152–3.
36. Pickartz T, Pickartz H, Lochs H, et al. Overlap syndrome of autoimmune pancreatitis and cholangitis associated with secondary Sjögren's syndrome. Eur J Gastroenterol Hepatol 2004;16(12):1295–9.
37. Garcia-Carrasco M, Ramos M, Cervera R, et al. Hepatitis C virus infection in 'primary' Sjogren's syndrome: prevalence and clinical significance in a series of 90 patients. Ann Rheum Dis 1997;56(3):173–5.
38. Shiboski CH, Shiboski SC, Seror R, et al. 2016 American College of Rheumatology/European League Against Rheumatism classification criteria for primary Sjogren's syndrome: a consensus and data-driven methodology involving three international patient cohorts. Ann Rheum Dis 2017;76(1):9–16.
39. Vivino FB, Carsons SE, Foulks G, et al. New treatment guidelines for Sjogren's disease. Rheum Dis Clin North Am 2016;42(3):531–51.
40. Sotoudehmanesh R, Anvari B, Akhlaghi M, et al. Methotrexate hepatotoxicity in patients with rheumatoid arthritis. Middle East J Dig Dis 2010;2(2):104–9.
41. Singh JA, Saag KG, Bridges SL Jr, et al. 2015 American College of Rheumatology guideline for the treatment of rheumatoid arthritis. Arthritis Care Res (Hoboken) 2016;68(1):1–25.
42. Ramos-Casals M, Tzioufas AG, Stone JH, et al. Treatment of primary Sjögren syndrome: a systematic review. JAMA 2010;304(4):452–60.
43. Vivino FB. The treatment of Sjogren's syndrome patients with pilocarpine-tablets. Scand J Rheumatol Suppl 2001;115:1–9 [discussion: 13].
44. Yamada H, Nakagawa Y, Wakamatsu E, et al. Efficacy prediction of cevimeline in patients with Sjogren's syndrome. Clin Rheumatol 2007;26(8):1320–7.
45. Silvestre-Donat FJ, Miralles-Jorda L, Martinez-Mihi V. Protocol for the clinical management of dry mouth. Med Oral 2004;9(4):273–9.
46. Ellepola AN, Samaranayake LP. Antimycotic agents in oral candidosis: an overview: 2. Treatment of oral candidosis. Dent Update 2000;27(4):165–70, 72-4.
47. Lindor KD, Gershwin ME, Poupon R, et al. Primary biliary cirrhosis. Hepatology 2009;50(1):291–308.
48. Zeron PB, Retamozo S, Bove A, et al. Diagnosis of liver involvement in primary Sjogren Syndrome. J Clin Transl Hepatol 2013;1(2):94–102.
49. Selmi C, Meroni PL, Gershwin ME. Primary biliary cirrhosis and Sjogren's syndrome: autoimmune epithelitis. J Autoimmun 2012;39(1–2):34–42.

Gastrointestinal and Hepatic Disease in Spondyloarthritis

Liron Caplan, MD, PhD[a],*, Kristine A. Kuhn, MD, PhD[b],1

KEYWORDS

- Spondyloarthropathies • Psoriatic Arthritis • Ankylosing Spondylitis
- Digestive system • Gastrointestinal diseases • Liver diseases

KEY POINTS

- Inflammatory bowel disease represents the most frequently encountered and well-described gastrointestinal manifestation of spondyloarthritis, affecting approximate 7% of axial spondyloarthritis clinically, with subclinical disease rates approaching 65%.
- Strong genetic and pathophysiologic associations have been identified between inflammatory bowel disease and spondyloarthritis, buoyed by recent intestinal microbiome studies.
- Nonalcoholic fatty liver disease (NAFLD) appears more frequently in psoriasis and psoriatic arthritis compared with the general population; the choice of therapies for psoriasis and psoriatic arthritis should reflect this association with NAFLD.

INTRODUCTION

Spondyloarthritis (SpA) refers to a collection of pathophysiologic and genetically related disorders whose manifestations co-occur in affected individuals. The manifestations include inflammatory arthritis of the axial skeleton and enthesitis as well as inflammatory disease of the eyes, skin, and gastrointestinal (GI) tract. Historically, SpA has primarily included ankylosing spondylitis (AS), reactive arthritis, psoriatic arthritis, undifferentiated arthritis, and enteropathic-associated arthritis (EAA; or inflammatory bowel disease [IBD]–associated arthritis), with the inclusion of SAPHO syndrome (synovitis, acne, pustulosis, hyperostosis, osteitis), uveitis, IBD, and psoriasis (all without arthritis) by some investigators.

[a] Medicine Service, Denver Veterans Affairs Medical Center, University of Colorado School of Medicine, Denver, CO, USA; [b] Department of Medicine, University of Colorado School of Medicine, 1775 Aurora Court, Campus Box B115, Aurora, CO 80045, USA
[1] Present address: 1775 Aurora Court, Campus Box B115, Aurora, CO 80045.
* Corresponding author. 1775 Aurora Court, Campus Box B115, Aurora, CO 80045.
E-mail address: Liron.Caplan@ucdenver.edu

Rheum Dis Clin N Am 44 (2018) 153–164
https://doi.org/10.1016/j.rdc.2017.09.004
0889-857X/18/Published by Elsevier Inc.
rheumatic.theclinics.com

For well more than 100 years, inflammatory arthritis has been associated with intestinal abnormalities, as physicians debated the pathophysiologic bases of these diseases. In the minutes of the British Medical Association's meeting for 1901, Dr EJ Cave reported "a case of rheumatoid arthritis produced by infection from a case of severe rectal ulceration."[1] In the decade that followed, several physicians and scientists began to explore the interaction of digestion and arthritis, some attributing the arthritis to diet,[2] GI infections, or an intestinal toxemia with "lasting and crippling lesions appearing only when the [primary microbic] infection, however slight, has long since subsided."[3] Interestingly, Dr Rea Smith[4] conjectured in 1922 that chronic arthritis deformans (ie, inflammatory arthritis) has its origin in "unbalanced or perverted intestinal flora," though he attributed the imbalance to local infections resulting from anatomic variations of the intestines.[4]

When inflammatory arthritis/SpA and IBD coincide, the disorder is frequently referred to as EAA. This entity has had many naming conventions but was clinically recognized at least as early as 1929 and pathologically described in the 1950s.[5,6]

EPIDEMIOLOGY
Spondyloarthritis

Estimates for the prevalence of SpA vary between 0.5% and 2.0% of the population (500 cases per 100,000 population).[7] Divergences in these values no doubt reflect differences in the selected disorders, their case definitions/classification criteria (which have changed over time), as well as underlying difference in the genetic and environmental forces responsible for the onset of disease. Given the typically indolent onset and challenging diagnosis of SpA, the incidence is much more challenging to assess because it is predicated on the ability to assign a specific diagnosis date. Nevertheless, the incidence for SpA has been determined for AS (range 0.5–10.6 per 100,000 population), psoriatic arthritis (range 0.1–8.0 per 100,000 population), and reactive arthritis (0.6–28.0 per 100,000 population).[6]

Inflammatory Bowel Disease

IBD represents the most frequently encountered and well-described GI manifestation of SpA. For this reason, it occupies the focus of this report. The prevalence for IBD is similar to that of SpA, with estimates of approximately 0.5% in North America (500 cases per 100,000 population).[8,9] In North America, the prevalence of ulcerative colitis (UC) slightly exceeds that of Crohn disease (CD); these two entities comprise the vast majority of IBD cases.[8,9] The annualized incidence of UC and CD has been reported as 6 to 10 per 100,000 population and 12 per 100,000 population, respectively.[9]

Few studies have simultaneously estimated the prevalence of both SpA as a whole and EAA in particular. An Italian study determined the prevalence of SpA to be 1.06% and IBD to be 0.09%,[10] whereas a Swedish study using a health registry estimated the prevalences at 0.55% and 0.02%, respectively.[11]

Frequency of Spondyloarthritis and Inflammatory Bowel Disease in Affected Populations

The prevalence of clinically apparent IBD among individuals with SpA has been estimated to be approximately 7%.[12] This estimate does not, however, reflect the high rates of subclinical (asymptomatic) inflammation apparent in patients with SpA, whether assessed by ileocolonoscopy[13] or capsule endoscopy.[14] Inflammatory lesions also appear in the biopsies of up to 65% of patients with SpA.[15,16] Likewise, a recent meta-analysis has estimated the prevalence of peripheral arthritis (13%), sacroiliitis (10%), and AS (3%) among individuals with IBD.[17]

Gastrointestinal Symptoms in Spondyloarthritis

Oral ulcers may be present with SpA complicated by concomitant CD as well as in reactive arthritis. Dysphagia is only very rarely present and may indicate the presence of severe cervical spine involvement from productive syndesmophytes or osteophytes. Hepatic steatosis, observed more frequently with psoriatic arthritis,[18] does not tend to cause symptoms.

Because intestinal symptoms may be subclinical, clinicians should be aware that more active SpA with less spinal mobility predicts the presence of inflammatory gut lesions.[19] Arthritis is found at a higher frequency in CD compared with UC and is more common in those with additional extraintestinal manifestations.[20]

PATHOGENESIS AND PATHOPHYSIOLOGY

Based on multiple lines of evidence, the *gut-joint hypothesis* has long suggested a connection between inflammation in both the intestine and spine. These findings include the following: (1) Up to one-third of patients with IBD will have SpA and there are high rates of colitis on histopathologic examination of patients with AS, as noted earlier.[15,16] (2) Genetic polymorphisms are shared between SpA and IBD. Consequently, first-degree relatives of patients with IBD have 3 times the relative risk of developing AS and vice versa.[21] (3) Gut-derived monocytes and T cells can be found within the joints of those with SpA.[22] (4) Intestinal microbiome studies in IBD and AS have shown significant dysbiosis (ie, a substantial alteration of the individual microbial species) in similar bacterial populations, as compared with healthy controls.[23–27] Thus, strong data exist to link intestinal microbiota and mucosal immune reactivity to joint pathophysiology.

Although HLA-B27 is the strongest genetic link to SpA; it confers less than 30% of the genetic risk, and its contribution to EAA is much less than in AS.[28] Given the overlapping clinical features between AS, psoriasis, and IBD, a recent genome-wide association study (GWAS) targeting these diseases aimed to identify shared genetic risk loci to better understand the overlapping pathways leading to these diseases.[29] The study confirmed the known common risk alleles between AS and IBD, including endoplasmic reticulum aminopeptidase 2, interleukin 23 receptor (IL-23R),[30,31] and fucosyltransferase 2, and revealed 3 novel shared loci. Others have shown that CARD15 (caspase recruitment domain-containing protein 15) polymorphisms linked to CD are found with similar frequency in a population of SpA with chronic gut inflammation[32] but not in those with SpA without intestinal inflammation. How the specific genetic polymorphisms contribute to disease is still under investigation, but most are hypothesized to result in altered bacterial antigen presentation and immune responses.[25] A better understanding of these genetic polymorphisms may shed light on pathways leading to arthritis, intestinal inflammation, or both.

Microbial dysbiosis within the intestine has been associated with both SpA[23,27,33,34] and IBD,[24,35] including in patients who are newly diagnosed and untreated.[25] However, the effect of dysbiosis on disease onset, progression, and recurrence is unclear.[36] Studies linking dysbiosis and disease in animal models have suggested that specific bacterial groups or their metabolites are protective against disease,[37–39] whereas others promote the development of T-helper 17 (TH17) cells[40,41] thought to mediate disease.[42] Relevant to SpA, in the HLA–B27/β2m–Tg rat model of spontaneous SpA and IBD, both inflammatory joint and gut disease do not appear among animals raised in a germ-free state,[43] whereas exposure to bacteria induces colitis.[44] In the B27 rat model, disease-specific dysbiosis occurs in parallel with metabolic and mucosal immune changes associated with developing inflammation,[45,46] further supporting the role of the microbiome in triggering altered T-cell responses relevant to the pathogenesis of SpA.

Although the specific mechanisms have yet to be defined, a general model of the gut-joint hypothesis is suggested by current data: Compounded by genetic polymorphisms, a state of microbial dysbiosis, and localized intestinal inflammation, a Th17 response and generation of autoreactive T and B cells is thought to emerge.[47–49] Locally activated lymphocytes and macrophages, expressing intestinal markers, such as invariant T-cell receptors,[50] IL-23R, interleukin-17a, $\alpha E\beta 7$, $\alpha 4\beta 7$, and CD163[22,47] then circulate to other tissues, such as the joint, where they engage self-antigens and initiate inflammation.

ANATOMIC DISTRIBUTION OF INVOLVEMENT FOR SPONDYLOARTHRITIS

Virtually the entire GI track may be involved in some manner among patients with SpA (**Table 1**). However, IBD represents by far the most common manifestation of GI pathology, with ulcerations possible along the full length of the digestive lumen in the presence of CD. The authors briefly summarize the data by organ:

Oral Cavity

Concomitant CD may present with oral ulcers in the setting of SpA. A cross-sectional study revealed high rates of focal sialadenitis in AS (58%) and SpA (41%) and lower unstimulated salivary flow rates in AS compared with a control cohort.[51] This study also demonstrated high rates of temporomandibular joint erosions by panoramic radiography in patients with SpA (38%) and AS (37%). Oral ulcerations may represent reactive arthritis in particular.

Esophagus

Esophageal involvement is rare in SpA, though large anterior cervical spine syndesmophytes (or, more likely, productive osteophytes) and craniovertebral junction disease may contribute to dysphagia, neck pain, or limited range of motion.[52,53]

Stomach

Gastric disease is not a common manifestation of SpA per se, though common treatments for axial SpA and peripheral SpA (nonsteroidal antiinflammatory drugs [NSAIDs] and sulfasalazine) are known to precipitate gastritis, gastric ulcers, and GI bleeding.[63,64]

Pancreas

Individuals with psoriasis and psoriatic arthritis seem to be at a higher risk of diabetes compared with the general population,[54] though this may not be true of AS.[55] Obesity and glucocorticoid use account for some, but not all, of this diabetes risk.

Liver

For hepatic abnormalities, distinguishing the complications of spondyloarthritides from the adverse drug reactions related to SpA treatment is challenging. As is the case with diabetes, nonalcoholic fatty liver disease appears more frequently in psoriasis and psoriatic arthritis compared with the general population.[18,56] As is also the case with diabetes, obesity accounts for a portion of the elevated risk.[57] Patients with psoriatic arthritis with more disease activity display higher-grade steatosis.[65] Minor transaminase elevation has been described in 26% of AS, which is high relative to controls.[66] Some have reported higher rates of hepatobiliary disease in UC compared with CD.[67]

Table 1
Anatomic distribution of the involvement for spondyloarthritis

Organ	Involvement	Evidence	Procedure	Citation
Mouth/pharynx	Ulcerative lesions from concomitant CD	N/A	Direct visualization, laryngoscopy	N/A
	Focal sialadenitis	Cross-sectional study	Symptom questionnaire, biopsy, salivary flow rates	Helenius,[51] 2005
Esophagus	Ulcerative lesions from concomitant CD	N/A	EGD	N/A
	Dysphagia & neck pain (cervical spine syndesmophyte)	Case series	EGD, lateral plain radiographs	Toussirot et al,[52] 2015
	Dysphagia (craniovertebral junction disease)	Case reports	EGD, lateral plain radiographs, cervical computer tomography	Albert & Menezes,[53] 2011
Stomach	Gastritis, gastric ulcers, GI bleeding (nonsteroidal antiinflammatory drugs, sulfasalazine)	Meta-analyses of randomized trials, observational studies	EGD	N/A
Pancreas	Diabetes	Observational cohort study	Glucose tolerance test	Dubreuil et al,[54] 2014; Sari et al,[55] 2007
Liver	Nonalcoholic fatty liver disease	Multiple observational cohort studies	Liver function tests, confirmatory imaging[a]	Madanagobalane & Anandan,[18] 2012; van der Voort et al,[56] 2014; Miele et al,[57] 2009
Gall bladder	Primary biliary cirrhosis, primary sclerosing cholangitis	Case reports	Liver function tests, confirmatory imaging,[b] liver biopsy, antimitochondrial antibody	Hirschfield et al,[58] 2013; Pineau et al,[59] 1997; Vargas et al,[60] 1994
Small intestine	Possible ulcerative lesions from concomitant CD; erythema, erosions	Cohort studies	EGD, capsule endoscopy	Eliakim et al,[14] 2005
Colon	Ulcerative/inflammatory lesions from CD, UC, celiac disease	Cohort studies and case reports	Colonoscopy	Shivashankar et al,[61] 2012
Rectum, anus	Ulcerative/inflammatory lesions from CD	Cohort studies	Sigmoidoscopy	Tabernero et al,[62] 2012

Abbreviations: NA, not applicable; EGD, esophagogastroduodenoscopy/upper endoscopy.
[a] Abdominal ultrasound, computed tomography, or MRI.
[b] Cholangiogram, magnetic resonance cholangiopancreatography.

Gallbladder

GWAS have identified possible risk alleles shared between primary biliary cirrhosis, primary sclerosing cholangitis, psoriasis, and AS.[58] However, only a few case reports have made these associations clinically.[59,60]

Small Intestine/Colon

In addition to the clinical overlaps described in the epidemiology section earlier, genomic studies have identified at least 20 loci shared between IBD and AS,[68] including both CD and UC.[69] The genetic overlap between AS and celiac disease is admittedly not as strong.[69] Patients with SpA with axial disease, older individuals, those with elevated SpA disease activity, and men are more likely to demonstrate microscopic gut inflammation than younger individuals or women with SpA.[19]

Several studies have suggested that patients with IBD should be screened for SpA if they complain of inflammatory low back pain or chronic low back pain beginning before 45 years of age. They should also be screened if they are found to be HLA-B27 positive or demonstrate sacroiliitis on imaging (often incidentally detected on computerized tomography of the abdomen).[70] Others have advocated for screening in the presence of arthritis, heel enthesitis, or dactylitis,[71] though these conditions are often difficult to assess reliably by nonrheumatologists; enthesitis and dactylitis are also relatively insensitive criteria.

Substantially fewer studies have examined screening approaches for identifying IBD in patients with SpA. The combination of serum C-reactive protein and serum or fecal calprotectin may point to the presence of IBD.[72] An interdisciplinary expert panel recently suggested IBD should be screened for in patients with SpA using an algorithm that includes rectal bleeding, chronic diarrhea, perianal disease, chronic abdominal pain, iron deficiency anemia or iron deficiency, fever, unexplained weight loss, and a family history of IBD.[71] This approach has not been corroborated.

UC, CD, and celiac disease can present with a microcytic anemia resulting from GI blood loss, abdominal pain, and frequent bowel movements. Although all 3 may present with bloody diarrhea, the diarrhea of ileal CD and celiac disease are classically nonbloody. Tenesmus is also associated with UC, more so than CD. The lesions of UC present as an uninterrupted inflammation restricted to the colon; CD can produce skip lesions anywhere along the GI tract.

DIAGNOSTIC EVALUATION
Differential Diagnosis

The differential diagnosis for spondylitic diseases with GI symptoms is extensive and may include CD and UC (both without and with true arthritis/EAA), nonsteroidal antiinflammatory enteropathy, Whipple disease, postenteritis reactive arthritis, celiac disease, spinal abscess, *Brucella* spondylitis and sacroiliitis, Behçet disease, sarcoidosis, leukemia/lymphoma, and familial Mediterranean fever. Diverticulitis, antibiotic-associated colitis, and small bowel malignancy are also considerations.

Diagnostic Testing

Serologic studies that include soluble tissue transglutaminase IgA, serum angiotensin converting enzyme, serum lysozyme, and amyloid A, may allow the clinician to rule out competing diagnoses. If the clinical scenario raises sufficient suspicion, it may be reasonable to send pyrin/MEFV gene mutation, and tissue *Tropheryma whipplei* polymerase chain reaction. Fecal calprotectin indicates the presence of large intestinal inflammation (resulting from neutrophil migration into the intestinal mucosa) and may suggest IBD[73]; but much like an erythrocyte sedimentation rate, fecal calprotectin does not specifically indicate the cause of inflammation. Anti–*Saccharomyces cerevisiae* antibodies may also suggest the presence of CD,[74] whereas perinuclear antineutrophil cytoplasmic antibodies without a positive antimyeloperoxidase antibody can suggest UC. In the case of celiac disease, patients may be positive for immunoglobulin A antiendomysial antibodies by immunofluorescence.

Plain radiography with dedicated views of the sacroiliac joints should be performed for evaluation of axial SpA and imaging of peripheral joints, as indicated by symptoms. Lateral views of the thoracic and lumbar vertebrae can be used to gauge the presence and degree of syndesmophyte formation. If these are nondiagnostic and patients have inflammatory back pain or a suggestive history (family history of SpA, uveitis, and so forth), the provider may consider MRI of the pelvis using T1 and short tau inversion recovery sequences.[75]

Diagnostic testing for GI disease may include upper and lower endoscopy, though capsule endoscopy may be more sensitive than ileocolonoscopy for the detection of small bowel lesions.[14] In pediatric patients, evaluation with magnetic resonance enterography may provide a method of evaluating for mild, or even subclinical, disease.[76] The diagnosis of UC, CD, and celiac disease is confirmed by biopsy. The findings of UC classically include excess tissue polymorphonuclear neutrophils, mucosal inflammation presenting as distortion, and inflammation of crypts, with crypt abscesses and goblet cell dropout. The histology of CD, in contrast, can extend the full thickness of the bowel wall, with ulcers, fistulas, stenosis, and non-necrotizing granuloma formation. Celiac disease typically manifests as villous atrophy with occasional elevated levels of intraepithelial lymphocytes.

DIGESTIVE AND HEPATIC ASPECTS RELATED TO TREATMENT OF SPONDYLOARTHRITIS

Given the elevated risk for diabetes in SpA, providers should use judicious use of glucocorticoids in these diseases and consider monitoring patients on glucocorticoids more closely (eg, weight gain, hemoglobin A1C, fasting glucose, and so forth). Sulfasalazine may be an ideal agent for patients with peripheral SpA with additional risk factors for diabetes, in light of preliminary data demonstrating a possible hypoglycemic effect with the use of this therapy.[77]

Appropriate liver function and viral hepatitis testing should be performed before initiation of hydroxychloroquine, leflunomide, methotrexate, and sulfasalazine.[78,79] Providers should exercise increased caution when prescribing methotrexate and leflunomide in the setting of concomitant hepatic disease. On the other hand, observational data have suggested a hepato-protective effect with tumor necrosis factor inhibitors.[80] Although some gastroenterologists prefer to forgo NSAIDs altogether in the setting of IBD, preliminary controlled trial data suggest low-dose NSAIDs, particularly celecoxib, may be used.[81]

SUMMARY

SpA can affect the digestive system and liver in several ways, most commonly presenting as IBD. The theories expounded more than 100 years ago linking intestinal pathology to arthritis seem to contain some element of truth, as revealed through recent investigations of dysbiosis. Clinicians have several diagnostic tools at their disposal to probe the potential causes of GI disease occurring in the setting of SpA.

ACKNOWLEDGMENTS

Both authors acknowledge that they have no financial and personal relationships with other people or organizations that could inappropriately influence the content of this article. Dr L. Caplan is supported by the US Department of Veterans Affairs (VA; HSR&D IIR 14-048-3; VA Innovators Network). Dr K.A. Kuhn is supported through National Institutes of Health (K08 DK107905), the Boettcher Foundation, and the Rheumatology Research Foundation. Drs L. Caplan and K.A. Kuhn have received project support from the Michelson Fund at the University of Colorado Foundation. However, the VA and University of Colorado Foundation had no role in the writing of this article or in the decision to submit the article for publication. The views expressed in this article are those of the authors and do not necessarily reflect the position or policy of the Department of Veterans Affairs.

REFERENCES

1. Cave EJ. Minutes of the British Medical Association meeting: the sections, medicine. The Lancet 1901 1901;158(4066):329.
2. Andrews CR, Hoke M. A preliminary report on the relation of albuminous putrefaction in the intestines to arthritis deformans (rheumatoid arthritis, osteoarthritis): its influence upon treatment. J Bone Joint Surg Am 1907;s2-5(1):61–72.
3. Warden CC. The toxemic factor in rheumatoid arthritis. Cal State J Med 1909;7(8): 299–301.
4. Smith R. The surgical relief of intestinal foci of infection in cases of arthritis deformans. Ann Surg 1922;76(4):515–8.
5. Bargen JA. Complications and sequelae of chronic ulcerative colitis. Ann Intern Med 1929;3(4):335–52.
6. Bywaters EGL, Ansell BM. Arthritis associated with ulcerative colitis: a clinical and pathological study. Ann Rheum Dis 1958;17(2):169–83.
7. Bakland G, Nossent HC. Epidemiology of spondyloarthritis: a review. Curr Rheumatol Rep 2013;15(9):351.
8. Hou JK, Kramer JR, Richardson P, et al. The incidence and prevalence of inflammatory bowel disease among U.S. veterans: a national cohort study. Inflamm Bowel Dis 2013;19(5):1059–64.
9. Loftus EV. Update on the incidence and prevalence of inflammatory bowel disease in the United States. Gastroenterol Hepatol (N Y) 2016;12(11):704–7.
10. De Angelis R, Salaffi F, Grassi W. Prevalence of spondyloarthropathies in an Italian population sample: a regional community-based study. Scand J Rheumatol 2007;36(1):14–21.
11. Haglund E, Bremander AB, Petersson IF, et al. Prevalence of spondyloarthritis and its subtypes in southern Sweden. Ann Rheum Dis 2011;70(6):943–8.
12. Stolwijk C, van TA, Castillo-Ortiz JD, et al. Prevalence of extra-articular manifestations in patients with ankylosing spondylitis: a systematic review and meta-analysis. Ann Rheum Dis 2015;74(1):65–73.
13. Leirisalo-Repo M, Turunen U, Stenman S, et al. High frequency of silent inflammatory bowel disease in spondylarthropathy. Arthritis Rheum 1994;37(1):23–31.
14. Eliakim R, Karban A, Markovits D, et al. Comparison of capsule endoscopy with ileocolonoscopy for detecting small-bowel lesions in patients with seronegative spondyloarthropathies. Endoscopy 2005;37(12):1165–9.
15. De Vos M, Mielants H, Cuvelier C, et al. Long-term evolution of gut inflammation in patients with spondyloarthropathy. Gastroenterology 1996;110(6):1696–703.

16. Mielants H, Veys EM, Cuvelier C, et al. HLA-B27 related arthritis and bowel inflammation. Part 2. Ileocolonoscopy and bowel histology in patients with HLA-B27 related arthritis. J Rheumatol 1985;12(2):294–8.

17. Karreman MC, Luime JJ, Hazes JMW, et al. The prevalence and incidence of axial and peripheral spondyloarthritis in inflammatory bowel disease: a systematic review and meta-analysis. J Crohns Colitis 2017;11(5):631–42.

18. Madanagobalane S, Anandan S. The increased prevalence of non-alcoholic fatty liver disease in psoriatic patients: a study from South India. Australas J Dermatol 2012;53(3):190–7.

19. Van Praet L, Van den Bosch FE, Jacques P, et al. Microscopic gut inflammation in axial spondyloarthritis: a multiparametric predictive model. Ann Rheum Dis 2013; 72(3):414–7.

20. Gionchetti P, Rizzello F. IBD: IBD and spondyloarthritis: joint management. Nat Rev Gastroenterol Hepatol 2016;13(1):9–10.

21. Thjodleifsson B, Geirsson AJ, Bjornsson S, et al. A common genetic background for inflammatory bowel disease and ankylosing spondylitis: a genealogic study in Iceland. Arthritis Rheum 2007;56(8):2633–9.

22. Rudwaleit M, Baeten D. Ankylosing spondylitis and bowel disease. Best Pract Res Clin Rheumatol 2006;20(3):451–71.

23. Costello ME, Ciccia F, Willner D, et al. Brief report: intestinal dysbiosis in ankylosing spondylitis. Arthritis Rheumatol 2015;67(3):686–91.

24. Frank DN, St Amand AL, Feldman RA, et al. Molecular-phylogenetic characterization of microbial community imbalances in human inflammatory bowel diseases. Proc Natl Acad Sci U S A 2007;104(34):13780–5.

25. Gevers D, Kugathasan S, Denson LA, et al. The treatment-naive microbiome in new-onset Crohn's disease. Cell Host Microbe 2014;15(3):382–92.

26. Scher JU, Ubeda C, Artacho A, et al. Decreased bacterial diversity characterizes the altered gut microbiota in patients with psoriatic arthritis, resembling dysbiosis in inflammatory bowel disease. Arthritis Rheumatol 2015;67(1):128–39.

27. Stoll ML, Kumar R, Morrow CD, et al. Altered microbiota associated with abnormal humoral immune responses to commensal organisms in enthesitis-related arthritis. Arthritis Res Ther 2014;16(6):486.

28. Ranganathan V, Gracey E, Brown MA, et al. Pathogenesis of ankylosing spondylitis [mdash] recent advances and future directions. Nat Rev Rheumatol 2017; 13(6):359–67.

29. Ellinghaus D, Jostins L, Spain SL, et al. Analysis of five chronic inflammatory diseases identifies 27 new associations and highlights disease-specific patterns at shared loci. Nat Genet 2016;48(5):510–8.

30. Burton PR, Clayton DG, Cardon LR, et al. Association scan of 14,500 nonsynonymous SNPs in four diseases identifies autoimmunity variants. Nat Genet 2007; 39(11):1329–37.

31. Duerr RH, Taylor KD, Brant SR, et al. A genome-wide association study identifies IL23R as an inflammatory bowel disease gene. Science 2006;314(5804):1461–3.

32. Laukens D, Peeters H, Marichal D, et al. CARD15 gene polymorphisms in patients with spondyloarthropathies identify a specific phenotype previously related to Crohn's disease. Ann Rheum Dis 2005;64(6):930–5.

33. Breban M, Tap J, Leboime A, et al. Faecal microbiota study reveals specific dysbiosis in spondyloarthritis. Ann Rheum Dis 2017;76(9):1614–22.

34. Tito RY, Cypers H, Joossens M, et al. Brief report: Dialister as a microbial marker of disease activity in spondyloarthritis. Arthritis Rheumatol 2017;69(1):114–21.

35. Frank DN, Robertson CE, Hamm CM, et al. Disease phenotype and genotype are associated with shifts in intestinal-associated microbiota in inflammatory bowel diseases. Inflamm Bowel Dis 2011;17(1):179–84.
36. Frank DN, Zhu W, Sartor RB, et al. Investigating the biological and clinical significance of human dysbioses. Trends Microbiol 2011;19(9):427–34.
37. Atarashi K, Tanoue T, Oshima K, et al. Treg induction by a rationally selected mixture of Clostridia strains from the human microbiota. Nature 2013; 500(7461):232–6.
38. Round JL, Mazmanian SK. Inducible Foxp3+ regulatory T-cell development by a commensal bacterium of the intestinal microbiota. Proc Natl Acad Sci U S A 2010; 107(27):12204–9.
39. Smith PM, Howitt MR, Panikov N, et al. The microbial metabolites, short-chain fatty acids, regulate colonic Treg cell homeostasis. Science 2013;341(6145): 569–73.
40. Ivanov II, Atarashi K, Manel N, et al. Induction of intestinal Th17 cells by segmented filamentous bacteria. Cell 2009;139(3):485–98.
41. Ivanov II, Frutos RL, Manel N, et al. Specific microbiota direct the differentiation of IL-17-producing T-helper cells in the mucosa of the small intestine. Cell Host Microbe 2008;4(4):337–49.
42. Harbour SN, Maynard CL, Zindl CL, et al. Th17 cells give rise to Th1 cells that are required for the pathogenesis of colitis. Proc Natl Acad Sci U S A 2015;112(22): 7061–6.
43. Taurog JD, Richardson JA, Croft JT, et al. The germfree state prevents development of gut and joint inflammatory disease in HLA-B27 transgenic rats. J Exp Med 1994;180(6):2359–64.
44. Rath HC, Herfarth HH, Ikeda JS, et al. Normal luminal bacteria, especially Bacteroides species, mediate chronic colitis, gastritis, and arthritis in HLA-B27/human beta2 microglobulin transgenic rats. J Clin Invest 1996;98(4):945–53.
45. Asquith MJ, Stauffer P, Davin S, et al. Perturbed mucosal immunity and dysbiosis accompany clinical disease in a rat model of spondyloarthritis. Arthritis Rheumatol 2016;68(9):2151–62.
46. Asquith M, Davin S, Stauffer P, et al. Intestinal metabolites are profoundly altered in the context of HLA-B27 expression and functionally modulate disease in a rat model of spondyloarthropathy. Arthritis Rheumatol 2017;69(10):1984–95.
47. Jacques P, Elewaut D. Joint expedition: linking gut inflammation to arthritis. Mucosal Immunol 2008;1(5):364–71.
48. Quaden DH, De Winter LM, Somers V. Detection of novel diagnostic antibodies in ankylosing spondylitis: an overview. Autoimmun Rev 2016;15(8):820–32.
49. Sorrentino R, Bockmann RA, Fiorillo MT. HLA-B27 and antigen presentation: at the crossroads between immune defense and autoimmunity. Mol Immunol 2014;57(1):22–7.
50. Gracey E, Qaiyum Z, Almaghlouth I, et al. IL-7 primes IL-17 in mucosal-associated invariant T (MAIT) cells, which contribute to the Th17-axis in ankylosing spondylitis. Ann Rheum Dis 2016;75(12):2124–32.
51. Helenius LMJ. Oral and temporomandibular joint findings in rheumatic disease [Thesis]. Helsinki (Finaland): Yliopistopaino; 2005.
52. Toussirot E, Mauvais O, Aubry S. Dysphagia related to esophagus compression by anterior cervical ossification in a patient with ankylosing spondylitis. J Rheumatol 2015;42(10):1922–3.
53. Albert GW, Menezes AH. Ankylosing spondylitis of the craniovertebral junction: a single surgeon's experience. J Neurosurg Spine 2011;14(4):429–36.

54. Dubreuil M, Rho YH, Man A, et al. Diabetes incidence in psoriatic arthritis, psoriasis and rheumatoid arthritis: a UK population-based cohort study. Rheumatology (Oxford) 2014;53(2):346–52.
55. Sari I, Demir T, Kozaci LD, et al. Body composition, insulin, and leptin levels in patients with ankylosing spondylitis. Clin Rheumatol 2007;26(9):1427–32.
56. van der Voort EA, Koehler EM, Dowlatshahi EA, et al. Psoriasis is independently associated with nonalcoholic fatty liver disease in patients 55 years old or older: results from a population-based study. J Am Acad Dermatol 2014;70(3):517–24.
57. Miele L, Vallone S, Cefalo C, et al. Prevalence, characteristics and severity of nonalcoholic fatty liver disease in patients with chronic plaque psoriasis. J Hepatol 2009;51(4):778–86.
58. Hirschfield GM, Chapman RW, Karlsen TH, et al. The genetics of complex cholestatic disorders. Gastroenterology 2013;144(7):1357–74.
59. Pineau BC, Pattee LP, McGuire S, et al. Unusual presentation of primary sclerosing cholangitis. Can J Gastroenterol 1997;11(1):45–8.
60. Vargas CA, Medina R, Rubio CE, et al. Primary biliary cirrhosis associated with ankylosing spondylitis. J Clin Gastroenterol 1994;18(3):263–4.
61. Shivashankar R, Loftus EV Jr, Tremaine WJ, et al. Incidence of spondyloarthropathy in patients with Crohn's disease: a population-based study. J Rheumatol 2012;39(11):2148–52.
62. Tabernero S, Marin-Jimenez I, Gomez F, et al. Factors associated to the presence of spondyloarthritis in patients with inflammatory bowel disease, AQUILES study. Inflamm Bowel Dis 2012;18(Supplement 1):S37.
63. Bhala N, Emberson J, Merhi A, et al. Vascular and upper gastrointestinal effects of non-steroidal anti-inflammatory drugs: meta-analyses of individual participant data from randomised trials. Lancet 2013;382(9894):769–79.
64. Nissila M, Lehtinen K, Leirisalo-Repo M, et al. Sulfasalazine in the treatment of ankylosing spondylitis. A twenty-six-week, placebo-controlled clinical trial. Arthritis Rheum 1988;31(9):1111–6.
65. Di Minno MN, Iervolino S, Peluso R, et al. Hepatic steatosis and disease activity in subjects with psoriatic arthritis receiving tumor necrosis factor-alpha blockers. J Rheumatol 2012;39(5):1042–6.
66. Robinson AC, Teeling M, Casey EB. Hepatic function in ankylosing spondylitis. Ann Rheum Dis 1983;42(5):550–2.
67. Mendoza JL, Lana R, Taxonera C, et al. Extraintestinal manifestations in inflammatory bowel disease: differences between Crohn's disease and ulcerative colitis. Med Clin (Barc) 2005;125(8):297–300 [in Spanish].
68. Parkes M, Cortes A, van Heel DA, et al. Genetic insights into common pathways and complex relationships among immune-mediated diseases. Nat Rev Genet 2013;14(9):661–73.
69. Cortes A, Hadler J, Pointon JP, et al. Identification of multiple risk variants for ankylosing spondylitis through high-density genotyping of immune-related loci. Nat Genet 2013;45(7):730–8.
70. Danve A, Deodhar A. Screening and referral for axial spondyloarthritis–need of the hour. Clin Rheumatol 2015;34(6):987–93.
71. Sanz Sanz J, Juanola Roura X, Seoane-Mato D, et al. Screening of inflammatory bowel disease and spondyloarthritis for referring patients between rheumatology and gastroenterology. Reumatol Clin 2017. [Epub ahead of print].
72. Cypers H, Varkas G, Beeckman S, et al. Elevated calprotectin levels reveal bowel inflammation in spondyloarthritis. Ann Rheum Dis 2016;75(7):1357.

73. Smith LA, Gaya DR. Utility of faecal calprotectin analysis in adult inflammatory bowel disease. World J Gastroenterol 2012;18(46):6782–9.

74. Walker LJ, Aldhous MC, Drummond HE, et al. Anti-Saccharomyces cerevisiae antibodies (ASCA) in Crohn's disease are associated with disease severity but not NOD2/CARD15 mutations. Clin Exp Immunol 2004;135(3):490–6.

75. Maksymowych WP. The role of MRI in the evaluation of spondyloarthritis: a clinician's guide. Clin Rheumatol 2016;35(6):1447–55.

76. Stoll ML, Patel AS, Punaro M, et al. MR enterography to evaluate sub-clinical intestinal inflammation in children with spondyloarthritis. Pediatr Rheumatol Online J 2012;10(1):6.

77. Haas RM, Li P, Chu JW. Glucose-lowering effects of sulfasalazine in type 2 diabetes. Diabetes Care 2005;28(9):2238–9.

78. Singh JA, Saag KG, Bridges SL Jr, et al. 2015 American College of Rheumatology guideline for the treatment of rheumatoid arthritis. Arthritis Rheumatol 2016;68(1):1–26.

79. Saag KG, Teng GG, Patkar NM, et al. American College of Rheumatology 2008 recommendations for the use of nonbiologic and biologic disease-modifying antirheumatic drugs in rheumatoid arthritis. Arthritis Rheum 2008;59(6):762–84.

80. Seitz M, Reichenbach S, Moller B, et al. Hepatoprotective effect of tumour necrosis factor alpha blockade in psoriatic arthritis: a cross-sectional study. Ann Rheum Dis 2010;69(6):1148–50.

81. Sandborn WJ, Stenson WF, Brynskov J, et al. Safety of celecoxib in patients with ulcerative colitis in remission: a randomized, placebo-controlled, pilot study. Clin Gastroenterol Hepatol 2006;4(2):203–11.

Gastrointestinal and Hepatic Disease in Systemic Lupus Erythematosus

 CrossMark

Brian N. Brewer, MD[a], Diane L. Kamen, MD, MSCR[b],*

KEYWORDS

- Lupus enteritis • Enteral vasculitis • Intestinal pseudo-obstruction
- Protein-losing enteropathy

KEY POINTS

- Lupus-associated enteritis is a rare feature of systemic lupus erythematosus (SLE) but has morbidity and mortality implications.
- Pathophysiology of lupus enteritis involves a vasculopathic process in the bowel wall with extension to the mesenteric plexus.
- Presenting signs and symptoms of lupus enteritis are often nonspecific but rarely present without other evidence of active SLE.

INTRODUCTION

Systemic lupus erythematosus (SLE) is a chronic, potentially severe, frequently disabling autoimmune disease with multiorgan involvement and a typically waxing and waning course. SLE is characterized by the production of a vast array of autoantibodies and is often considered the prototypical autoimmune disease. SLE has the potential to affect virtually every organ, including the gastrointestinal (GI) system, but most commonly presents with musculoskeletal, cutaneous, renal, cardiovascular, hematologic, and/or central nervous system involvement. In contrast with other autoimmune diseases, such as systemic sclerosis and inflammatory bowel disease (IBD), GI system disease activity is rare among patients with SLE. However, for that minority of patients, SLE activity involving the GI system can be severe and even life threatening.

Disclosure: All authors acknowledge that they have no financial or personal relationships with other people or organizations that could inappropriately influence the content of this article. Dr D.L. Kamen is supported by funding from the National Institute of Arthritis and Musculoskeletal and Skin Diseases, NIH under award number K24 AR068406.
[a] Department of Internal Medicine, Augusta University-University of Georgia, 108 Spear Road, Athens, GA 30602, USA; [b] Division of Rheumatology and Immunology, Medical University of South Carolina, 96 Jonathan Lucas Street, Suite 916 e, Charleston, SC 29425, USA
* Corresponding author.
E-mail address: kamend@musc.edu

Rheum Dis Clin N Am 44 (2018) 165–175
https://doi.org/10.1016/j.rdc.2017.09.011
0889-857X/18/© 2017 Elsevier Inc. All rights reserved.

rheumatic.theclinics.com

This article reviews the types of GI system involvement associated with SLE. It includes GI manifestations directly caused by SLE disease activity as well as those occurring in patients with SLE but not directly attributable to active disease. This article is focused on the clinical manifestations of SLE-related GI involvement, with less emphasis on the therapies, which are covered elsewhere in this issue.

WHO IS AT RISK FOR SYSTEMIC LUPUS ERYTHEMATOSUS GASTROINTESTINAL INVOLVEMENT?

The onset of SLE can emerge at any age, but it most often occurs in young women between puberty and menopause. The incidence and severity of SLE is also disproportionately higher among certain racial and ethnic groups, such as people of African descent who live in North America or Europe.[1] In spite of its high impact on individual lives as well as high societal cost, little is known about the cause of SLE.

The clinical symptoms and laboratory manifestations of SLE are extremely diverse. Early diagnosis can be difficult because of the insidious onset of predominantly nonspecific constitutional symptoms (eg, fatigue, joint pains, and low-grade fever). This delay between symptom onset resulting from inflammation, subsequent diagnosis, and initiation of treatment can result in the development of organ system damage. The intent is to identify, when possible, and distinguish between active inflammatory features and features seen in long-standing disease caused by damage.

GI symptoms are common and can occur in approximately half of people with SLE, often triggered by an underlying infection or by medication adverse effects.[2] The most prevalent GI symptoms are nonspecific, such as nausea and vomiting, anorexia, and abdominal pain.[3] Other clinical clues are often needed to distinguish between GI manifestations stemming from an infection, medication side effects, active SLE, and/or a comorbid GI-related medical condition.

DEFINING LUPUS ENTERITIS

By definition, lupus enteritis encompasses a wide spectrum of GI involvement. Lupus enteritis, as part of the British Isles Lupus Assessment Group (BILAG) disease activity index, is defined as either vasculitis or inflammation of the small bowel, with supportive imaging and/or biopsy findings.[4] Abdominal pain is the most common presenting symptom of lupus enteritis, although presenting symptoms vary in character and severity (**Fig. 1**). Studies show a range of 0.2% to 5.8% of patients with SLE affected

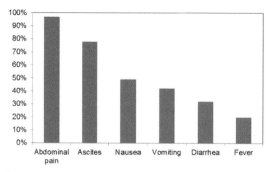

Fig. 1. Incidence of symptoms at presentation with lupus enteritis. (*From* Janssens P, Arnaud L, Galicier L, et al. Lupus enteritis: from clinical findings to therapeutic management. Orphanet J Rare Dis 2013;8:67.)

by lupus enteritis.[5] The median age of onset is 34 years and it develops, on average, 34.3 months after the diagnosis of SLE; 85% of patients are female.

GI activity arising in isolation without additional manifestations of active SLE is highly unusual, because other organ systems typically show evidence of ongoing involvement. Consequently, higher scores on disease activity measurements, such as the BILAG or SLE Disease Activity Index (SLEDAI), are common for individuals affected by SLE enteritis. For example, 65% of SLE enteritis cases also carry a concomitant diagnosis of lupus nephritis, which contributes to the score on both instruments.

Although the wide differential diagnoses for patients with SLE presenting with GI symptoms complicate matters, it is important to identify lupus enteritis in a timely manner because of its rare but serious course. For instance, the mortality among patients with SLE with acute abdominal pain is 11%.[5] There may also be subclinical presentations that go undiagnosed, as suggested by an autopsy study showing 60% to 70% of patients with SLE with evidence of peritonitis, despite only 10% being recognized clinically.[6]

PATHOGENESIS AND PATHOPHYSIOLOGY

Oral ulcers are a classic and common manifestation of SLE. The 3 principal pathologic and pathophysiologic components of lupus enteritis are lupus mesenteric vasculitis, intestinal pseudo-obstruction, and protein-losing enteropathy. Pancreatitis and hepatobiliary involvement are more rarely encountered.

Oral Ulcers

The characteristic oral ulcers of SLE are painless, involve the upper (hard) palate, and are unrelated to systemic complement levels or levels of autoantibodies.[7] These ulcers affect 25% to 50% of patients with SLE,[8] and are a component of the classification criteria for SLE, both for the American College of Rheumatology 1982 Revised Criteria as well as the Systemic Lupus International Collaborating Clinics Criteria,[9,10] assuming they occur in the absence of other causes of ulcers. Other oral manifestations include hyperkeratotic lesions and lichenoid inflammatory mononuclear infiltrates appearing as macules and plaques on direct visualization.[11]

Lupus Mesenteric Vasculitis

The term lupus enteritis was initially used to distinguish true mesenteric vasculitis from other causes of intra-abdominal manifestations of SLE-associated GI complications. Typically, true mesenteric vasculitis involves small vessel arteritis or venulitis.[12] Variance in appropriate nomenclature of the disorder has led to some confusion in describing the condition. Lupus arteritis, lupus enteritis, GI vasculitis, intra-abdominal vasculitis, and acute GI syndrome have all been used to describe the same entity.[13] Primary concern for untreated disease is for development of bowel wall infarction, ischemia, or perforation.[13] These complications have a high rate of associated mortality. The underlying cause for the enteric vasculitis continues to be unknown.

Reports vary regarding the prevalence of increased antiphospholipid antibody levels, incidence of thrombosis, as well as systemic disease activity during episodes of lupus enteritis. The current understanding of these thrombotic events relates inflammation of the blood vessels to immune complex deposition as well as complement activation, leading to endothelial cell and platelet activation.[2] Pathology reports from thromboses complicating lupus enteritis have been nonspecific. These reports show findings of multisegmental involvement in multiple vascular territories.[14]

Typically the jejunum and ileum are the GI tract locations most commonly involved. Macroscopic examination reveals edematous, hyperemic, or ischemic bowel wall with or without infarction.[14] Microscopic (histologic) examination is consistent with infiltration of the submucosal and muscular layers and necrotizing vasculitis with pan-mural predominant eosinophilic, neutrophilic, or mixed infiltrate.[14]

Intestinal Pseudo-obstruction

Intestinal pseudo-obstruction is defined as ineffective propulsion in the intestinal tract. This entity may be a misnomer, because manometry studies reveal more frequent GI involvement in the esophageal and gastric portions of the GI tract.[15] Pathologic processes featured with intestinal pseudo-obstruction include intestinal vasculitis leading to visceral smooth muscle damage. Typical involvement not only implicates the smooth muscle but also involves the enteric nerves, leading to visceral autonomic nervous system dysfunction, further compromising GI motility.[16] Patients are subject to an increased risk of developing urinary tract infections. However, urinary tract infections can also be associated with impaired gastric motility independently of intestinal pseudo-obstruction. Main areas of involvement include the lower third of the esophagus as well as the antrum and duodenum.

Protein-losing Enteropathy

Protein-losing enteropathy is defined as profound edema with hypoalbuminemia secondary to excessive protein loss from the GI tract. There are 3 main pathophysiologic mechanisms that have been proposed, and all 3 involve impairment of the permeability of the gut wall. The first mechanism is vasculitis leading directly to increased intestinal vessel permeability.[17] The second mechanism is complement conversion leading to cytokine-mediated damage and vasodilation. The third proposed mechanism is intestinal lymphangiectasia. In order to establish the diagnosis of protein-losing enteropathy, decreased dietary protein intake and excessive urinary losses must be ruled out.[18]

Association with Inflammatory Bowel Disease

Case reports and case series from around the world indicate an infrequent association between IBD and SLE. However, overlapping symptoms can make differentiating the two diagnoses challenging.[19] Observational studies have shown a prevalence of ulcerative colitis in SLE at 0.4%, which is comparable with general population controls.[20] With regard to Crohn disease, the prevalence has been estimated at 0.7% to 0.3% of patients with SLE,[20] which, in contrast with ulcerative colitis, suggests a possible association between SLE and Crohn.

Reports of SLE among patients with IBD are confounded by the possibility of tumor necrosis factor inhibitor (TNFi)–induced lupus reactions. Because TNFi are the most common class of biologic used for IBD, it is difficult to discern whether characteristics of SLE represent drug-induced lupus/lupuslike syndrome or the systemic inflammatory disease unrelated to therapy. The pathophysiologic mechanism of drug-induced lupus is thought to invoke dysregulation of apoptosis and exposure of nuclear antigens.[21] Increased antinuclear antibody (ANA) levels are commonly found in this patient population; however, symptoms of drug-induced lupus correlate more strongly with the presence of anti–double-stranded DNA (dsDNA) antibodies. A review found that 11% to 26% of adalimumab-treated patients with IBD had a positive ANA test, whereas 45% of infliximab-treated patients had a positive ANA test.[22]

Association with Celiac Disease

Prior investigations have revealed a possible association between SLE and celiac disease. Celiac disease has an approximately 1% prevalence in the general population,[23] and has a tendency to coexist with other autoimmune conditions, including rheumatoid arthritis and type 1 diabetes, among other diseases.[24] There seems to be overlap in disease presentation as well as autoantibody positivity, as manifest through high ANA titers and human leukocyte antigen serotypes. There is also similar immune system activation in the form of increased soluble interleukin-2 receptor and soluble intercellular adhesion molecule-1 levels.[24] These clinical and biomarker overlaps feed the speculation of an association between SLE and celiac disease. Results from an epidemiologic study identified an increased prevalence of celiac disease in an SLE population, compared with age-matched and sex-matched controls (0.8% compared with 0.2%).[24] However, continued exploration on a verifiable clinical association is ongoing.

Lupus-Associated Pancreatitis

Rates and definitions of pancreatitis among SLE cohorts vary across studies. Variations in laboratory assays may produce increased levels of pancreatic enzymes without clinical symptoms compatible with pancreatitis. Estimates of prevalence range from 0.7% to 4% of patients with SLE. Some investigators report that, in up to 22% of the SLE population, pancreatitis is the initial presentation of SLE.[2] It is typically more prevalent in the first few years following the onset of SLE symptoms. Vasculitis leading to tissue necrosis, antiphospholipid-associated thrombosis of pancreatic arterioles and arteries, and intimal thickening with immune complex deposition in the wall of the pancreatic arteries are possible underlying pathophysiologic causes of pancreatitis related to SLE.[2] Other causes of pancreatitis, including azathioprine-induced pancreatitis, must be ruled out before diagnosis. Some investigators suggest a possible correlation between the presence of anti-La antibodies and the risk of pancreatitis.

Associated Hepatobiliary Manifestations

Increased transaminase levels/transaminitis have been found among patients with SLE with a frequency of between 15% and 55%.[25] As has been noted in several articles in this issue, many of the medications used for SLE therapy can affect the liver and involve routine monitoring of liver enzyme tests as standard of care. Medications such as nonsteroidal antiinflammatory drugs (NSAIDs), methotrexate, azathioprine, mycophenolate, and corticosteroids are possible causes.[25] Other SLE-associated conditions include viral hepatitis, hemolysis, myositis, venous congestion, and veno-occlusive disease, especially in the setting of antiphospholipid antibody syndrome. Autoimmune hepatitis and primary biliary cirrhosis should be considered if antimitochondrial antibodies and increased alkaline phosphatase level are present.

With regard to biliary disorder, 2 main associated disorders are typically considered for patients with SLE: primary sclerosing cholangitis and autoimmune cholecystitis. The underlying mechanism is thought to be subclinical vasculitic damage of the intramural capillary network.[3] This condition may eventually progress to acute acalculous cholecystitis.

Serositis

Abdominal serositis (lupus peritonitis) is seen in 10% of patients with SLE, although the 1982 revised criteria for classification of SLE limit consideration of serositis to pleural and pericardial surfaces.[9] In almost all cases, SLE is simultaneously active in other organ systems (**Table 1**).[26]

Table 1
Anatomic distribution of gastrointestinal involvement among patients with systemic lupus erythematosus

Organ	Involvement	Evidence	Citation
Mouth/pharynx	Oral ulcers	Review article	Sultan et al,[8] 1999
Esophagus	Dysphagia Esophageal dysmotility Gastric reflux Bullous epidermolysis Ulcerative esophagitis	Review article	Ebert & Hagspiel,[3] 2011; Witt et al,[25] 2006; Jackson,[27] 2015
Stomach	Peptic ulcer disease Gastric enteritis Dyspepsia	Review article	Ebert & Hagspiel,[3] 2011; Jackson,[27] 2015
Pancreas	Acute pancreatitis	Review article	Alves et al,[2] 2016; Jackson,[27] 2015
Liver	Hepatomegaly Type 1 autoimmune hepatitis Steatosis Nodular regenerative hyperplasia	Review article	Alves et al,[2] 2016; Ebert & Hagspiel,[3] 2011
Gall bladder	Primary sclerosing cholangitis Autoimmune cholangiopathy Acute acalculous cholangitis	Review article	Ebert & Hagspiel,[3] 2011
Small intestine	Celiac disease Mesenteric vasculitis Protein-losing enteropathy Cytomegalovirus enteritis Intestinal pseudo-obstruction	Case control	Alves et al,[2] 2016; Ebert & Hagspiel,[3] 2011; Dahan et al,[24] 2016
Colon	Crohn disease Bowel perforation Pneumatosis cystoides intestinalis Benign pneumoperitoneum	Review article	Ebert & Hagspiel,[3] 2011; Shor et al,[20] 2016
Rectum, anus	Ulcerations	Case study	Yau et al,[28] 2014
Other	Appendicitis Primary lupus peritonitis Splenomegaly Ascites	Review article	Ebert & Hagspiel,[3] 2011

DIAGNOSTIC EVALUATION

The main modality for diagnosis of SLE-associated mesenteric vasculitis revolves around imaging. Typically, computed tomography (CT) of the abdomen is the test of choice, with a recent study describing 98% of images showing bowel wall edema and 71% showing abdominal bowel wall enhancement (termed the double-halo or target sign). Another 71% of images associated with this study showed engorgement and increased visibility of the mesenteric vessels (comb sign[14]; **Fig. 2**) In addition, attenuation of the mesenteric fat can also be a feature. Serology and inflammatory markers in SLE-associated mesenteric vasculitis are typically nonspecific. The mean C-reactive protein level has been reported as 2.0 mg/dL with low complement levels noted in 88% of the study population.[2] ANA testing was positive in 92% with a positive dsDNA antibody present in 74% of the study population. Anti-RNP, anti-SSA, and anti-Sm was positive in 28%, 26%, and 24% respectively.[2] Proteinuria (>0.5 g/24 h or 2+ on dipstick) was found in 47% of patients with SLE. An association

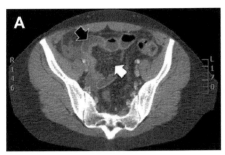 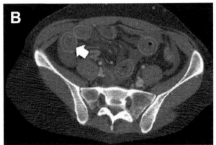

Fig. 2. Abdominal CT findings of lupus enteritis. (*A*) Comb sign. Engorgement and increased visibility of the mesenteric vessels. (*B*) Target sign. Enhancement and thickening of bowel wall. (*From* Janssens P, Arnaud L, Galicier L, et al. Lupus enteritis: from clinical findings to therapeutic management. Orphanet J Rare Dis 2013;8:67.)

with antiphospholipid antibodies (of concern because of concurrent mesenteric thrombosis) remains in dispute.[14]

For intestinal pseudo-obstruction, a combination of imaging and manometry may clarify the diagnosis. Imaging, in the form of abdominal plain radiographs, is usually sufficient to reveal evidence of intestinal obstruction. Follow-up endoscopy frequently does not reveal a specific structural cause of the obstruction.[16] As mentioned earlier, the lower third of the esophagus, the gastric antrum, and duodenum are particularly susceptible to pseudo-obstruction.

The diagnostic evaluation for protein-losing enteropathy is most definitive when based on technetium-99m (99m Tc)–HSA (human serum albumin) scintigraphy and fecal alpha1-antitrypsin assays. A low serum albumin level should be attributed to protein-losing enteropathy only after the clinician has ruled out excessive urinary losses (which may be present in SLE glomerulonephritis) or decreased protein intake. Firm laboratory cutoffs for classifying the source of protein loss do not exist; however, levels of serum albumin less than 22 g/L and urinary protein of less than 0.84 g/dL show high specificity and positive predictive value for identification of protein-losing enteropathy.[17] Correlations with anti-SSA positivity and hypercholesterolemia have also been described. However, the evidence for 99m Tc-HAS scintigraphy and fecal alpha1-antitrypsin is more specific than the aforementioned biochemical tests. In a study of 67 cases with 99 m Tc-HAS scintigraphy, protein leakage was identified in all cases, with 58 cases revealing the anatomic location of the leakage.[18] In 49 of the cases, the area of leakage was in the small intestine. The investigators also subjected 24 of the participants to a 24-hour stool collection, and in all cases a positive fecal alpha1-antitrypsin clearance was present.[18] Ultrasonography and CT studies are also useful for identifying bowel wall obstruction and ascites.

When evaluating the differential diagnosis for GI symptoms in patients with SLE, endoscopy is commonly used to complete a thorough diagnostic evaluation. Endoscopy with pathologic biopsy evaluation assists in the diagnosis of IBD as well as celiac disease. Direct biliary evaluation is typically at the discretion of a specialist. Initial abdominal imaging in the emergency department typically consists of either abdominal ultrasonography or CT of the abdomen, because these modalities can narrow the broad differential posed by nonspecific GI symptoms.

PHYSICAL EXAMINATION FINDINGS

Very few physical examination findings are specific to GI disease among patients with SLE. For example, mucocutaneous ulcerations involving the nose and mouth are common in the general population. However, in SLE, as noted earlier, the ulcerations tend to be painless and frequently involve the hard palate, buccal mucosa, or vermillion border (**Fig. 3**). Erythematous lesions often have edema and petechiae of the hard palate.[8] Most GI conditions present with traditional signs and symptoms of biliary and hepatic disease, and without features unique to SLE. Patients with peritonitis as a manifestation of SLE-related serositis can present with findings mimicking an acute abdomen and rarely have evidence of ascites on examination.

GASTROINTESTINAL ASPECTS RELATED TO TREATMENT OF SYSTEMIC LUPUS ERYTHEMATOSUS

The pharmacologic therapies for SLE are recognized for their potential to induce GI and hepatobiliary adverse drug reactions. These reactions are summarized here.

NSAIDs are used in SLE, particularly for symptomatic management of inflammatory joint pain, pericarditis, and pleuritis. They are usually taken as needed; however, some patients take them on a daily scheduled basis. NSAIDs, particularly nonselective cyclooxygenase-2 inhibitors, can lead to gastritis as well as ulcerations in the mucosa of the stomach and subsequent GI bleeding. In addition, these medications can lead to a reversible increase in hepatic enzyme levels.[29]

Corticosteroids are also used for early bridging therapy in SLE, as well as for flares. Prolonged administration necessitates monitoring for hyperlipidemia, fatty liver disease, and complications of central obesity.[29]

Hydroxychloroquine is generally a well-tolerated first-line therapy for patients with SLE, although it, too, has the possibility of producing GI adverse effects. These effects include abdominal cramping, nausea, vomiting, and diarrhea.[29] Azathioprine may cause similar GI adverse effects to hydroxychloroquine and has been associated with pancreatitis. Methotrexate for SLE can occasionally cause hepatotoxicity and, very rarely, cirrhosis. Its administration is contraindicated in most forms of chronic hepatitis.[30] Patients on methotrexate should be cautioned regarding alcohol intake.

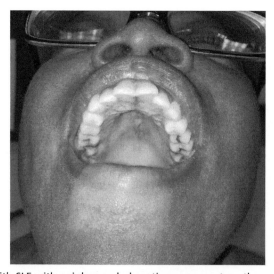

Fig. 3. Patient with SLE with painless oral ulcerations apparent on the upper palate.

Cyclosporine and cyclophosphamide are both associated with GI intolerance. Patients on cyclosporine require routine liver enzyme measurement to monitor for hepatotoxicity. Both medications may benefit from antiemetic coadministration for improved tolerance.[29]

MANAGEMENT OF THE DIGESTIVE/HEPATIC MANIFESTATIONS

GI manifestations primarily related to SLE activity follow the general tenets of SLE medical management: immunosuppressive therapy should be tailored to the severity of organ involvement. For potentially organ-threatening or life-threatening GI involvement, high-dose corticosteroids are indicated. The dose and duration required for control of GI disease have never been examined through a randomized controlled trial, so current practice is governed by observational data and expert opinion.

For SLE-related mesenteric vasculitis, glucocorticoid therapy can range from 40 mg/d to 1 mg/kg/d. Dose and delivery is based on severity of symptoms as well as tolerance of oral intake. Case reports vary dramatically in their reported duration of glucocorticoid use, from 1 to 34 days.[14] In cases with concomitant systemic disease (neurologic involvement, nephritis), cyclophosphamide has been used successfully with dosages ranging from 500 mg/m^2 to 750 mg/m^2 intravenously. Time to symptom resolution averaged around 7 to 10 days.[14] Maintenance therapy has consisted of varying regimens of azathioprine, mycophenolate mofetil, and (less frequently) hydroxychloroquine. Other maintenance therapeutic considerations include tacrolimus and rituximab. Tacrolimus was also shown to be effective in recurrent refractory lupus enteritis in a case study.[31]

As is the case for mesenteric vasculitis, first-line medications for intestinal pseudo-obstruction are also glucocorticoids. Dosage and duration of therapy from case reports have varied, ranging from 5 mg/d of prednisone to 1 mg/kg/d of methylprednisone. Symptoms typically improved in 7 to 10 days with improvement in manometry between 3 to 8 weeks.[15] Four out of 5 cases reported in a case series showed complete remission at 48 months.

Dosages of 1 mg/kg/d of intravenous glucocorticoid or prednisone oral equivalent have also been used in protein-losing enteropathy. Cyclophosphamide, mycophenolate mofetil, and methotrexate have also been used with some success.[17] In addition, diets high in protein and medium-chain triglycerides have been thought to be helpful in protein-losing enteropathy.[18] Resolution was considered complete if serum albumin level was greater than 35 g/dL and partial if greater than 30 g/dL.[17]

Surgical emergencies should be ruled out at the time of acute presentation. Such emergencies include bowel infarction, perforation, or ischemia. In addition, specialty care should be considered for advanced hepatobiliary manifestations.

SUMMARY

GI disease may complicate SLE and is an important cause of morbidity and mortality. Oral ulcers are a cardinal feature of SLE. Distinguishing GI involvement from active SLE versus other causes is critical because therapy ranges from aggressive immunosuppression for lupus enteritis, to lowering immunosuppression while starting antimicrobial therapy in settings in which infection is the cause. Treatment strategies for GI and hepatic disease in SLE are based on limited data (primarily small, uncontrolled series and case reports) and the experience from other connective tissue disorders. Continued investigations into the pathogenesis and treatment of SLE-related GI and hepatic involvement are needed to improve morbidity and mortality outcomes for patients with SLE.

REFERENCES

1. Kaul A, Gordon C, Crow MK, et al. Systemic lupus erythematosus. Nat Rev Dis Primers 2016;2:16039.
2. Alves SC, Fasano S, Isenberg DA. Autoimmune gastrointestinal complications in patients with systemic lupus erythematosus: case series and literature review. Lupus 2016;25(14):1509–19.
3. Ebert EC, Hagspiel KD. Gastrointestinal and hepatic manifestations of systemic lupus erythematosus. J Clin Gastroenterol 2011;45(5):436–41.
4. Isenberg DA, Rahman A, Allen E, et al. BILAG 2004. Development and initial validation of an updated version of the British Isles Lupus Assessment Group's disease activity index for patients with systemic lupus erythematosus. Rheumatology (Oxford) 2005;44(7):902–6.
5. Koo BS, Hong S, Kim YJ, et al. Lupus enteritis: clinical characteristics and predictive factors for recurrence. Lupus 2015;24(6):628–32.
6. Takeno M, Ishigatsubo Y. Intestinal manifestations in systemic lupus erythematosus. Intern Med 2006;45(2):41–2.
7. Urman JD, Lowenstein MB, Abeles M, et al. Oral mucosal ulceration in systemic lupus erythematosus. Arthritis Rheum 1978;21(1):58–61.
8. Sultan SM, Ioannou Y, Isenberg DA. A review of gastrointestinal manifestations of systemic lupus erythematosus. Rheumatology (Oxford) 1999;38(10):917–32.
9. Tan EM, Cohen AS, Fries JF, et al. The 1982 revised criteria for the classification of systemic lupus erythematosus. Arthritis Rheum 1982;25(11):1271–7.
10. Petri M, Orbai AM, Alarcon GS, et al. Derivation and validation of the Systemic Lupus International Collaborating Clinics classification criteria for systemic lupus erythematosus. Arthritis Rheum 2012;64(8):2677–86.
11. Lopez-Labady J, Villarroel-Dorrego M, Gonzalez N, et al. Oral manifestations of systemic and cutaneous lupus erythematosus in a Venezuelan population. J Oral Pathol Med 2007;36(9):524–7.
12. Lee CK, Ahn MS, Lee EY, et al. Acute abdominal pain in systemic lupus erythematosus: focus on lupus enteritis (gastrointestinal vasculitis). Ann Rheum Dis 2002;61(6):547–50.
13. Yuan S, Ye Y, Chen D, et al. Lupus mesenteric vasculitis: clinical features and associated factors for the recurrence and prognosis of disease. Semin Arthritis Rheum 2014;43(6):759–66.
14. Janssens P, Arnaud L, Galicier L, et al. Lupus enteritis: from clinical findings to therapeutic management. Orphanet J Rare Dis 2013;8:67.
15. Perlemuter G, Chaussade S, Wechsler B, et al. Chronic intestinal pseudo-obstruction in systemic lupus erythematosus. Gut 1998;43(1):117–22.
16. Wang JL, Liu G, Liu T, et al. Intestinal pseudo-obstruction in systemic lupus erythematosus: a case report and review of the literature. Medicine (Baltimore) 2014; 93(29):e248.
17. Chen Z, Li MT, Xu D, et al. Protein-losing enteropathy in systemic lupus erythematosus: 12 years experience from a Chinese academic center. PLoS One 2014; 9(12):e114684.
18. Al-Mogairen SM. Lupus protein-losing enteropathy (LUPLE): a systematic review. Rheumatol Int 2011;31(8):995–1001.
19. Yamashita H, Ueda Y, Kawaguchi H, et al. Systemic lupus erythematosus complicated by Crohn's disease: a case report and literature review. BMC Gastroenterol 2012;12(1):174.

20. Shor DB, Dahan S, Comaneshter D, et al. Does inflammatory bowel disease coexist with systemic lupus erythematosus? Autoimmun Rev 2016;15(11):1034–7.
21. Beigel F, Schnitzler F, Paul Laubender R, et al. Formation of antinuclear and double-strand DNA antibodies and frequency of lupus-like syndrome in anti-TNF-alpha antibody-treated patients with inflammatory bowel disease. Inflamm Bowel Dis 2011;17(1):91–8.
22. De Rycke L, Baeten D, Kruithof E, et al. The effect of TNFalpha blockade on the antinuclear antibody profile in patients with chronic arthritis: biological and clinical implications. Lupus 2005;14(12):931–7.
23. Denham JM, Hill ID. Celiac disease and autoimmunity: review and controversies. Curr Allergy Asthma Rep 2013;13(4):347–53.
24. Dahan S, Shor DB, Comaneshter D, et al. All disease begins in the gut: celiac disease co-existence with SLE. Autoimmun Rev 2016;15(8):848–53.
25. Witt M, Zecher D, Anders HJ. Gastrointestinal manifestations associated with systemic lupus erythematosus. Eur J Med Res 2006;11(6):253–60.
26. Man BL, Mok CC. Serositis related to systemic lupus erythematosus: prevalence and outcome. Lupus 2005;14(10):822–6.
27. Jackson NM. GI tract complications. Washington, DC: Lupus Foundation of America; 2015.
28. Yau AH, Chu K, Yang HM, et al. Rectal ulcers induced by systemic lupus erythematosus. BMJ Case Rep 2014;2014 [pii:bcr2014205776].
29. Klippel JH. Primer on rheumatologic disease. New York: Springer; 2008.
30. Hellmann DB, Imboden JB Jr. Rheumatologic, immunologic and allergic disorders. In: Papadakis MA, McPhee SJ, Rabow MW, editors. Current medical diagnosis and treatment 2017. New York: McGraw-Hill Education; 2016.
31. Shirai T, Hirabayashi Y, Watanabe R, et al. The use of tacrolimus for recurrent lupus enteritis: a case report. J Med Case Rep 2010;4(1):150.

Moving?

Make sure your subscription moves with you!

To notify us of your new address, find your **Clinics Account Number** (located on your mailing label above your name), and contact customer service at:

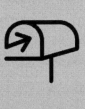

Email: journalscustomerservice-usa@elsevier.com

800-654-2452 (subscribers in the U.S. & Canada)
314-447-8871 (subscribers outside of the U.S. & Canada)

Fax number: 314-447-8029

Elsevier Health Sciences Division
Subscription Customer Service
3251 Riverport Lane
Maryland Heights, MO 63043

*To ensure uninterrupted delivery of your subscription, please notify us at least 4 weeks in advance of move.

Printed and bound by CPI Group (UK) Ltd, Croydon, CR0 4YY

11/05/2025

01866603-0001